Managing Complex Cases in Gastroenterology

W. Harley Sobin • Kia Saeian
Patrick Sanvanson

Editors

Managing Complex Cases in Gastroenterology

A Curbside Guide

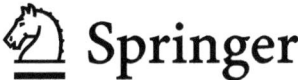

Editors
W. Harley Sobin
Division of Gastroenterology and
Hepatology
Medical College of Wisconsin
Milwaukee, WI, USA

Kia Saeian
Division of Gastroenterology and
Hepatology
Medical College of Wisconsin
Milwaukee, WI, USA

Patrick Sanvanson
Division of Gastroenterology and
Hepatology
Medical College of Wisconsin
Milwaukee, WI, USA

ISBN 978-3-031-48948-8   ISBN 978-3-031-48949-5   (eBook)
https://doi.org/10.1007/978-3-031-48949-5

This Springer imprint is published by the registered company Springer Nature Switzerland AG
The registered company address is: Gewerbestrasse 11, 6330 Cham, Switzerland

Paper in this product is recyclable

Preface

This book was designed to help gastroenterologists take care of their patients with challenging problems. Every day in practice we face patients with issues that are not simple to master. Oftentimes, we search out some guidance from "the experts," and, if they are available, we will curbside them, either by phone or in person.

This text is written from the standpoint of a community gastroenterologist curbsiding his academic cohorts with his challenging cases. We present a patient with a difficult GI problem and ask the academic expert how he, or she, would manage the case. We have provided over a hundred examples of problem cases and asked the experts at the Medical College of Wisconsin (MCW) for help in their management. These cases run the gamut, including general GI, motility disorders, inflammatory bowel disease, advanced therapeutics, hepatology, and disorders of gut–brain interaction.

The main objective of this book is to compile the most clinically useful questions, present them to experts who frequently deal with these problems, and then wrap up their knowledge within one clinically useful text. If a community gastroenterologist had endless access to an academic panel of GI experts, these are the questions they might ask. There are hundreds of useful clinical pearls between the pages of this book which should help anyone taking care of patients with GI problems. We want to thank the academic GI team at the Medical College of Wisconsin who, with their hundreds of years of accumulated experience, share their invaluable counsel.

While the text may be targeted particularly toward practicing community gastroenterologists, it certainly can be of benefit to GI fellows in training, academic gastroenterologists, and general internists and surgeons with a strong interest in gastroenterology as well as APPs.

Of course, these opinions shouldn't be accepted as the only choice for your patient. Indeed, in some cases, we share several opinions for managing the same condition. But any decision-making in your individual patient should be done in the context of the latest developments, and specific medical details of your particular patient. But we hope this text will serve as a useful adjunct in managing your more difficult patients.

Disclaimer—the cases presented in this text are hypothetical composites and don't represent specific individuals.

We would like to acknowledge the substantial help of Pilar Kuderer and Clarissa Marsh in the preparation of this text. They were assisted by Emma Kiefer and Kari Warren.

W. Harley Sobin
Kia Saeian
Patrick Sanvanson

Milwaukee, WI

Contents

Contributors

Helmut Ammon Division of GI and Hepatology/Department of Medicine—GI, Medical College of Wisconsin, Milwaukee, WI, USA

Poonam Beniwal-Patel Medicine, Gastroenterology/Hepatology Division, Medical College of Wisconsin, Milwaukee, WI, USA

GI and Hepatology Division, Medical College of Wisconsin, Milwaukee, WI, USA

William Berger Division of Gastroenterology and Hepatology, Medical College of Wisconsin, Milwaukee, WI, USA

Keely Browning Madison Medical Affiliates, Milwaukee, WI, USA

Department of Gastroenterology, Medical College of Wisconsin, Milwaukee, WI, USA

Phillip Chisholm Department of Medicine, GI/Hep Division, Medical College of Wisconsin, Milwaukee, WI, USA

Kulwinder Dua Division of Gastroenterology and Hepatology, Department of Medicine, Medical College of Wisconsin, Milwaukee, WI, USA

GI and Hepatology Division, Dept. of Medicine, Medical College of Wisconsin, Milwaukee, WI, USA

Francisco Durazo Division of Gastroenterology and Hepatology, Department of Medicine, Medical College of Wisconsin, Milwaukee, WI, USA

Francis Edeani Division of Gastroenterology and Hepatology, Department of Internal Medicine, Medical College of Wisconsin, Milwaukee, WI, USA

James Esteban Division of Gastroenterology and Hepatology, Department of Medicine, Medical College of Wisconsin, Milwaukee, WI, USA

Salina Faidhalla Department of Medicine Division of Gastroenterology and Hepatology, Medical College of Wisconsin, Milwaukee, WI, USA

Jose Franco Department of Medicine-Division of Gastroenterology and Hepatology, Medical College of Wisconsin, Milwaukee, WI, USA

Ben George Division of Hematology and Oncology, Department of Medicine, Medical College of Wisconsin, Milwaukee, WI, USA

Jon Gould Department of Surgery, Medical College of Wisconsin, Milwaukee, WI, USA

Veronica Loy Division Gastroenterology and Hepatology, Department of Medicine, Medical College of Wisconsin, Milwaukee, WI, USA

Srivats Madhavan Department of Medicine, Division of Gastroenterology and Hepatology, Medical College of Wisconsin, Milwaukee, WI, USA

Benson Massey Division of Gastroenterology and Hepatology, Department of Medicine, Medical College of Wisconsin, Milwaukee, WI, USA

Ling Mei Department of Medicine, GI/Hepatology Division, Medical College of Wisconsin, Milwaukee, WI, USA

Matt Mohorek Department of Gastroenterology, GI Associates, Wauwatosa, WI, USA

Jim Nelson Department of Medicine, Division of Gastroenterology and Hepatology, Medical College of Wisconsin, Milwaukee, WI, USA

Wilfredo Pagani Division of Gastroenterology and Hepatology, Medical College of Wisconsin, Milwaukee, WI, USA

Amir Patel Dept. of Medicine, Division of Gastroenterology and Hepatology, Medical College of Wisconsin, Milwaukee, WI, USA

Division of Gastroenterology and Hepatology, Department of Internal Medicine, Medical College of Wisconsin, Milwaukee, Milwaukee, WI, USA

Krupa Patel Methodist Medical Group, Dallas, Texas, USA

Elizabeth Pieper Department of Gastroenterology and Hepatology, Froedtert Hospital, Milwaukee, WI, USA

Kia Saeian Division of Gastroenterology & Hepatology, Medical College of Wisconsin, Milwaukee, WI, USA

Patrick Sanvanson Division of Gastroenterology and Hepatology, Department of Medicine, Medical College of Wisconsin, Milwaukee, WI, USA

Preetika Sinh Division of Gastroenterology and Hepatology Medical College of Wisconsin, Milwaukee, WI, USA

Zachary Smith Division of GI and Hepatology, Department of Medicine, Medical College of Wisconsin, Milwaukee, WI, USA

W. Harley Sobin Division of Gastroenterology and Hepatology, Medical College of Wisconsin, Milwaukee, WI, USA

Achutan Sourianarayanane Division of Gastroenterology and Hepatology, Department of Medicine, Medical College of Wisconsin, Milwaukee, WI, USA

Daniel Stein Division of Gastroenterology and Hepatology, Department of Internal Medicine, Medical College of Wisconsin, Milwaukee, WI, USA

Juan Trivella Division of Gastroenterology and Hepatology, Department of Medicine, Medical College of Wisconsin, Milwaukee, WI, USA

Part I
General GI

Chapter 1
Introduction to the General GI Section

W. Harley Sobin

In the General GI section, we start with the case-based management of complicated eosinophilic esophagitis. The use of PPIs, budesonide, fluticasone, and dupilumab are outlined. Dosage and prolonged duration of therapy are discussed. Management of severe strictures and fibrostenotic disease is outlined.

Next is a case discussing the diagnosis and management of oropharyngeal dysphagia, including how to direct the correct questions in taking a history and how to work with your speech therapist.

In reviewing achalasia, the author discusses the tendency to misdiagnose achalasia as GERD. He differentiates the management of types 1, 2, and 3 achalasia and discusses the advantages of Heller myotomy and POEM. Diagnosis and management of achalasia in the elderly are discussed, as are the diagnosis of pseudoachalasia and difficulties in diagnosing achalasia in someone on opioids.

Multiple examples of motility disorders of the esophagus including non-achalasia cases are provided. Some of the issues discussed include the evaluation of a patient with chest pain and dysphagia; use of esophageal manometry in diagnosing motility disorders; diagnosis and treatment of jackhammer esophagus and ineffective esophageal motility disorders; opioid-induced esophageal motility disorders; and the diagnosis and treatment of corkscrew esophagus.

There are case examples of some of the intricacies in the treatment of GERD and pH testing in the diagnosis and management of GERD. There is a review of various options to treat refractory GERD, as well as the management of patients with functional heartburn and reflux hypersensitivity.

W. H. Sobin (✉)
Division of Gastroenterology and Hepatology, Medical College of Wisconsin,
Milwaukee, WI, USA
e-mail: hsobin@mcw.edu

© The Author(s), under exclusive license to Springer Nature
Switzerland AG 2023
W. H. Sobin et al. (eds.), *Managing Complex Cases in Gastroenterology*,
https://doi.org/10.1007/978-3-031-48949-5_1

An esophageal surgeon, using case examples, discusses the complex decisions about whether to operate in GERD. He reviews the benefits of the LINX and Toupet procedures over the Nissen fundoplication; who is a candidate for magnetic sphincter augmentation (MSA), performing an MRI in someone with an MSA; surgical management of GERD in the obese patient; and issues with transoral incisionless fundoplication (TIF).

There are case examples of Barrett's esophagus with and without dysplasia. Surveillance guidelines in patients with Barrett's with and without dysplasia are discussed. Endoscopic modalities for the treatment of dysplasia are reviewed, as well as the pros and cons of performing ablation, techniques of performing ablation, and EMR of esophageal nodules. Newer techniques for screening and diagnosing Barrett's are outlined.

Case examples of problems in the management of PEG tubes are discussed including: dealing with a PEG tube that won't stop draining; PEG tube tracts that won't close; dealing with clogged G tubes and J tubes; techniques for placing a G-J tube; controversies in placing a PEG in someone who has ENT cancer; avoiding complications inserting PEG tubes; and how to manage those complications should they occur. Issues with replacing a PEG tube are discussed, as are the management of a prematurely pulled-out PEG tube and managing a buried bumper.

Case examples of the diagnosis of pernicious anemia (PA) are provided. Pathophysiology of autoimmune metaplastic atrophic gastritis (AMAG), surveillance for gastric cancer in AMAG, HP, and the development of environmental metaplastic atrophic gastritis (EMAG) are discussed, as are the distinctions between EMAG and AMAG and techniques of gastric mapping and its use in PA, AMAG, and EMAG.

In the section on subepithelial lesions and NETs, we provide case examples of gastric submucosal lesions and how to determine their etiology. The management of gastric GISTs, neuroendocrine tumors of the gut, and treatment of a small rectal carcinoid are reviewed. There are three types of gastric carcinoids, and their evaluation and treatment are outlined.

There is a chapter on viewpoints on managing common clinical GI disorders from a practitioner with over 50 years of "real-world" experience. He discusses case examples of difficulties managing: chronic constipation, IBS-D, gastroparesis, GERD, microscopic colitis, fecal incontinence, and diverticulitis.

A case of severe SIBO and its management is discussed. Clinical findings, diagnosis, pathophysiology, predisposing mechanisms, and antibiotic choice are reviewed. How should you manage a patient with SIBO where antibiotics are no longer working?

A case of a patient with a functional GI disorder who has an abnormal breath test is discussed. Problems with interpretation of breath tests, a comparison of glucose and lactulose breath tests, and the benefit of adding scintigraphy to breath testing are highlighted. The problem of frequent false positive breath tests is delved into and explained. A strong case for limiting breath testing to patients who have a predisposing reason to have SIBO is made.

Unusual causes of abdominal pain and controversies in the diagnosis of chronic abdominal pain are the subject of another chapter. Case examples of difficult-to-make diagnoses in the determination of an etiology of chronic abdominal pain are reviewed. These include acalculous cholecystitis, median arcuate ligament compression syndrome, disorders of gut-brain interaction, narcotic bowel syndrome, microscopic colitis, chronic mesenteric ischemia, sphincter of Oddi dysfunction, endometriosis, chronic abdominal wall pain, epiploic appendagitis, porphyria, sclerosing mesenteritis, and abdominal migraine. Conflicts about ordering CT scans for chronic abdominal pain are discussed. The peculiar circumstance of peptic ulcer disease and cholecystitis first presenting as complicated disease in previously asymptomatic elderly and RA patients is highlighted.

Case examples of patients with-acute mesenteric insufficiency, mesenteric vein thrombosis, chronic mesenteric ischemia, non-occlusive mesenteric ischemia, colon ischemia, and median arcuate ligament syndrome are reviewed. Difficulties in diagnosis and management are discussed.

There are case examples that describe the pros and cons of cold snare and hot snare polypectomy. Other topics discussed in the chapter on polypectomy include the use of cold snares for removing large laterally spreading granular tumors; choice of snare in doing a polypectomy in a patient receiving anticoagulation; use of clips in cold snare vs hot snare polypectomies; and whether or not to hold anticoagulation or antiplatelet agents prior to elective colonoscopy. There is also a discussion of injection technique and other recommended maneuvers in EMR, including a review of obstacles encountered. The authors also discuss which polyps to send to the surgeon; endoscopic features that suggest deep submucosal invasion; management of pedunculated polyps, including polyps with a thick stalk; and how to deal with post-polypectomy bleeding.

In a chapter on rectal incontinence, the authors provide case examples describing the management of passive, urge, and seepage incontinence. They describe the best techniques for rectal examination in the incontinent patient. They extensively discuss the evaluation of fecal incontinence and examples of etiologic causes. This includes diagnosing fecal incontinence due to overflow and its management. Managing diarrhea in fecal incontinence is extensively reviewed including the use of biofeedback therapy, surgery, and sacral nerve stimulation in various patients with incontinence. Incontinence in the post-stroke patient is discussed, as is managing the patient with intermittent involuntary seepage.

In the chapter on diverticulitis, we provide case examples discussing controversies in the management of diverticulitis including whether all patients need to receive antibiotics; how to manage smoldering diverticulitis; when to recommend elective surgery; and how to avoid recurrent diverticulitis. The entities of symptomatic uncomplicated diverticular disease (SUDD) and segmental colitis associated with diverticulosis (SCAD) and their management are reviewed.

There are case studies that demonstrate when (and how) to evaluate a pancreatic cyst, including the use of EUS and FNA, the analysis of amylase and CEA in cyst fluid, and the evaluation of pancreatic IPMNs. Other subjects reviewed include how to evaluate the patient with idiopathic recurrent pancreatitis, how to diagnose and manage pancreas divisum, sphincter of Oddi dysfunction, and autoimmune pancreatitis.

Case studies diagnosing and evaluating etiologies for chronic pancreatitis in alcohol abusers and those without a history of alcohol use are reviewed. The utility of the secretin-stimulated MRCP is discussed as are the management of chronic pain in chronic pancreatitis and the management of pancreatic stones.

In a section on GI oncology, the author provides case studies demonstrating the use of chemotherapy in colon cancer, Lynch syndrome, EGJ adenocarcinoma, and pancreatic cancer. Different management for right-sided vs. left-sided colon cancer is discussed. The different approaches to chemotherapy, immunotherapy, and surgical therapy in Lynch syndrome are reviewed. There is a wide-ranging discussion of different responses to chemotherapy and immunotherapy in different GI cancers.

There are case studies reviewing the management of refractory benign esophageal strictures, the use of stents in benign and malignant esophageal strictures, and the role of stents in extrinsic malignant esophageal obstruction. Issues concerning the diagnosis and staging of pancreatic cancer and the diagnosis of pancreatic cancer when preliminary tests are negative are discussed.

A PharmD specializing in GI pharmacology provides case studies analyzing the use of GI drugs in treating EOE, HP, HBV, HCV, IBS, IBD, pancreatic insufficiency, and autoimmune hepatitis. Issues concerning the use of budesonide and fluticasone are discussed. Obstacles with patients using quadruple therapy for HP are outlined. Many more challenges are reviewed. Important drug-drug interactions, drug-food interactions, drug toxicity, and insurance coverage are highlighted.

Chapter 2
Eosinophilic Esophagitis

Patrick Sanvanson

Case 1 A 28-year-old man presents with a food impaction after eating a turkey sandwich. He has a history of food sticking over the last couple of years but has always gotten it down by swallowing water. He tends to cut his food into small pieces, but this time he swallowed a too large piece of meat. On endoscopy, he appears to have a mildly narrowed esophagus; it has multiple rings and some longitudinal furrows. The piece of chicken is removed with a Roth net. Biopsies show 80 eos/hpf in the upper and lower esophagus.

He is placed on pantoprazole but feels like food continues to stick intermittently.

Would you agree with that initial treatment and how would you proceed now?

Yes, it sounds like he has a classic presentation of eosinophilic esophagitis with greater than 15 eosinophils per high-power field. Obviously, you have the other components with the rings and the furrows, but those won't necessarily make the diagnosis of eosinophilic esophagitis (EOE).

The histologic diagnosis seems pretty clear for EOE, and the history of food impaction is one of the more common presentations of eosinophilic esophagitis. They placed him on a PPI right away, which I agree with. There is usually a delay in diagnosis of EOE, and in this case, it sounds like he's had symptoms going on for the last couple of years.

After starting pantoprazole, his symptoms are not completely relieved. The question I ask in patients with incomplete relief is as follows: Is he compliant with the pantoprazole, and is he taking it correctly?

P. Sanvanson (✉)

Division of Gastroenterology and Hepatology, Department of Medicine, Medical College of Wisconsin, Milwaukee, WI, USA

e-mail: psanvans@mcw.edu

© The Author(s), under exclusive license to Springer Nature
Switzerland AG 2023
W. H. Sobin et al. (eds.), *Managing Complex Cases in Gastroenterology*,
https://doi.org/10.1007/978-3-031-48949-5_2

I always like to bring these patients back into the clinic, to explain the disease EOE, and to inform them that they have one of the more common complications, which is a food impaction. I let him know that this is a medical condition that we can manage but can't necessarily cure and then to also give him insight into the therapy itself.

So, he's been placed on proton pump inhibitor therapy, and the question is as follows: Why do EOE patients respond to this? Is it because you're managing acid reflux and that's stimulating the disease, or is it because you're blocking eotaxin-3 expression, which subsequently has an effect on eosinophil recruitment?

Obviously, PPIs have been used extensively to treat EOE, but this patient is having inadequate relief. So, we question what dose he's on, how long he's been on the medication, whether he is compliant with the medication dosing, and how is he taking the pantoprazole, before we conclude that he hasn't necessarily responded to PPI therapy.

Do you normally start with pantoprazole or a different PPI and what dose do you like to start with?

It varies and is generally dependent on insurance coverage. Numerous PPIs have been tried with EOE. If I'm using pantoprazole, I will usually start with 40 mg twice a day. I usually err on the side of using high-dose PPI. This may be supra-therapeutic, but I just don't want to underdose these patients. If I'm using omeprazole, I would also use 40 mg twice a day. So, the key is that whatever PPI you choose, always make sure to err on the side of the higher dose, just so you don't underdose them prior to their repeat endoscopy.

There have been studies looking at the potency of different PPIs, but these were based on GERD data, not EOE data, so, we can't be sure this extrapolates to EOE. However, in GERD, pantoprazole is considered one of the least potent acid-suppressing PPIs, while rabeprazole and dexlansoprazole are the most potent. Omeprazole and esomeprazole are in the middle.

.

The patient is taking pantoprazole 40 mg bid and has been taking it on an empty stomach a half hour before meals for the past 8 weeks. While there might be mild improvement, he is still complaining of dysphagia.

What would you do, would you repeat endoscopy, would you dilate the esophagus, and would you start him on steroids?

In terms of symptoms, it's always hard with EOE patients, because I feel like their symptoms vary so much from person to person, and a lot of these patients no longer know what normal is.

In making therapeutic decisions, symptoms can be confusing, and so I usually like to guide my decision-making on endoscopic evaluation with biopsies. So, I like to treat the patient for 8–10 weeks, and then, at that point I would go in and do another EGD and get repeat biopsies of the esophagus.

I don't typically dilate on that follow-up endoscopy. However, if there is an isolated ring in the distal esophagus at the GE junction level, I will often dilate those patients on the subsequent EGD. Also, if I am dealing with a narrow caliber esophagus where the only scope I can advance is an ultrathin endoscope, I feel those patients are at very high risk of food impaction, so, I will frequently do a bougie dilation on the follow-up EGD.

However, if there is no severe narrowing, only a mild diffuse narrowing, where the esophageal diameter is well above 12 mm, and they're able to chew their food and get it down, I will not dilate at the 8-week follow-up. In those patients, I will give them more chances to respond to additional medical therapy. The reason I try to defer dilation as long as possible is that we've seen many patients that have been on medical therapy, and once you get their inflammation under control, the esophagus starts to remodel and a lot of their stricturing disease just goes away. I'm not necessarily hesitant to dilate their esophagus, but if it's not absolutely necessary, I'd rather avoid it. With any type of procedure, there are potential complications, and in terms of dilating patients with EOE, the initial reports were concerning due to an increased perforation risk. However, those initial concerns have been mitigated.

However, it is clear that a lot of EOE patients may experience significant chest discomfort and chest pain post-dilatation. So, if I'm going to dilate them, I warn them ahead of time that if we do dilate you, you might experience some degree of chest discomfort post-procedure.

However, not everyone is comfortable dilating EOE. You mustn't be too aggressive with dilation, start with lower caliber dilators, and then slowly move your way up. Using these precautions, the risk is fairly low. You have to realize, in treating EOE that this is not a condition that is going to lead to cancer or shorten someone's life, so it is well worthwhile to be conservative, to go out of your way to avoid a perforation. This is one of the reasons why I'm not too aggressive with dilation.

How will the results of endoscopy and biopsy on that second EGD affect your management plans?

Obviously, the main thing is measuring the response to therapy. So, you are looking for histologic improvement, and you are evaluating endoscopic improvement with regard to stricturing and narrowing. These are important, along with symptom improvement as well.

With our biopsies, the goal, from a histologic standpoint, is to have essentially zero eosinophils per high-power field, but typically, we accept less than 15 eosinophils per high-power field as an adequate goal for response. However, there are some patients where I'll start up PPI therapy after the initial endoscopy showed an eosinophil count of 100/hpf, and they may go down to 14 eos/hpf with treatment, and I say, okay, that's an adequate response.

However, then you have subsets of patients that present with a low-grade eosinophilia like 25 eos/hpf, and now they've down to 13 or 14. So you'll wonder, if that is really a significant response, or not, but usually we are also taking into account any improvement in symptoms or endoscopic appearance.

If their response to therapy is suboptimal and the patient doesn't have a decrease in their eosinophil count to less than 15 eos/hpf, what do we do next? Then, you started talking about alternate therapies. Our other therapies involve making a decision between using topical steroids versus doing an elimination diet. As of May 2022, there is another therapy, the newly approved dupilumab.

So, I always give my patients the option of choosing between elimination diet versus topical steroids. Unfortunately, none of the topical steroids are FDA-approved therapies. The two most commonly used are budesonide and fluticasone which have been found to be relatively equivalent in terms of clinical response.

Unfortunately, a lot of our guidance on steroid choice depends on cost. I don't necessarily have a favorite, budesonide, or fluticasone. I base it more on the cost to the patient and the convenience of taking the particular regimen. From the standpoint of topical steroids, the goal is to decrease the inflammation within the esophagus.

If I'm using budesonide, I start at 1 mg twice a day. If we can get their insurance to cover a compounded version of budesonide, it is much simpler for the patient to use this, but, unfortunately, a lot of insurance companies don't cover the compounded version, which makes the use of budesonide much more difficult. Those patients have to compound their own budesonide. They take respules of budesonide, which are designed for use with nebulizers in asthma, mix the liquid medicine in these respules with a high viscosity agent, usually sucralose or honey, and then swallow the admixture. You can see how that's pretty cumbersome for a lot of patients to take and requires a patient who is very motivated and compliant.

The other option is fluticasone, which is administered by inhaler, but you have to educate the patient to spray it in their mouth and not inhale it into their lungs. There have been studies that show a number of patients make that mistake. So, it's key to educate patients on how to take fluticasone properly. From a dosing standpoint, I recommend two puffs at 220 µg per puff, i.e., 440 µg twice a day. Occasionally, I will go up to 880 µg twice a day in patients who are initial non-responders. Some patients who are initial non-responders will respond to 880 µg bid. Once I start steroids, I'll usually wait 8–10 weeks then re-biopsy the esophagus and assess the response.

The response rate to elimination diets is thought to be above 50%. Obviously, this requires a very dedicated patient that they have to be extremely compliant with the diet. It requires working closely with our GI dietician as well. When we start an elimination diet, we also repeat endoscopy after each manipulation to gauge response to the withdrawal of a particular food group. When we decide to reintroduce a particular food, we also repeat endoscopy to gauge response. I will explain the elimination diet strategy to see if this is something the patient wants to pursue. In addition to being on a strict diet, the other challenging factors are the cost and the time required for multiple endoscopies to assess response.

In addition, our Wisconsin patients are not thrilled about the idea of restricting wheat and dairy, the two major food groups that are frequently eliminated. I do have a number of patients that are on elimination diets, but unfortunately these are the select few who are very compliant people that are willing to put in the time and the work to do the elimination diet. However, if somebody has some hesitancy, they feel like they can't do it, we try our other options.

Pantoprazole is continued at 40 mg BID. The patient opts to be placed on ste-roids, and fluticasone is started at 440 mg bid. Repeat endoscopy with biopsy is done 8 weeks later and shows histologic response. Symptomatically, the patient is doing very well with much-improved swallowing.

How long will you maintain PPIs and steroids?

We have learned that these patients will need some type of long-term mainte-nance of whatever therapy they're on, as EOE is a chronic illness. We know that when they stop the therapies most people will have a recurrence of the esophageal eosinophilia and, then, subsequently, the scarring and other classic findings of EOE.

From a PPI standpoint, if they're doing well on twice a day dosage, I'll decrease it to once a day and see how they do from a symptom standpoint. If they're doing fine, I won't repeat the endoscopy, but if they're not doing well, I may consider repeating the biopsies.

Topical steroids are a little trickier. I usually keep them on some type of long-term therapy. However, we know that if you decrease the maintenance dose of budesonide or fluticasone from their initial induction dose, then probably about 25–50% of people will have a recurrence of their esophageal eosinophilia. So, we have some shared decision-making to decide whether to lower the dose. If patients are happy, and they're doing well on their current regimen, I give them the option of maintaining their current dose of topical steroids without taper.

We do see some problems with steroid compliance since it's a twice-daily regi-men. If it's very cumbersome for the patient, I may decrease it from twice a day to once a day and see how they do, but we do know from randomized, placebo-controlled studies that a lot of these patients, essentially 50% or more, may have a recurrence of their esophageal eosinophilia within 6-month time.

It sounds like you are keeping most people on these medicines indefinitely

Exactly, assuming that they're getting some benefit from them, I always compare it to blood pressure issues. Typically, when people have hypertension, unless you get rid of some other factor, it becomes a lifelong management issue. With EOE, there may be some things that we can modify, like diet, that may help maintain remission. Unfortunately, most of the studies suggest a recurrence of eosinophilia and recurrence of symptoms once you stop their maintenance therapy.

In which cases will you use dupilumab therapy?

Dupilumab is basically the first FDA-approved medication for EOE. It's obvi-ously a systemic therapy that should target some of these remodeling pathways and inflammatory pathways and hopefully prevent fibrostenotic disease. There are a number of other agents in the pipeline that are coming out as well.

Dupilumab is thought to work by inhibiting signaling of interleukin 4 and 13. It's a monoclonal antibody against IL-4 receptor. Historically, it's been approved for other disease processes, including atopic dermatitis, asthma, chronic rhinosinusitis, and now EOE. The data are quite strong in terms of response of esophageal eosino-philia, the classic endoscopic findings of EOE, and symptom improvement as well.

The population, for sure, that may benefit from this treatment are those who are refractory to PPIs and steroids. Patients who find budesonide or fluticasone too cumbersome to take may also be good candidates. Right now, we have to see where dupilumab lands in terms of insurance coverage. Dupilumab is given as one injection once a week. We do have a number of patients that are refractory to PPI therapy and topical steroid therapy who will be considered for dupilumab therapy in the near future.

What would be very interesting is to use dupilumab in our EOE patients who also have eosinophilic asthma or atopic dermatitis. I think these patients should be perfect candidates, where you try to reduce the medications they're on, save them money, and hopefully give them back some more quality of life. In the long term, if you can treat multiple illnesses with the same medication, it would be a significant advantage.

So, I think that if patients fail to respond to combination therapy, then you should at least introduce the idea of using dupilumab therapy.

Besides for dysphagia, what other symptoms do you tend to see in your EOE patients?

I think there are variable presentations, but the other common complaint besides dysphagia is heartburn. The hard part in that scenario is deciding whether the heartburn is due to the EOE or is it reflux-related. Sometimes, that requires additional investigations to figure that out.

Another symptom we occasionally see is nausea, which is probably more common in the pediatric population. Our pediatric colleagues are more likely to see EOE presenting with food intolerance and weight loss in their patients.

We occasionally see bloating, although not that commonly. Regurgitation is more often seen with reflux disease than with eosinophilic esophagitis. However, if someone has an EOE-related stricture, then they're more likely to have esophageal reflux and other related issues depending on the severity of the stricture.

However, once again, these EOE patients have varied symptoms that don't necessarily correlate with the severity of their endoscopic findings. Some patients have a wide-open esophagus yet have severe symptoms, while other patients may have close to a pinhole esophagus and will have essentially no symptoms. So, evaluating symptoms is important but can be misleading.

Case 2 Another patient, a 32 year-old man, presents with a food impaction. He has a known history of EOE but got lost to follow-up 10 years ago, shortly after diagnosis. He has had progressive dysphagia which he has managed by cutting his food into small pieces, avoiding tough meats, like steak, no salads. In spite of this, food is frequently getting stuck, and now, he presents to the ER because a piece of sausage got stuck and he was unable to vomit it out. On endoscopy, the esophagus is quite narrow. The food stuck in the mid-esophagus is able to be removed. The endoscope is unable to be passed all the way down the esophagus because it is too narrow.

How do you manage a patient who has a long duration of untreated EOE and has developed significant narrowing, significant fibrosis?

I've seen a number of patients that have had more fibrostenotic disease. It's presumed that there is more fibrosis because the disease has been persisting untreated for a longer period of time. EOE starts as an inflammatory process, and then over time, the inflammation progresses and develops into more and more fibrotic disease.

I think the pathophysiology is probably fairly similar to patients with more acute presentations. EOE starts as an immune response to some type of antigen stimulus, whether it's a food or whether it's environmental, with probably some degree of a genetic abnormality involved as well.

We do know that in a long term, some patients will develop a narrow caliber esophagus, as a result of tissue remodeling and fibrosis. Subsequently, there is a change in the mechanical properties of the esophagus, where fibrosis leads to issues with decreased distensibility and dysmotility.

The medical treatment of these patients is similar to those with a normal caliber esophagus. However, because of the severe narrowing of the esophagus, I may modify the particular medicine regimens that they're on. I might give lansoprazole, which is available as an oral dissolvable formulation. I may also prescribe a capsule version of omeprazole, rather than the pill form, where you open up the capsule and put the medicine in applesauce and swallow that just to make certain that they're actually able to get their pills down and get an adequate trial of the medication.

In addition, if there is severe narrowing, with an extremely narrow caliber esophagus, I'll frequently have to go down with an ultrathin endoscope and begin gradual dilation over a guidewire. When I dilate, I am not too aggressive, starting off. I've had patients that come in with a 5-mm esophagus. I may do a 21 French bougie dilation, which is about 7 mm. Initially, we might tell them to stay on a liquid diet, or more of a pureed type of diet, as opposed to swallowing solid foods. One of the more important parts of education is to make sure that the patient takes his time with eating, chewing his food extremely well, and drinking a lot of liquid in-between bites as well.

If it is the very narrow esophagus, how often would you repeat dilation?

A stricture from EOE acts differently than a GERD-related stricture. In a tight GERD-related stricture, we might bring them back weekly, but in an EOE-related stricture I want to give their medications time to work. I feel that, with a lot of these EOE patients, once you treat the inflammatory component of the disease with your medication, the dilations are more effective, compared to long-standing peptic, GERD-related strictures.

So, if they're able to tolerate something liquid and perhaps other foods as well, usually I'll try to go 8 weeks between dilations. If, however, the patients contacting me say they're not doing well, they're miserable, and everything is getting stuck, then I'll bring them back earlier, at 4-week intervals. However, I've never really had to dilate them more frequently than that.

A part of the reason is that I just want to see what their response to therapy is. A lot of times, patients are able to tolerate some type of diet once they're on medical therapy, they're maintaining their weight, and they're able to maintain their hydration. However, it's also important with EOE patients that every time you see them you try to confirm compliance with medication. I had a patient that came in with an extremely narrow caliber esophagus. I did six or seven dilations on him, and he just wasn't improving. He wasn't responding to PPI therapy, and he wasn't responding to topical steroid therapy. We even tried switching his steroid formulations, and there was still no improvement. Then, after multiple ED visits, he finally confessed that he was not complying with taking his meds the way he was instructed. Once he started complying with the medication instructions, there was rapid remodeling of the esophagus and I was quickly able to dilate him sufficiently.

Chapter 3
Oropharyngeal Dysphagia

Patrick Sanvanson

A 78-year-old man with a history of Parkinson's disease is complaining of dyspha-gia. A swallowing evaluation suggests that he has oropharyngeal dysphagia. Despite maneuvers by the speech therapist, he continues to have problems.

How do you manage patients with oropharyngeal dysphagia?

You always need to know the underlying pathophysiology of the dysphagia.

Is it stroke-related? Is it related to a neuromuscular issue, like ALS, or Parkinson's disease? We also see some patients that have head and neck cancer, and they've had surgical therapy or radiation therapy that has resulted in dysphagia. So, you always want to consider whether the underlying condition can be rehabilitated and whether improvement is possible? If you're dealing with ALS, you're very limited from a therapy standpoint because the disease progresses, which is often the case in Parkinson's disease as well. On the other hand, you have some stroke patients that may have a significant degree of rehabilitative potential. When there are no obvious explanations for the dysphagia, we may be witnessing idiopathic oropharyngeal dysphagia, and these patients may present in a variety of ways with various rehab potential.

However, whenever I have a patient who says they have difficulty swallowing, I always ask them, "Do you feel like you have coughing when you swallow? Do you ever feel like things go down the wrong pipe? Have you ever felt that you needed to have the Heimlich maneuver, because you were unable to breathe when these epi-sodes were occurring?"

There are other patients who may be completely asymptomatic but present with aspiration pneumonia. Obviously, the most important thing that we want to avoid

P. Sanvanson (✉)
Division of Gastroenterology and Hepatology, Department of Medicine,
Medical College of Wisconsin, Milwaukee, WI, USA
e-mail: psanvans@mcw.edu

© The Author(s), under exclusive license to Springer Nature
Switzerland AG 2023
W. H. Sobin et al. (eds.), *Managing Complex Cases in Gastroenterology*,
https://doi.org/10.1007/978-3-031-48949-5_3

with these patients is aspiration, because that can lead to significant morbidity and mortality. Oropharyngeal dysphagia is a very common disease, with significant costs to the healthcare system. In evaluating these patients, I think the thing that's key is to have a close relationship with your speech therapist and to understand what the patient's video swallow study shows.

So, if you're worried that a patient has oropharyngeal dysphagia, the typical first approach will be to do a video swallow study to see if they have any penetration above the vocal cords or if they have any aspiration. Then, if they do, what is the consistency of the food that is aspirated? Do they have liquid aspiration? Do they have aspiration of pudding? Do they aspirate thicker liquids? Do they have aspiration for solid foods as well? And sometimes, from that standpoint, initial management is to try to determine if there are certain foods that can be tolerated without aspirating. If so, the speech therapist can work with the patient to see if they can modify the consistency of some of the other foods. If the patient aspirates liquids, then they can be taught to thicken up the liquid that they're taking in. If they cannot swallow any foods without aspirating, then you have to talk about whether or not alternate delivery of nutrition is necessary, including enteral feeding or G-tube placement to get you through the initial phases of the oropharyngeal dysphagia.

The speech therapists are good at teaching certain maneuvers that patients can do to limit their aspiration risks. One of these is the Shaker exercise, which requires a head lift, to try to strengthen some of the pharyngeal swallowing musculature. This maneuver can also help with upper esophageal sphincter opening. Obviously, the limitation of many of these exercises is that you have to have a patient who is capable of following instructions. If the patient is neurologically devastated, that's less of an option.

Also, if you have a patient with restricted neck mobilization, because they have had a big spinal surgery or other type of neurosurgery, this also limits your ability to do certain swallowing exercises, including the Shaker exercises. Then, there are things down the pipeline that hopefully will address some of these issues. We are doing research protocols in our laboratory, working with a swallow resistance exercise device, which is a pressure collar that people wear. Patients basically practice swallowing against resistance. In some of the initial data, we're able to improve aspiration and penetration in a subset of individuals who wear this collar, including some with Parkinson's disease. These are all areas of study where hopefully we can modify the swallowing mechanism, find a way to strengthen their musculature to delay the disease progression, and prevent or delay aspiration.

However, in patients who have persistent aspiration, we consider PEG tubes. Although PEG tubes are not necessarily the best thing in demented patients that have oropharyngeal dysphagia, they may be options for patients that have ALS, Parkinson's disease, and some stroke patients to hopefully maintain their nutritional status.

Chapter 4
Achalasia

Benson Massey

Case 1 *A patient is referred to your surgeon by a community gastroenterologist requesting a fundoplication for chronic gastroesophageal reflux. The gastroenterologist thinks the surgeon should consider doing a Toupet procedure because his patient, in addition to having chronic reflux esophagitis, has ineffective esophageal motility. The surgeon, concerned about the presentation, is asking you to review the case, wondering if he has been misdiagnosed.*

This is a 40-year-old man with a long history of heartburn and regurgitation. This has been going on for a couple of years and is getting worse. He has lost about ten pounds over the past couple of months. The patient frequently has regurgitation after eating, and over time, the patient has transitioned to a softer and more liquid diet. He avoids eating for several hours before bedtime. In fact, he occasionally induces vomiting before going to bed because, on occasion, he has woken up in the middle of the night regurgitating liquid, occasionally solid material.

His gastroenterologist did an EGD that showed some retained liquid and superficial ulceration in the distal esophagus, all of which he interpreted as reflux esophagitis. The GE junction was somewhat tight, which he interpreted as a reflux stricture. He dilated the stricture using a TTS balloon (to 18 mm), with minimal symptomatic improvement. The patient has been taking PPIs long term, and yet his symptoms keep getting worse.

The gastroenterologist has previously sent patients to this surgeon for anti-reflux surgery with great results. He knows that the surgeon likes to have manometry done beforehand. His GI practice still uses older water-infusion manometry catheters, and his experience doing manometry is somewhat limited. He goes ahead and

B. Massey (✉)
Division of Gastroenterology and Hepatology, Department of Medicine, Medical College of Wisconsin, Milwaukee, WI, USA
e-mail: bmassey@mcw.edu

performs the procedure, after placing the manometry catheter without using fluo-roscopy. His interpretation of the study is that there is clearly decreased pressure in the esophagus with limited, if any peristalsis. He is unable to detect a lower esopha-geal sphincter zone. He interpreted this to mean that the LES was nonfunctional, blown-out.

When the patient comes to see you, he brings the manometry tracing which you review. Looking at the tracing, you suspect that the probe never passed the LES and never entered the stomach. Without being able to evaluate the LES, you are not sure if you are dealing with GERD in a patient with ineffective motility or if the patient may have Type 1 achalasia.

How often do you see patients being diagnosed with GERD, who actually have achalasia?

First, it can be very difficult to distinguish GERD from achalasia by history, and there is a lot of overlap, particularly in early achalasia. We use dysphagia for solids and liquids as a marker of achalasia, but early on in achalasia there may just be dysphagia for solids. This may be very hard to distinguish from the symptoms of someone with a peptic stricture or even something like eosinophilic esophagitis. So, the symptom overlap may confuse the diagnosis early on.

Second, because, achalasia is several orders of magnitude less frequent than GERD, anyone who's coming in with esophageal symptoms, even if they seem a little weird, like dysphagia for solids and liquids, they're still more likely to have GERD than they are achalasia, just a priori without doing any investigation at all.

Interestingly, the reliability of the clinical history for diagnosing GERD is poor. If you look at the Diamond study [1], done some years ago, which looked at primary care doctors trying to determine whether a patient had GERD based on symptoms, their decision-making was not much better than flipping a coin (sensitivity and specificity of 63%, based on the history when you're using actual acid exposure as the gold standard). Gastroenterologists don't do much better. The sensitivity and specificity of their history are about 67% and 70% which still mean that about a third of the time they got it wrong [1].

So, with GERD and achalasia both being tricky diagnoses, unless someone pres-ents with advanced achalasia where they're having really obvious features, such as an esophagus that is massively filled with liquid in a manner that really gets your attention, I think it's really a bit of a challenge.

There are a few clinical clues that may help distinguish the two. First, the patient described here is regurgitating. When you have achalasia and you regurgitate, the stuff tastes the same coming up as when it goes down. When GERD patients regur-gitate, it will taste sourer, unless the patient is on vigorous PPI therapy for reflux, in which case the regurgitation may not taste acidic.

An endoscopic technique to help determine whether achalasia is present is to inflate the esophagus with a lot of air, watch if the GEJ opens up, and then inflate the stomach with a lot of air and retroflex and see if the GE junction opens up. In achalasia, the GEJ stays shut; in GERD, it tends to open wide. In fact, if you look from below, in retroflex, it's hard to keep the stomach insufflated in GERD because so much air is leaking back up through the opening (that's only in very end-stage conditions like systemic sclerosis, where there is a very hypotensive LES).

So, it's a pretty accurate sign if you see the GEJ opening up, and the patient is belching air, that the patient doesn't have achalasia (if they've not already had surgery).

Another thing you can do, if you're unsure whether you're dealing with GERD or achalasia, is to combine your endoscopy with a BRAVO study. If your EGD is unrevealing and the Bravo returns negative, then you're not dealing with GERD, and you have to really start thinking about another diagnosis like achalasia.

You decide to repeat the manometry yourself. You pass the probe into the stomach with fluoroscopic guidance. On the tracing, you note absent peristalsis, but the IRP is only borderline elevated, with some decreased relaxation. You still think this is likely achalasia, but you want more convincing evidence.

What other tools can help define whether the patient has achalasia?

When you're dealing with someone with absent contractility, the question is as follows: Is this achalasia or is this a scleroderma-like dead esophagus? Is that possibly borderline high IRP in supine swallows really due to high deglutitive residual tone in the LES? To help determine whether an elevated IRP may be clinically important, you should also do the manometry sitting up as well as supine. If the IRP is normal on swallows while sitting, the high IRP during supine swallows should be disregarded.

When the IRP is also elevated during sitting swallows, there can still be a concern that this reflects muscle activity of the diaphragmatic crura (particularly in patients with obesity or lung disease) or could reflect a structural problem (e.g., a paraesophageal hernia or tight fundoplication wrap). This is where provocative pharmacologic testing during manometry using amyl nitrite can help with the diagnosis. Amyl nitrite completely abolishes smooth muscle tone in the esophageal body and LES for around 30 s. If the nadir pressure at the esophagogastric junction after amyl nitrite falls over 10 mmHg lower than the IRP on swallows, then you have impaired LES relaxation. If there is really no change with amyl nitrite, then the cause of the pressure is not smooth muscle tone in the LES.

Do you rely on the timed barium esophagram to help make a diagnosis of achalasia?

No, I don't think that the timed barium esophagram is as helpful in making a diagnosis of achalasia as it is in measuring the response to therapy. The timed barium esophagram can show you a delay in esophageal emptying, but it can't differentiate whether the delay is due to decreased esophageal contractions or to EGJOO or a combination of the two. We feel we get much more information by doing an impedance study at the time of manometry. Using impedance, if liquid is not emptying normally, I can determine whether it relates to decreased squeeze of the esophageal body, or increased resistance at the GEJ, or elevation of gastric pressure (in an obese patient there is elevation of intragastric pressure that may delay esophageal emptying). I can also assess the height of the fluid column remaining in the esophagus at different times, when the patient is in a seated position.

After you evaluate your manometry and impedance studies, you are convinced the patient has achalasia. How do you approach the management of the different types of achalasia?

For patients with spastic achalasia, the type 3 achalasia, we often try pharmacologic therapy first, a calcium channel blocker, like nifedipine or sublingual hyoscyamine, and many of them will get relief from pharmacology alone. In a number of these patients, the dysphagia is caused more by spastic contractions than outflow obstruction. We find that a number of these patients will respond to low-dose sublingual hyoscyamine. Even though it doesn't normalize the motility, they get symptomatic relief without needing to do an intervention on the GEJ and spastic contractions in the esophageal body.

In type 2 achalasia, I would not try pharmacologic therapy because it will decrease pan-pressurization and you need that pressure to help empty the esophagus.

I would also avoid doing a POEM in type 2 because you still have intrinsic motility that can help empty the esophagus in a non-peristaltic fashion, and you destroy that with a POEM. When you're doing a POEM, you are essentially creating a scleroderma-like esophagus, and you're getting rid of all motility. What you need in a type 2 is to get rid of the EGJOO either with a Heller myotomy or pneumatic dilation. There is usually enough remaining intrinsic esophageal motility that the reduction in LES tone produced by pneumatic dilation should be sufficient to relieve symptoms in type 2. However, the reduced esophageal body contractility in type 1 (end-stage achalasia) usually requires a more complete ablation of the LES tone, which necessitates a myotomy.

In type 1, I am worried less about a POEM ablating esophageal body contractility, because it is already essentially absent. However, the concern for increased reflux after POEM remains.

People talk about pan-pressurization (in type 2 achalasia) as if it is a bad thing. I think it is a good thing, a driving force that can help to empty the esophagus. So, if the esophagus is pan-pressurized to 30 mm of mercury, and you can reduce the pressure at the LES to 10 mm of mercury, now you've got a 20-mm mercury driving pressure to empty out the esophagus. The difficulty comes when there's not sufficient esophageal squeeze pressure and then you have to really obliterate all the tone at the LES, allowing things to empty by gravity.

However, when you obliterate all tone at the GEJ, you also knock out your anti-reflux barrier. With a Heller, you can restore some of that by also performing a Dor or Toupet anti-reflux procedure, but with a POEM you can't. I have some concerns about the POEM long term. I think there's the potential for a lot of reflux damage that can accumulate over time, including Barrett's esophagus and possibly associated neoplasia.

One of the things to watch out for post-achalasia treatment is that patients will feel great when you see them 1 or 2 months after their initial therapy. Some gastroenterologists mistakenly tell their patients not to come back unless they're having problems. That's not a good idea. Many patients, especially after a POEM, will have significant reflux. Many patients will put on a lot of weight since they're able to eat a lot better now that their obstruction is relieved. As a result, they develop even more reflux related to weight gain, and many will develop reflux esophagitis and even reflux strictures. Also, pills are more likely to lodge unawares in the esophagus of these patients, so they are more prone to pill injury from NSAIDS, etc. Therefore, I think you have to monitor these patients long-term and continue to re-educate them regarding potential problems.

I also think that with the surgical myotomy in type 2 achalasia, the surgeons should try to disrupt as little of the muscle in the esophageal body above the LES as possible. There is an understandable tendency to err on the side of cutting higher into the esophageal body, to avoid the disaster of an incomplete myotomy of the LES. We're starting to see an increased number of patients who have a blown-out esophagus, years after their surgery because too much esophageal muscle has been destroyed.

Case 2 *An 82-year-old woman is referred to you for dysphagia. She has had dysphagia for 6 months that has been getting progressively worse. It was initially for solids, but now she has dysphagia for liquids as well. Her community gastroenterologist did an EGD that showed a corkscrew esophagus. The LES was somewhat tight and seemed to have a birds-beak appearance. The scope easily passed the zone of resistance at the LES and popped into the stomach. He did a TTS dilation of the LES, and the swallowing improved for about a week, and then, swallowing got worse.*

He suspects the patient may have a variant of achalasia and wants your opinion. He thinks she probably is a candidate for Botox. While he thinks a pneumatic dilation would help her, he is reluctant because of her age and asks your opinion.

You examine the patient. She is somewhat frail and fairly immobile. She is reluctant to have esophageal manometry.

Would you ever inject Botox without a manometry documenting achalasia?

I don't want to empirically treat someone for achalasia without manometry. There are different presentations and different types of achalasia. Some have spastic contractions, and some have a dead and scleroderma-type esophageal body. You manage these differently.

For the patient who complains that they don't want to go through an esophageal manometry because they are afraid of the catheter placement being painful, we will place the catheter at the time of endoscopy while they are sedated, so it should not be a problem.

Do you ever see 80-year-old patients presenting with a new diagnosis of achalasia?

I do see achalasia being diagnosed in patients who are in their 70s and 80s. Of course, many patients have had their disease for years before the diagnosis is made. I've seen some patients where I have looked back in their old X-ray jacket and saw a dilated esophagus on a CAT scan done years before symptom onset that was not appreciated at the time.

Of course, when you diagnose achalasia in elderly, frail patients there is a reluctance to send them to surgery because of the higher risk of postoperative complications. They're also reluctant to have the patient get a pneumatic dilation for the same reason, because there's a 2% risk of potential perforation. So, you inject Botox and the patient does great.

However, when you decide to treat the older patient with Botox because it is less invasive are you just delaying the inevitable? They do great for, at best, a year, and then you inject them again. After a while, you've injected a lot of Botox down there, the patient develops antibodies, and the Botox stops working. In addition, all that Botox may or may not cause fibrosis which surgeons aren't too happy about.

So, if the patient survives long enough to outlast the Botox what are you going to do? You've got to do something, but it's going to be at higher risk. When you decide whether you should start Botox on an elderly patient, that is a challenging decision that your present self has to make, that your future self is going to have to live with. So, they're now five years older, and the Botox is not working. You have to do something more substantial, but now they're only a poorer surgical candidate.

In this case the patient received a TTS dilation that helped very briefly. What do you think about doing an empiric TTS dilation in a patient with achalasia?

I actually think it is a good idea. A number of patients with achalasia also have a stricture at the GEJ. Empirically, dilating the stricture can improve their dysphagia, and some of them may not need further treatment for their achalasia for a long time. It may be hard to tell that they've got a stricture down there, and you can't see the stricture because the LES isn't relaxing. However, I do have any number of achalasia patients who, in addition to their achalasia, have a stricture at the GE junction. You won't know it unless you pass a 60 French bougie across there or inflate a TTS 20-mm balloon.

I've had some patients with achalasia that probably had the condition for 10 or 20 years without bothersome symptoms, and then, they get a stricture, and that's the thing that tips them over. If I dilate the stricture, they can live with the achalasia. I wouldn't do that in a 20-year-old, but a 70-, 80-year-old, if you can find a stricture and dilate it, and they get symptomatic relief I wouldn't treat their achalasia any further, although they still need to be followed and their symptoms monitored.

We don't really know how Botox works to relieve symptoms in achalasia. We assume that it works on the motility of the sphincter, but is it possible that it works more on the sensory component? I had a guy this last year who was in his nineties with well-documented achalasia. We treated him with Botox, and his symptoms of dysphagia and regurgitation got dramatically better, but then we noticed that he also had iron deficiency anemia. I'm not too excited about working up iron deficiency anemia in a 90-year-old, but then, 2 or 3 weeks later he started having black stool. He was on an antiplatelet agent for heart disease, and his blood count was dropping more. So, we felt we had to do a colonoscopy, but we didn't find anything. So, what was causing this dark stool? Did he have something concerning down in his small bowel?

At that point, he's saying his swallowing is doing great, because of the Botox, and so we decided to do a capsule endoscopy, which he swallowed without difficulty. It was a 12-h capsule, and then, we went to read the images and the capsule sat in the esophagus for 11 h. Then, it finally came out, but he felt no dysphagia at all. Clearly, the esophagus wasn't emptying correctly, and he just didn't feel it.

Case 3 *A 64-year-old woman with a history of small cell lung cancer that has been in remission is referred with dysphagia. Dysphagia started about a month earlier and rapidly worsened. She is now having marked difficulty swallowing solids and liquids.*

A CT scan shows a mildly dilated esophagus but no suggestion of metastatic disease in the region of the esophagus or stomach. An EGD is performed that shows a birds-beak-type LES with increased resistance, but eventually the scope successfully pops through. No lesions are seen in the esophagus and cardia, etc. A TTS dilation is performed without prolonged clinical benefit. You suspect the patient has pseudoachalasia.

What are some of the markers that make you suspect pseudoachalasia?

Historical markers for pseudoachalasia include older age, more rapid onset of symptoms, and more substantial weight loss. A clue during endoscopy is that it may be more difficult to get the scope through the GEJ. In idiopathic achalasia, the GEJ may not open with air insufflation alone, but you can easily advance the scope through the sphincter into the stomach. One of the markers of pseudoachalasia is significant difficulty advancing the scope into the stomach. There may be tumor infiltrating the GEJ which may be difficult to visualize.

Are there manometric distinctions that can help differentiate between idiopathic achalasia and pseudoachalasia?

Idiopathic achalasia is very uncommon, pseudoachalasia is extremely uncommon, and pseudoachalasia as a paraneoplastic phenomenon is extremely rare. To tell you whether there are manometric findings that can help distinguish pseudoachalasia from achalasia is difficult because there are so few cases to evaluate. It might be possible there will be different responses to pharmacologic provocative maneuvers, but at this point we really have insufficient data to tell, and there are so few cases out there.

Case 4 *A 43 year-old man presents to his community gastroenterologist with dysphagia of one-month duration. He has dysphagia for solids and liquids. He has been taking high doses of Percocet for months after a back injury. The gastroenterologist does an EGD that suggests achalasia. He does a manometry that is consistent with achalasia. He sends the patient to you because he refers all his pneumatic dilations to you.*

Do you approach the diagnosis of achalasia differently in patients on opiates?

If you look at patients with type 3 achalasia and patients with EGJOO, there is an increased number of people in these cohorts who take high doses of narcotics. If you look at their responses to pharmacologic provocative testing during manometry, the responses to amyl nitrite and CCK are different in patients who have opiate-associated achalasia from those patients with idiopathic achalasia.

We only see this clinical picture in patients who are taking high doses of narcotics, at least 30 milliequivalents of morphine daily, not just one or two Percocet a day. Even before we knew about the connection of achalasia with opiates, we realized that patients on opiates did not get as good a result with achalasia therapy as patients who were not on opiates. The symptomatic outcomes were especially poor in people who appeared to have type 3 achalasia who were treated with ablative therapies.

On the other hand, we have seen that if you can get these patients completely off opiates, many of them will get total relief from their symptoms. So, that becomes the goal.

For whatever reason, we are seeing fewer of these patients than before, perhaps because community gastroenterologists have been made aware of this connection and they're explaining to their patients that the opiates are the problem. Anyway, when we see patients like this, we will not refer them for surgery until they've gone off narcotics. If they do that, symptoms will resolve in most patients.

One thing about my approach to treating opiate-induced esophageal dysmotility is that I don't want to be overly aggressive in patients who have symptoms that are simply a nuisance and not a threat to life (e.g., not having substantial weight loss or recurrent pneumonias). I am loath to recommend a POEM to someone whose condition is potentially reversible upon stopping opiates or dropping to a lower dosage, because the POEM creates a scleroderma-like esophagus, something that can't be reversed.

Reference

1. Dent J, Vakil N, Jones R, Bytzer P, Schöning U, Halling K, Junghard O, Lind T. Accuracy of the diagnosis of GORD by questionnaire, physicians and a trial of proton pump inhibitor treatment: the Diamond Study. Gut. 2010;59(6):714–21.

Chapter 5
Other Motility Disorders of the Esophagus and Achalasia

Francis Edeani

Case 1 *The patient is a 35-year-old woman who presents with a history of occasional chest pain which is clearly related to meals, definitely worse when eating. The pain is described as an ache or a cramp. She also has the sensation of food sticking intermittently, both solids and liquids. Her symptoms are exacerbated when she is stressed. Her physical exam is normal. An EKG is normal. She is treated with PPIs for one month without relief.*

How do you evaluate a patient with chest pain and dysphagia during swallowing?

Dysphagia to solids and liquids suggests a motility disorder of the esophagus. We generally start with the simplest test—an esophagram. This is noninvasive, provides a "roadmap" and can give a general idea about esophageal motility, shows the presence of strictures or rings, and may provide some information about the mucosal lining. Challenge with a barium tablet or marshmallow can sometimes reproduce the patient's symptoms and can demonstrate stasis of the food bolus.

The gold standard test for esophageal motility disorders is esophageal manometry. EGD is typically performed as a complementary test to assess for lesions due to reflux esophagitis, eosinophilic esophagitis, infectious esophagitis (such as CMV, HSV, candida in immunocompromised patients), esophageal strictures, rings or webs, and malignancy. A tight esophagogastric junction during EGD may suggest the presence of an esophageal outflow obstruction motility disorder. If the EGD with biopsies is normal, esophageal manometry is performed. In patients with high probability for esophageal motility disorder as determined by findings on

F. Edeani (✉)
Division of Gastroenterology and Hepatology, Department of Internal Medicine, Medical College of Wisconsin, Milwaukee, WI, USA
e-mail: fedeani@mcw.edu

esophagram (bird-beak appearance, esophageal spasms, dysmotility, etc.), a manometry catheter can be placed during EGD. Esophageal dilation should be performed if a ring or stricture is present.

Aren't the manometry results altered by the sedation?

Earlier studies raised concerns about the potential impact of sedation on esophageal motility. However, recent studies have failed to show any significant differences in esophageal motility between post-sedated and unsedated studies.

We avoid the use of topical lidocaine spray to numb the oropharynx because this may affect safe swallowing during manometry and may potentially affect esophageal motility.

In this case, the EGD was normal, and biopsies returned negative for EOE. The manometry revealed a normal pressure LES that relaxed normally, with an IRP of 8. Esophageal peristalsis was coordinated, but contractions were of increased amplitude. Out of ten swallows, the distal contractile integral (DCI) was over 8000 on four swallows with the highest reaching 10,000.

The DCI represents the vigor of esophageal contractions based on pressure measurements from multiple sensors across the body of the esophagus. The IRP is a measure of LES relaxation pressure computed by measuring the pressures of any 4 s with the lowest pressures over a 10-s window.

Findings in this case are consistent with Jackhammer esophagus. The Chicago Classification v 4.0 states that if at least 20% of swallows have a DCI > 8000, this is consistent with Jackhammer esophagus. In this case, 40% were higher than 8000.

In Jackhammer, the forceful contractions produce luminal occlusion which can cause dysphagia and chest pain.

How does Jackhammer differ from nutcracker esophagus and esophageal spasm?

Nutcracker is a terminology that isn't used anymore. In the past, nutcracker esophagus was used to refer to patients who had multiple swallows with a DCI > 5000 but <8000. However, subsequently it was noted that many asymptomatic individuals have DCIs > 5000, so this term has been removed from the Chicago classification.

Esophageal spasms, which are non-peristaltic contractions, are characterized by short distal latency, defined by the time from initiation of the swallow to the bolus reaching the distal esophagus in less than 4.5 s.

In these cases, the lower esophageal sphincter may not have enough time to relax before the bolus arrives and the food bolus gets stuck, which can cause chest pain and/or the sensation of dysphagia. This rapid emptying is also seen in patients with type 3 achalasia where most contractions are spastic.

How do you treat patients with Jackhammer esophagus?

Jackhammer esophagus represents hypercontractile peristalsis, and so, we use medications that cause smooth muscle relaxation. We typically start with peppermint oil and, if ineffective, calcium channel blockers. Patients on calcium channel blockers should be monitored for side effects such as hypotension, lightheadedness, and headache. For peppermint, we recommend two Altoids three times a day, before meals. If this is ineffective, we can add hyoscyamine 2.5 mg (two tablets) SL before each meal. If that doesn't work, we may go to diltiazem 30–90 mg 4 times daily. Nifedipine has been used in the past at a dose of 10 mg three times daily 20 min before meals, but sublingual formulations should be avoided as this can cause an exaggerated drop in blood pressure. If symptoms improve or resolve with calcium channel blockers, we decrease the dose to once daily or take only as needed.

For patients who do not improve with the above, a trial of neuromodulators is recommended. We recommend a low-dose tricyclic antidepressant such as amitriptyline or nortriptyline, taken at bedtime. Symptoms are reassessed after 3 months.

Are Botox injections useful?

Botox may be useful for hypercontractile and impaired relaxation disorders of the lower esophageal sphincter but is not used for hypercontractile disorders of the esophageal body. We don't use Botox injections along the length of the body of the esophagus like we do with the LES in achalasia. In achalasia, we are simply knocking out the LES. In Jackhammer, we can't afford to knock out all peristalsis by injecting along the length of the esophagus; we might go from having too strong contractions to no contractions and create a more serious problem. Patients with Jackhammer esophagus may improve over time allowing for discontinuation of smooth muscle-relaxing medications. For the same reason, POEM is not being used in Jackhammer esophagus.

Case 2 A 45-year-old woman is referred for difficulty with swallowing that has been present for 6 months. She is aware of the sensation of solid food sticking and liquids going down slowly. The symptoms are slowly getting worse. She has no smoking or drinking history. She has been getting increased heartburn. An EGD is done which appears normal, and biopsies return negative for EOE. A timed esophagram shows mild-to-moderate esophageal dysmotility. Manometry reveals a normal LESP with normal relaxation, with an IRP of 9. However, esophageal contractions show low amplitude.

How do you approach a patient with dysphagia and low-amplitude contractions?

This is a very common finding when we do manometry to investigate dysphagia.

In patients with a LES that relaxes appropriately, we divide swallows of low amplitude into weak contractions, where the DCI is <450, and failed contractions where the DCI is <100. The diagnosis of ineffective esophageal motility (IEM) is used if 50% or more swallows have a DCI < 100, or 70% have a DCI < 450. The most recognized finding with IEM is gastroesophageal reflux. The lack of effective esophageal contractions interferes with the clearance of gastric refluxate, as well as the ingested bolus.

While ineffective or absent contractility is seen in scleroderma, this is not really part of the differential for our patient, who has a normal LES. In scleroderma, the LES is hypotensive at baseline, predisposing to severe reflux. Ineffective esophageal motility can occasionally be seen in other mixed connective tissue diseases.

Occasionally, we are asked whether GERD produces decreased esophageal motility. There is no evidence to support this. GERD can be associated with dysphagia, related to the inflamed mucosa. PPIs can help relieve dysphagia in this instance, but there is no evidence that esophageal motility is altered by GERD or administration of PPIs.

IEM is poorly understood, but it is very common in patients investigated with manometry for dysphagia. Many asymptomatic controls can have a degree of ineffective motility.

Case 3 *A 38-year-old man has a history of difficulty swallowing. He is on chronic opiates for a bad back, taking three Percocet a day. He smokes 1 PPD and has 2–3 drinks a day. He denies heartburn, nausea, and vomiting. His dysphagia started several months earlier. He has problems swallowing solids and liquids that have gradually worsened. His physical exam is unremarkable. An EGD is negative for any stricture, and biopsies are negative for EOE. Manometry shows simultaneous contractions, with no true peristalsis. Overall pressure measurements are low during swallowing, but there is an elevated LESP that does not relax appropriately on swallowing, with an IRP of 20.*

How would you evaluate and manage this patient?

This patient appears to have opioid-induced esophageal motility disorder. The absence of coordinated esophageal contractions along with a hypertonic LES that does not relax adequately with swallowing is suggestive of achalasia. However, the diagnosis of achalasia should not be made in patients on opioids because these drugs can cause a similar motility disorder.

The mechanism of opioid-induced esophageal motility disorders is not completely understood. Stimulation of μ opioid receptors has been associated with symptoms of dysphagia and heartburn. Opioids decrease esophageal peristalsis and affect function of the LES through impairment of nitric oxide pathway. We don't want to send the patient for unnecessary achalasia surgery when the syndrome may be caused by opiates.

The management in this case requires getting the patient off opioids and repeating the manometry if symptoms persist. If the pattern persists then the patient has true achalasia, but in most cases the manometry will normalize off opioids. We don't know the true incidence of opioid-induced dysphagia, but it would appear to be relatively uncommon considering the number of patients on chronic opioids and the small proportion of these patients that present with dysphagia. However, in evaluating patients with swallowing disorders, getting them off opioids may alleviate their symptoms.

Case 4 *A 30-year-old man presents with dysphagia for solids and liquids going on for three months. He has lost 12 pounds over that time. No history of opiate use, no smoking, and drinks only occasional alcohol. On EGD, he has a tight LES, but the scope passes through with a gentle pop as it is gently advanced into the stomach. Manometry is performed and demonstrates incomplete relaxation of the LES, with an IRP of 17, absent esophageal peristalsis, and no pan-pressurization.*

How would you manage this patient?

This appears to be a classic type 1 achalasia. The patient is in the expected age range for achalasia, 25–60 years old. The history of dysphagia with solids and liquids is suggestive of esophageal motility disorder. This patient is also not on opioids. The high IRP and failed esophageal body peristalsis all meet the criteria for type 1 achalasia.

We recommend a timed barium esophagram in our patients with achalasia, which can serve as a baseline for comparison with follow-up studies in the future.

Treatment of type 1 achalasia is directed at disrupting the LES as there is no peristalsis. The least invasive treatment is a trial of smooth muscle-relaxing medications such as peppermint and calcium channel blockers. Botox may relieve dysphagia with efficacy lasting from a few weeks to several months. Repeat Botox injections can be performed, but patients develop antibodies, and the efficacy of repeated injections decreases.

Other treatments for achalasia depend on the age, comorbidities, and expected life expectancy of the patient. Pneumatic dilation can relieve dysphagia for up to 5 or more years, but the potential complication is esophageal perforation. Therefore, pneumatic dilation should only be considered in a patient who is a candidate for cardiothoracic surgery in the unfortunate event of esophageal perforation.

Heller myotomy and POEM are other therapies for patients who are surgical candidates. POEM is less invasive and recovery is quicker, but there is a small risk of esophageal perforation, and all patients will have esophageal reflux post-op. Because of the universal problem with reflux after a POEM, most centers will place all their patients on PPIs post-op and attempt to de-escalate over time.

There is much more experience with the Heller myotomy, which has been performed for decades. Because the Heller myotomy is typically combined with a fundoplication, reflux is not as prevalent a problem compared with POEM postoperatively.

The choice between pneumatic dilation, Heller myotomy, and POEM in patients who are surgical candidates depends on local expertise. In our center, most patients have had Heller myotomy, but the number getting a POEM is increasing.

In this patient, we mentioned that pan-pressurization was absent. What would it mean if pan-pressurization was present?

This would be consistent with type 2 achalasia, where the LES does not relax, and contractions occur in all segments of the esophageal body simultaneously, leading to pressurization of the esophageal lumen. An accurate diagnosis of the achalasia subtype has implications for the treatment options. For instance, patients with type 3 achalasia should have POEM or long Heller myotomy with proximal extension of myotomy.

Case 5 An 85-year-old woman, who is chronically ill, presents with food impaction. EGD is performed, and there is soft food sitting in a corkscrew-shaped esophagus. After the food is removed, the LES zone appears mildly tight, but the scope *could pop into the stomach. Dilation with a TTS balloon is performed, but there is not much symptomatic improvement. Manometry is performed (somewhat limited), and the LES pressure is elevated and does not relax, with an IRP of 16. There is no normal esophageal peristalsis.*

How would you manage the case of a patient with corkscrew esophagus where the LES does not relax appropriately?

This patient sounds like she may have type 1 achalasia. However, in patients presenting with findings of achalasia in this age range, we need to rule out pseudo-achalasia. It's important to make sure that there is no GEJ cancer causing obstruction and would also perform a chest radiograph to rule out any mediastinal mass. Once we've ruled out pseudoachalasia, we would generally treat a patient like this with Botox. This may provide some dysphagia relief for a few to several months, before needing to repeat injection. As we mentioned earlier, pneumatic dilation should be avoided unless the patient were a candidate for cardiothoracic surgery should a complication occur. This patient also would not be a great candidate for a POEM or Heller myotomy because of her age and frailty. Medical therapy can be considered although this is the least effective treatment option. Long-acting nitrates such as isosorbide dinitrate 5 mg may be administered sublingually 10–15 min before meals. Sublingual nitroglycerine 0.4 mg is an alternative. PDE5 inhibitors (e.g., sildenafil), anticholinergics (e.g., atropine), and beta-adrenergic agonists (e.g., terbutaline) have been used for treatment of achalasia, but there are limited data on their efficacy. If the patient is already on an anti-hypertensive that is not a calcium channel blocker, you could consult with her primary care physician about switching her medication to a calcium channel blocker.

We encounter a number of elderly patients with corkscrew esophagus some of whom present with food impactions. Is this simply an aging process of the esophagus?

Corkscrew esophagus is a radiographic finding on barium esophagram characterized by non-peristaltic contractions and may reflect esophageal spasm. However, most patients with esophageal spasm do not have corkscrew morphology on esophagram. Age-related esophageal dysmotility is a nonspecific finding on esophagram and is termed presbyesophagus. With advancing age, more people develop changes in esophageal motility including an increase in the number of simultaneous contractions, lower amplitudes of contraction, and diminished LES relaxation. Patients may remain asymptomatic early on, but later some will develop dysphagia and even food impactions.

Chapter 6
GERD

Patrick Sanvanson

Case 1 *A 35-year-old man with a BMI of 28 is referred to you with a history of chronic heartburn. He doesn't smoke. He has only one to two drinks on weekends. He stops eating 2 h before bedtime and elevates the head of his bed. Despite this, he has ongoing heartburn. He started taking over-the-counter omeprazole at bedtime and initially had limited response. He spoke to his primary care doctor who corrected the timing of the PPI, and taking it before breakfast worked much better. As soon as he stopped the omeprazole, his heartburn came right back again. Rather than simply continuing the omeprazole, his primary care doctor referred him to you.*

Would you accept the diagnosis of GERD in this case? Or are there other conditions you would consider? How would you manage this?

He has a pretty classic presentation of GERD, with chronic heartburn. He takes the medication and responds pretty well to it. Initially, he was taking it incorrectly, at nighttime. We usually tell our patients to try to take PPIs 30 min before breakfast when the proton pumps are the most active to be able to expose more of the proton pumps to the drug.

In terms of risk factors for Barrett's esophagus, he is overweight. On the other hand, he is young, under 50 years old, and has no alarm symptoms like dysphagia or weight loss. We usually don't recommend endoscopy looking to rule out Barrett's esophagus in someone who is 35. All things considered, he's probably at less of a risk for Barrett's esophagus right now.

I think the other thing that is always important in taking care of these patients is to instruct them early on about lifestyle factors, including trying not to eat late at night, elevating the head of your bed, and weight loss. The medications we give

P. Sanvanson (✉)
Division of Gastroenterology and Hepatology, Department of Medicine, Medical College of Wisconsin, Milwaukee, WI, USA
e-mail: psanvans@mcw.edu

© The Author(s), under exclusive license to Springer Nature Switzerland AG 2023
W. H. Sobin et al. (eds.), *Managing Complex Cases in Gastroenterology*,
https://doi.org/10.1007/978-3-031-48949-5_6

decrease gastric acid, but they do nothing for esophageal clearance. They do nothing to correct a hiatal hernia. The lifestyle measures will help decrease the volume of refluxed material.

In this case, when the patient stops the drug, his symptoms come right back. At that point, I have a discussion with him about potential next steps. For some patients I will say, "It's okay, it sounds like you have reflux disease. You respond well to the therapy, so we can just keep you on the 20-mg dose of PPI." Unfortunately, at this time, he will need to stay on the PPI indefinitely unless some other risk factors are modified. Hopefully, decreasing his weight may help with some of the reflux that he's having.

Some patients don't like to be on medications long term, and that's understandable. So, in those patients, I might give them the option of potentially doing a scope, looking for erosive esophagitis. Seeing that they have erosive esophagitis or a hiatal hernia may be more of a reason to keep them on medication long term, since they have structural findings that will continue to promote reflux and evidence of esophageal damage already present.

Endoscopy can also be helpful in excluding alternate diagnoses, like eosinophilic esophagitis (EOE). Do we need to do an endoscopy simply to rule out Barrett's esophagus in this gentleman? No. Usually, we don't recommend screening for Barrett's esophagus at the age of 35. American College of Gastroenterology guidelines for screening for Barrett's esophagus recommend it be limited to men with chronic reflux symptoms and two or more risk factors including age > 50, Caucasian race, presence of central obesity, a history of smoking, and a family history of Barrett's esophagus or esophageal adenocarcinoma. Unfortunately, I've had patients who were in their twenties that I've diagnosed with Barrett's esophagus.

In considering whether to endoscope this patient, it is unlikely that he has Barrett's esophagus, but I might give him the option, particularly if he feels like he doesn't want to be in therapy long term.

If you decide to do an endoscopy, do you want the patient off of PPIs?

Yes, I try to stop PPIs at least two months beforehand, because that way I feel like you're not masking anything, you're not masking erosive esophagitis, and you're not masking EOE. Then, if there is no evidence of Barrett's esophagus, and there is no erosive esophagitis, then we are managing a non-erosive reflux disease patient. They may have reflux that isn't causing esophagitis, or they may have functional heartburn or esophageal hypersensitivity. Regardless, when dealing with non-erosive disease, it's less essential to be on medication, except from a quality-of-life standpoint.

If you do the endoscopy and it's grossly normal, are you prepared to do pH testing at that time?

It depends on how severe their symptoms are. If they're tolerating their symptoms pretty well, and the endoscopy is completely normal, then I wouldn't necessarily do pH testing. If their symptoms are mild, we might just suggest taking an H2 blocker, which is quite safe.

But if the patient wants to see if they truly have reflux disease, or you want to determine if this is functional heartburn, or esophageal hypersensitivity, at that point I do offer pH testing. Unfortunately, pH testing is not the most sensitive testing in the world.

We do know that probably around 70% of patients with heartburn don't have evidence of erosive changes on endoscopy. So, from that standpoint, all we can tell him is he doesn't have reflux diseases causing damage or ulceration of their esophagus.

If they do want further evaluation to see if this is truly reflux disease, the next option would be doing pH testing, whether it's catheter-based pH testing or it's a wireless Bravo pH testing.

Which do you prefer in terms of pH testing?

It all depends on the patient. I think they both have their benefits. When I do pH testing to determine if reflux is occurring, then I stop their PPI therapy for at least 7 days and test off therapy.

If somebody is unable to tolerate any catheter within their nose for a 24-h time period, they make the decision for you, and you do a Bravo study. However, if you have previously done an endoscopy and you want to save the patient the cost of another endoscopy, and if they're able to tolerate a catheter in their nose, then choosing a catheter-based test is prudent.

The Bravo device might be advantageous if you have a patient with nonspecific symptoms like chest pain that occurs intermittently, not daily. A Bravo study usually gives you 96 h worth of data. The pH catheter just studies 24 h of data. So, in that scenario, a Bravo study may be more likely to capture the event in question.

On the other hand, occasionally we'll have patients that come in with some vague symptoms like a globus sensation or some kind of cough-related issue, and we want to answer the question whether these symptoms are reflux-related. There are two advantages to the pH catheter device compared to the Bravo. The pH catheter has two sensors, so it can measure acid levels proximally and distally. The Bravo just measures at one location, usually 6 cm above the LES. In addition, the pH catheter measures impedance, so it can detect reflux of liquid that is non-acid, as well as acid.

So, using the pH catheter with its proximal sensor and impedance monitoring, we can determine whether there are proximal reflux events that correspond with coughing or globus.

Then once again, if the patient just can't tolerate a catheter within their nose for 24 h, we have to use the Bravo and recognize that the data collection has its limitations. So, it depends on the patient and the clinical scenario, and then, we give them our recommendation of which test we think will give us the higher yield for what we're looking for.

Now, we've discussed doing pH studies off PPIs. Occasionally, we will do the studies on PPI to assess the patient's response to therapy. If the patient is still symptomatic, in spite of taking PPIs, doing the pH study while on therapy can be beneficial to determine whether the patient is having residual acid reflux, and if you're using the pH catheter, you can also see if they are having non-acid reflux.

How do you approach patients who are complaining of heartburn waking them at night, who are taking a PPI once a day in the morning?

We know that PPIs work very well at healing erosive esophagitis, and when patients complain of ongoing heartburn in spite of PPIs, there are two things I question. Is the diagnosis of GERD correct? Is the patient on a PPI regimen with sufficient potency?

However, if somebody's complaining more about nocturnal symptoms, for example, they feel like they wake up in the middle of the night choking on acid or coughing. In these patients, it's very important to stress lifestyle factors. So, elevating the head of the bed and not eating late at night, usually at least 2 h before lying down, are essential.

Then, if that is not working, I will often add an H2 blocker like famotidine at bedtime. The main reason I do that is because a lot of nocturnal reflux events are thought to be histamine-driven. So, frequently, H2 blockers are a little bit more effective for nighttime reflux. Unfortunately, there may be tachyphylaxis after extended H2 blocker use, where patients over time become tolerant to the medication, and it has less efficacy. So that's always a concern.

Then, another option, although it's not currently commercially available (until a new manufacturer starts delivering it), is a device for patients who have supra-esophageal reflux symptoms, where you think they're coughing at night because of acid going above the level of the upper esophageal sphincter (UES). This is an upper esophageal sphincter assist device that was developed at the Medical College of Wisconsin. It was initially known as the Reza band, but is now known as the reflux band. This band applies some pressure at the level of the upper esophageal sphincter to prevent acid going above the UES. This may be an option for a subset of patients, although certain patients can't tolerate anything around their neck while they sleep. The nice thing about the reflux band is that it's not a medication, and it's quite safe. When you stop using it, you just go back to your baseline. So, there's no dependency that occurs.

Have you ever used nighttime omeprazole-bicarbonate (Zegerid)?

It's an option that I've only used in a small set of patients. More often, what I'll do is try to switch them to a more potent PPI to see if that's more effective. In addition to that, I may give them a double dose where they take the second dose 30 min before dinner time. Or, if they have predominantly nighttime symptoms, stop the morning dose and simply prescribe their PPI 30 min before dinner. I will also occasionally use dexlansoprazole (Dexilant), which is a PPI with a longer half-life.

Have you ever done genetic testing for the CYP2C19 polymorphism to see if they were rapid metabolizers?

No, usually I just increase the dose or give one of the more potent PPIs, including rabeprazole or dexlansoprazole. Then, if somebody is not responding to double-dose higher potency PPI, I will want to perform pH testing on medication to determine whether they have residual acid reflux.

While there may be some patients who are more likely to be nonresponders because of genetic polymorphisms, more commonly you wonder if that is just one contributing factor. Other factors that might exacerbate reflux include structural ones like a hiatal hernia, or perhaps, there's some dietary noncompliance issues, or perhaps, there are other modifiable factors like weight. Then, there is also a subset of our patients that have some degree of esophageal hypersensitivity or functional heartburn that might cause them to be nonresponders.

So, before I go down that line of considering genetic testing, I think the key is always to see (1) whether or not you're treating the right condition, (2) whether you're suppressing acid sufficiently, with pH testing, and (3) seeing if there's a symptom correlation with events, which might suggest hypersensitivity.

However, at this point, I'm not doing the genetic polymorphism tests. I think that as genetic testing becomes more available and, hopefully, cost-efficient, I may want to add in these tests. Right now, from my experience, I just don't know how it's going to impact clinical practice. I feel that even if they are hyper-metabolizers, at the end of the day, you're probably just going to increase the dose of PPI or change to the more potent agent, regardless.

Case 2 *The patient is a 40-year-old white woman who has been taking OTC PPIs for months without relief from heartburn. An EGD is performed, and the results are normal and biopsies negative. You decide to do a Bravo procedure to evaluate whether the symptoms are reflux-related. The Bravo procedure is done off PPI and reveals the time with pH < 4 is only 2%, a negative study. However, a symptom log was reviewed, and the patient did note episodes of symptoms that did correlate with isolated reflux episodes.*

How would you approach this situation?

Yes, this is a very difficult group of patients. The most important thing is that these are patients who you definitely want to avoid sending for anti-reflux surgery.

When dealing with patients who have esophageal hypersensitivity or functional heartburn, there are not a lot of well-defined therapies to use. From the standpoint of understanding their symptoms, I think it is always important to tell these patients that although their symptoms may feel like severe reflux disease, their esophagus is NOT severely damaged, and the pH testing demonstrates that they are not refluxing large amounts of acid into their esophagus.

There are some patients that have reflux hypersensitivity who may respond to a larger dose of acid-reducing medication, PPI therapy. Further suppressing their acid levels below the normal level may actually help with some of their reflux symptoms, whether it's heartburn or regurgitation, or whatever.

However, a lot of the time, with many of these patients, we consider what other options are available. A lot of the strategies aim to work on the esophageal sensitivity levels. We turn to medications that have been used for other neuropathic conditions or visceral hypersensitivity issues as well. The ones that I have the most experience within this population are low-dose tricyclic antidepressants (TCAs), whether it's nortriptyline, amitriptyline, or imipramine.

We've had some success using these as adjunctive agents in terms of altering the sensory threshold to esophageal hypersensitivity. We also try dietary therapies trying to limit trigger foods in patients whose symptoms are worsened with particular foods.

Sometimes, we've tried diaphragmatic breathing techniques in this patient population as well. Hopefully, in the future, we will develop some targeted therapies, because a lot of the therapies we're using now are neuromodulating agents that are used for other purposes and extrapolated to the esophagus.

It is known that TCAs and SSRIs can help with symptom improvement by increasing the sensory threshold for pain perception. People have done some esophageal balloon distension studies. They've done esophageal acid perfusion studies, and some of these neuromodulating agents have been shown to be beneficial in patients who have esophageal hypersensitivity or functional heartburn.

Comments on Case 2: Dr. Sobin

This patient clearly does not have increased acid reflux but appears to have **reflux hypersensitivity**. I give patients the "princess and the pea" analogy to explain their heightened sensitivity. These patients are distinguished from those who have normal 24-h pH testing and no correlation between symptoms and pH reflux episodes. This is so-called **functional heartburn**. In both these instances, we think there is a functional component to their symptoms.

In reflux hypersensitivity, I would continue a PPI even though 24-h acid levels are not increased, seeing how the patient's symptoms are exacerbated when there are episodes of reflux. If the symptoms are severe, I might turn to a central neuromodulator. Trazodone and SSRIs have been used and found effective in treating functional esophageal syndromes, although large population studies are lacking. SSRIs have been found more helpful in treating functional esophageal disorders than other functional disorders of gut-brain interaction. Tricyclics may also be tried, as noted by Dr. Sanvanson.

Chapter 7
Refractory GERD

W. Harley Sobin

Case 1 *A 41-year-old white man with a BMI of 26 presents with a history of chronic acid reflux symptoms for the past year. He has frequent heartburn and intermittent regurgitation. He has taken occasional OTC Prilosec. You put him on esomeprazole, 40 mg a day, and see him back in 1 month. Despite therapy, he has ongoing heartburn.*

Is it surprising to you that the symptoms of heartburn aren't gone after a month of therapy?

Many people assume that PPIs universally clear up GERD symptoms, but only 60% of patients with GERD, at best, will become asymptomatic after a month of PPI therapy.

When patients aren't responding to PPIs what is the checklist you go through?

I always review whether they are actually taking the medicine and timing it appropriately. Many people take their PPIs with meals or HS which leads to poor results. I consider alternative diagnoses: Could the patient have pill esophagitis—are they taking minocycline, doxycycline, potassium pills, or alendronate? Might there be an underlying motility disorder—either gastroparesis exacerbating GERD or achalasia masquerading as GERD? Could it be eosinophilic esophagitis—is there a history of food impactions or multiple allergies?

He had mistakenly been taking his PPI HS, so, instead, he starts to take his esomeprazole 30 min before breakfast and presents a month later with almost the exact same complaints.

W. H. Sobin (✉)
Division of Gastroenterology and Hepatology, Medical College of Wisconsin,
Milwaukee, WI, USA
e-mail: hsobin@mcw.edu

© The Author(s), under exclusive license to Springer Nature
Switzerland AG 2023
W. H. Sobin et al. (eds.), *Managing Complex Cases in Gastroenterology*,
https://doi.org/10.1007/978-3-031-48949-5_7

So now it has been 2 months since starting daily PPI and he is still symptomatic. How would you proceed?

At that time, I would investigate further with an EGD. However, I would want to do the study off PPIs; if I do it on PPIs, I may get misleading information. Although I will be looking for endoscopic evidence of reflux esophagitis, I realize that the majority of patients with true reflux do not have erosive esophagitis on their index endoscopy, only about 30% do. If I see erosive esophagitis, I have my diagnosis, but since the majority of reflux patients have NERD (non-erosive reflux disease), I would be prepared to do a pH study if the endoscopy is normal. I would have the BRAVO probe ready to go. I would also do biopsies to rule out eosinophilic esophagitis, etc.

You instruct him to taper his PPI off over a week to avoid acid rebound, and then, he stays off it for a month. His symptoms go back to baseline. An EGD is performed, and on EGD, the esophageal mucosa appears normal. Esophageal biopsies are negative for EOE, Barrett's esophagus, etc. The BRAVO probe is introduced and shows time with pH < 4 of 10%, a positive result.

How would you manage this?

At this time, I would go to bid PPI 30 min before breakfast and before dinner. In one study of pH results in patients with refractory heartburn, the pH results were abnormal on one PPI daily in 31% of patients, but only 7% in patients on two PPI daily [1].

If patients don't respond sufficiently to this, I will add an H2 blocker at bedtime. This works well in many patients, but eventually a lot of them develop tachyphylaxis.

The other thing I might do is switch PPIs. There is a gradation of potency of different products which goes-pantoprazole is weakest, omeprazole and esomeprazole, somewhat stronger, rabeprazole and dexlansoprazole-the strongest.

In addition, there are patients who may have a genetic polymorphism in CYP2C19. They may be hyper-metabolizers of PPIs who will do better on rabeprazole than most of the other PPIs. Esomeprazole should do better as well.

Another trick, in patients who suffer from nocturnal heartburn is giving Zegerid, which is immediate release, not enteric coated, omeprazole-bicarbonate. This does not have to be taken before meals; it may be taken at bedtime.

A common problem is that patients may have improvement in their heartburn but still suffer from regurgitation. These patients generally have a significant anatomic defect, hiatal hernia, etc. I will reemphasize to these people the importance of elevating the head of their beds and other anti-reflux measures.

Are there other medical regimens that may improve regurgitation?

Taking baclofen before meals may be efficacious. Baclofen is a GABA-B agonist, and GABA-B inhibits TLESRs. However, most patients don't tolerate baclofen well, certainly long term.

The patient does not respond to protonix 40 mg bid and nighttime famotidine. He is switched to rabeprazole and finds dramatic improvement. He is able to discontinue his ranitidine and go to once daily rabeprazole before breakfast.

Patient 2 *A 38-year-old woman with chronic heartburn and regurgitation. Three months earlier, she had an EGD because of melena at which time she was found to have a hiatal hernia, reflux esophagitis (LA grade A), and a small duodenal ulcer. Biopsies were negative for Barrett's esophagus and HP. She was started on PPIs. After 2 months, the heartburn has improved, but she complains of severe regurgitation. A repeat EGD is performed that demonstrates healing of the esophagitis and duodenal ulcer. However, her LES appears quite lax, and she has a 3-cm sliding hiatal hernia.*

How would you approach this patient?

I think she is probably going to require anti-reflux surgery to fix the hernia and correct the reflux. Our surgeons do Nissen, Toupet, and LINX procedures to correct these hernias. Their philosophy is outlined in the next chapter.

Reference

1. Charbel S, Khandwala F, Vaezi MF. The role of esophageal pH monitoring in symptomatic patients on PPI therapy. Off J Am Coll Gastroenterol ACG. 2005;100(2):283–9.

Chapter 8
Surgery for GERD

Jon Gould

Case 1 A 40-year-old man, with 10 years of medically refractory reflux, remains on omeprazole. Despite omeprazole, he has severe regurgitation. When he stops omeprazole, he has severe heartburn as well.

Workup reveals a 4-cm hiatal hernia, normal esophageal motility, and a positive pH study with good symptom correlation. He has avoided having GERD surgery because of horror stories on the Internet about difficulties swallowing, not being able to vomit after surgery, or having severe gas bloat.

Most patients with GERD are being treated medically. In a case like this, the patient is really suffering despite medical therapy. Overall, is surgery underused?

Tons of patients suffer from this condition; GERD is a really common disease. Medical therapy with PPIs is frontline treatment, it's used frequently. It's accessible to patients. They can prescribe it for themselves. Primary care doctors hand it out frequently. We all prescribe it.

However, there are data that suggest that if you look at people who truly have a well-established GERD diagnosis, who are on a PPI, as many as one-third of those people are not completely satisfied with their treatment. We end up operating on a very small subset of those patients, less than 1% of people who would meet surgical criteria, which means symptoms of GERD refractory to medical therapy. We've got a small subset of people getting surgical therapy, and we've got a lot of people that are treading water, feeling like there's got to be something better, but they're not ready to commit to surgery.

J. Gould (✉)
Department of Surgery, Medical College of Wisconsin, Milwaukee, WI, USA
e-mail: jgould@mcw.edu

W. H. Sobin et al. (eds.), *Managing Complex Cases in Gastroenterology*,
https://doi.org/10.1007/978-3-031-48949-5_8

Fundoplication outcomes can be excellent when done properly in the appropriate patient. However, a lot of patients who have GERD interventions end up back on PPIs. There are doctors who tell their patients to avoid fundoplication because they only last a few years, and there are surgeons who have an opinion that these things never fall apart. The truth is somewhere in the middle. These procedures are intended to be lifelong interventions, but in the end, the bottom line is that you fail on some people.

We can do an intervention, but the patient may be left with side effects. In the end, are they better off? In some cases, no. There are some surgical failures. These repairs can work for a while and then fall apart. There are some bad outcomes. The wrong procedure might be done on the wrong patient.

The operations are not always as effective as we want them to be. So, we've got this issue. We've got a prevalent disease with a lot of people who are suffering, who aren't completely happy with their current treatment. However, they're not ready to make the next leap because they don't feel like there's an ideal option for them.

The good news is that newer techniques and learning from past mistakes allow us to have better surgical results.

You mention surgical repairs coming apart. Do the sutures loosen? Is that what is happening here?

We used to think that the sutures that we placed in the hiatus were tearing and the repair was disrupting. Now, we think that the repair doesn't disrupt, and it dilates over time. The hiatus stretches out, and then, the stomach herniates through there.

So now, what people are trying to do is close it tight enough that when it stretches, it doesn't stretch too much. You make it tight enough to prevent recurrence but not so tight that you get symptoms.

So, I tighten it to where I think it's about right. My way of doing it is a little different from the next guy. It's very much art, and it's judgment. For what it's worth, good judgment comes from having bad judgment a few times.

The 40-year-old patient described above seems to be a good candidate for surgery. He has a 10-year history of symptoms, severe regurgitation in spite of PPIs, and a disordered anatomy. I have always thought that the recommended surgical therapy for these patients was a Nissen. If the patient had disordered esophageal motility, you would do a Toupet instead. In this case the motility looks normal so would you do a Nissen?

No, we had a multi-society GERD Consensus Conference [1] with GI and surgery societies participating, and we reviewed a lot of data comparing Nissen with Toupet. We looked at a lot of different outcomes that matter, including hiatal hernia recurrence over time, dysphagia requiring an intervention, gas-bloat symptoms, inability to vomit, and recurrence of reflux symptoms at 1 year. What the data showed is that patients did better with a partial wrap (Toupet) than a complete wrap (Nissen). Our panel recommended that adult patients with GERD would benefit more from a partial wrap than a complete wrap. We shouldn't be doing as many Nissens as we do.

These studies also show that esophageal motility does not make much of a difference. If your motility is normal, a partial wrap has fewer side effects, with equal

GERD outcomes to a full wrap. If your motility's abnormal, same statement, it probably doesn't matter as much as we once thought. The only exception is those cases with extreme dysmotility and real aperistalsis.

The bottom line is that the Toupet is better than the Nissen. The problem is that surgeons in the USA haven't been trained to do Toupets, and they only learn how to do Nissens. We're the only country in the world that does Nissens. Last month, I did my first Nissen in the last 5 years, and I've completely switched to partial wrap fundoplication.

You mention esophageal manometry. Do you think everyone should get an esophageal manometry prior to GERD surgery?

The guidelines say you should, and it's nice to have a baseline, in case things don't go well. However, as I just pointed out, it doesn't make as big a difference as we once thought, unless there is severe aperistalsis. That being said, I do them in about 75% of cases.

What do you think about the LINX anti-reflux system, in comparison with fundoplication?

I'm a fan. It's an early technology, but so far, the data suggest that GERD may be better treated with magnetic sphincter augmentation (MSA) than fundoplication.

So far, in terms of symptom recurrence, and perioperative complications, the data suggest better outcomes with MSA. This includes dysphagia, which is counter-intuitive, because the biggest problem with the LINX is concern about dysphagia. When we look out over a longer time interval, at more than 2 years, quality of life measures favor MSA.

The great thing about LINX is that it's very easy to put in. The dissection is very minimal compared to what you have to do for a wrap. You can put it in, and if there are problems, you can take it out very easily. There are way fewer decision points, and the technique is very standardized. There's an established technique that's taught to every surgeon.

I think the physics at the diaphragm is different for a LINX than for a fundoplication. You don't have this big bulky wrap pushing on the diaphragm. You've got a magnet that's sitting there without any tension. It's not pushing as hard, and it eventually gets encapsulated in some scar tissue that helps hold it into place. So, you don't see the same rate of anatomic failures in hiatal hernias after a LINX that you do after a fundoplication. What I say is "let's do the least invasive option that leaves us as many options as we can possibly still have on the table."

What if you do a LINX and it's not working well, is it permanently embedded? And what about erosions with the LINX?

Most of the failures we see are people who develop dysphagia that doesn't improve. There is also a very small incidence of erosions about 0.2%. Most of the erosions occurred on devices that were overly tight. The philosophy over time has changed from making it tight to the point where you can see the things squeezing the esophagus to actually having it loose enough that it doesn't compress at all.

In terms of managing dysphagia, if you go in to remove the device a year later, you find that every bead has a perfectly formed scar on top of it. It's like a little capsule that you touch with a little cutter, and the magnet pops out and you grab the magnet and you just ride around each side and you cut the wire.

However, what we've found is that even though you've removed the device, there's scar tissue remaining that changes the compliance there. When you take it out and don't do anything, the dysphagia is gone and about 75% of people don't get the reflux back.

Do you take all patients with post-op dysphagia from the LINX back to surgery?

No, there's a reversal time frame, and at first, you need to try and ride it out. Some people will react to the implant with scarring, and you try to dilate it. You might also prescribe a brief course of oral steroids to soften up the scar tissue.

You would try to manage it with dilation and steroids for a few months. If people are struggling, asking to get them out, I would try to wait at least 2 or 3 months, unless there's a major issue. Most of these people will improve sufficiently to avoid surgery.

The patient under discussion has a 4-cm hiatal hernia. I thought that the LINX was approved only for patients with a hiatal hernia under 3 cm. Does that mean a LINX is contraindicated in this patient?

The original MSA studies only looked at patients with small hiatal hernias. Large hernias were a relative contraindication because they were not studied in the pivotal and premarket trials conducted to attain original FDA approval. Now, appropriate studies have been done with larger hernias, and currently, the FDA indications for LINX include larger hernias.

If that's the case, would you prefer to do an MSA for most of your GERD operations?

To be a candidate, the patient can't have any MSA contraindications, which include a BMI > 35, ineffective motility (IEM) on manometry, baseline dysphagia that is moderate or worse, or an allergy to nickel. Insurance is a frequent obstacle, Medicare and Medicaid don't cover it; private insurance is about 50/50.

All else being equal, I would say that the MSA is simpler, more likely to be performed without an overnight hospital stay, easily reversible, and may have a lower failure rate. When MSA fails, Toupet is an option—not the other way around in my opinion, so MSA saves options in the event of a failure. In the short term, however, MSA is more likely than Toupet to cause dysphagia.

The advantages of the Toupet include that it is universally covered; it's okay in patients with IEM and dysphagia, and there's no foreign body/implant, no worries about MRI.

In my opinion, both are good options. All else being equal, I think a patient who meets criteria and has access to either may be better off with the MSA due to the long-term thoughts and preservation of options as described.

What are the concerns regarding MSA and MRIs?

The current generation of LINX is compatible with a 1.5 TESLA MRI. About 90% of the MRIs done in this country utilize an MRI 1.5 T or weaker. Most of the bone and joint and spine MRIs are all 1.5. However, some of the breast indications use a 3 Tesla MRI, and those functional brain MRIs are 7.

If you use an MRI that's stronger than the device is compatible with, it depolarizes the magnets. So instead of attracting each other, they repel, and people get their reflux back. That's usually the worst thing that happens.

Patients are educated and given a card. You would be amazed that someone could have an operation and have a magnet implanted in their body, and then when they go to get an MRI, they check the form saying "no implants." I've had it happen to two of my patients who didn't follow our warnings.

Case 2 *A 45-year-old man with a BMI of 22 has a long history of GERD well controlled on PPI. His only symptom is heartburn, and it is totally relieved with PPI. He had an EGD that showed a small hiatal hernia with a mildly lax lower esophageal sphincter and Grade A esophagitis.*

He is concerned about continuing PPIs long term because he read on the internet that PPI use can cause cancer and dementia and wonders whether he should just proceed with a hiatal hernia repair?

How do you feel about operating on patients whose symptoms are well controlled on PPIs?

When I see people that are well controlled on PPIs but say that they want to get off them, I'll have a debate with them about whether that's the right thing to do. Because if their symptoms are completely under control, there's a chance they'll do worse with surgery. I may give them a side effect from an operation that might ultimately fail.

Of course, there's potential downsides to PPIs, but things have been blown out of proportion. For the patient who uses the C word (cancer), who doesn't have Barrett's or dysplasia on endoscopy, I tell them that's simply not a big concern. There's downsides to an invasive intervention. So, I'll actually talk those people back.

I think that a patient who's well managed medically on a PPI, who has symptoms under control, whose quality of life as it relates to their GI symptoms is acceptable to them is best left alone. Now, I might meet them in the future to discuss surgery if things change, but for now I would counsel against surgery.

On the other hand, if I'm dealing with a patient whose main complaint is regurgitation, a PPI is not going to fix that. Most people with bad regurgitation have a significant hiatal hernia. They have an anatomic issue.

Case 3 *A 38-year-old woman has a long history of severe reflux. She has a BMI of 40. On EGD, she has a 1-cm hiatal hernia. PPIs are not controlling her symptoms.*

How do you manage GERD in the obese patient?

If a patient with a BMI of 40 has medically refractory reflux, the best GERD operation that I can do for them is a gastric bypass. We call it an esophageal disconnect instead, which is because many insurance companies will deny it if we call it a bypass, claiming that they don't cover cosmetic operations for obesity. So, I have to get a medical doctor on the phone and tell him or her what I'm trying to accomplish.

We can usually get it covered if we call it a disconnect and have a peer-to-peer review.

The reason it works so well is that we make a small pouch, about a 20-cc gastric pouch, and there are very few parietal cells in there. Obviously, there's no biliopancreatic secretions that can get in there. There's no pepsin that can get in there. So that's how it works to prevent reflux. Of course, this patient is obese and will lose weight, which is a factor for all these other things.

So, a gastric bypass or a disconnect is good in the high BMI patients. We know that BMI is a risk factor for hiatal dilation leading to fundoplication failure. We also prefer a gastric bypass for GERD in some patients with scleroderma and others with profound motility problems. A bypass doesn't rely on a valve that's tight enough to prevent reflux, but not so tight that they'll have a swallowing problem that gets worse. It just diverts all that caustic stuff.

Case 4 *A 63-year-old female, is 5 years status post an endoscopic TIF (transoral incisionless fundoplication). Her symptoms prior to surgery were heartburn and regurgitation refractory to medical therapy. She had a positive pH test, with no hiatal hernia. Following the TIF, her symptoms resolved for 3 months, but after that her symptoms came back, and they pretty quickly returned to baseline.*

What is your impression of the new surgical-endoscopic hybrid procedure, the *transoral incisionless fundoplication (TIF)*?

The word on the street is that because you're doing it endoscopically, you don't burn any bridges whatsoever and that you leave everything on the table. You haven't done anything to harm the patient, and you have every option that you would want to have in your back pocket if that should fail.

However, the issue with TIF has always been that if a patient has a hiatal hernia, it's hard to do a wrap, have it in the chest, and have it work at all. So now people are doing the cTIF, where they go in laparoscopically or robotically, fix the hernia, and then close all the incisions and step back and do a blind endoscopic TIF.

However, our Consensus Conference reviewed the data and found that as time goes by the failure rate of a TIF is going to exceed the failure rate of a fundoplication. Therefore, we recommended that adult patients with GERD would get greater benefit from fundoplication than TIF.

We need to come up with an endoscopic treatment for medically refractory reflux; we have to do it. Of all the things that are out there, TIF is really the closest thing I think, to what we do in surgery. We're not there yet.

In terms of the ease of a redo, if the TIF fails, I find that these are really hard things to undo. The people that claim that it's easy are cutting corners and putting wraps on top of TIFs. However, this stuff is bound to fail. The only technique that works is to do a minimally invasive hernia repair with takedown of the TIF and conversion to a Toupet. It's really hard to remove all those TIF anchors. I would rather redo a fundoplication any day of the week than someone who had a TIF.

Reference

1. Slater BJ, Collings A, Dirks R, Gould JC, Qureshi AP, Juza R, Rodríguez-Luna MR, Wunker C, Kohn GP, Kothari S, Carslon E. Multi-society consensus conference and guideline on the treatment of gastroesophageal reflux disease (GERD). Surg Endosc. 2023;37(2):781–806.

Chapter 9
Barrett's Esophagus

Kulwinder Dua and Wilfredo Pagani

Case 1 *A 60-year-old Caucasian man is referred to your office for Barrett's esophagus. He was diagnosed with Barrett's esophagus when he had an EGD for hematemesis during a vacation in Florida 1 year ago. The EGD revealed a small duodenal ulcer, which was the source of the bleeding. Biopsies were negative for helicobacter pylori, but he was also found to have C4M5 Barrett's esophagus. There was intestinal metaplasia without dysplasia on biopsy. He has been on PPIs, feels fine, and is without heartburn. He was told that he should follow up with a local gastroenterologist in 1 year.*

Would you repeat the endoscopy at this time?

When deciding on surveillance frequency, it is important to consider the length of the segment of BE and whether dysplasia is present or not. In those patients with non-dysplastic Barrett's esophagus (NDBE), the most recent guidelines recommend assigning a surveillance interval of 3 years for those who have a long segment of NDBE (≥3 cm) and a 5-year interval for those with a short segment of NDBE (<3 cm) [1]. So, I would repeat the endoscopy in two more years, not now.

K. Dua (✉)
Division of Gastroenterology and Hepatology, Department of Medicine, Medical College of Wisconsin, Milwaukee, WI, USA
e-mail: kdua@mcw.edu

W. Pagani
Division of Gastroenterology and Hepatology, Medical College of Wisconsin, Milwaukee, WI, USA
e-mail: wpagani@mcw.edu

© The Author(s), under exclusive license to Springer Nature
Switzerland AG 2023
W. H. Sobin et al. (eds.), *Managing Complex Cases in Gastroenterology*,
https://doi.org/10.1007/978-3-031-48949-5_9

What is your recommendation regarding surveillance vs. treatment if a patient is found to have dysplasia, and what would be the timing if you decided on surveillance alone?

There are three pathological determinations of dysplasia—low grade, high grade, and indeterminate. If dysplasia is diagnosed, a second pathologist with expertise in BE should review the diagnosis. In patients with confirmed dysplasia by a second expert pathologist [1, 2], the surveillance frequency is guided by the grade of dysplasia. Patients with high-grade dysplasia (HGD) should not be offered surveillance; they need to undergo endoscopic eradication therapy or surgery. In patients with low-grade dysplasia (LGD), there is a lot of debate about whether surveillance or ablation should be performed.

Therefore, the current guidelines for LGD recommend shared decision-making with the patient regarding the risks and benefits of endoscopic eradication therapy vs surveillance. In a patient who chooses to pursue surveillance, an endoscopy in 6 months should be performed and then annually if LGD remains present.

In cases where the pathologist is unable to discern if there is dysplasia or if the histologic findings are due to inflammatory changes, a diagnosis of indeterminate for dysplasia is given. Again, a second expert pathologist should review the diagnosis. In patients with a confirmed diagnosis of indeterminate for dysplasia, current guidelines recommend performing a surveillance endoscopy 6 months after diagnosis and then annually if indeterminate for dysplasia remains present.

What endoscopic approaches are available for treatment?

Endoscopic eradication therapy (EET) is recommended by all GI societies for patients with HGD or intramucosal cancer (IMC), and it can also be used in LGD to prevent progression [1, 2]. EET includes endoscopic mucosal resection (EMR) for visible lesions and ablation therapies, which include thermal ablation and cryotherapy ablation [2].

Photochemical ablation which was used in the past has fallen out of favor, mainly because it was expensive, caused increased discomfort in patients, and was not very effective. The most studied and established ablative treatment is radiofrequency ablation (RFA) with studies showing rates of complete eradication of intestinal metaplasia of 54–100% and rates of complete eradication of dysplasia of 80–100%. There are multiple RFA catheters with different sizes which can provide circumferential RFA vs focal RFA therapy.

Another thermal ablation therapy used in the treatment of BE is argon plasma coagulation (APC) [4]. APC is a contact-free technique that uses ignited ionized argon gas to achieve tissue ablation. Hybrid APC is an alternative technique that involves a submucosal fluid injection prior to performing APC to reduce the depth of thermal injury and minimize post-ablation stricture formation [5].

Finally, cryotherapy ablation can also be performed with liquid nitrogen-based cryotherapy or balloon-based nitrous oxide therapy which also appears to be effective [6]. RFA continues to be the most used ablation technique [1] given its extensive data confirming its safety and effectiveness, with the use of cryotherapy ablation techniques for those patients who fail RFA or experience increased discomfort with RFA.

Case 2 *A 62-year-old man has an EGD performed because of chronic heartburn. He is found to have Barrett's C3 M3, and biopsies show low-grade dysplasia. He is treated with PPIs for 6 months, and a repeat endoscopy still shows low-grade dysplasia confirmed by a second pathologist.*

Will you invariably recommend ablation?

I think there is no question but that ablation should be performed for high-grade dysplasia. I think the management of low-grade dysplasia is less clear-cut. There are certainly studies that show that low-grade dysplasia will occasionally turn into high-grade dysplasia in some patients.

However, here's the problem. I talk to the patient, and I tell them, "You have got low-grade dysplasia. Because of that you are not a candidate to have repeat surveillance endoscopies every 3 years. No, now I need to scope you again in 3 or 6 months to begin with, and then, we need to do more extensive, quad biopsies every 1 cm. If your low-grade dysplasia remains low grade on repeat, then I will repeat again in 6 months, and if biopsies are stable, maybe spread it out to 1 year. As long as you have low-grade dysplasia, we will be doing this every year. If it turns into high grade, we must treat it."

"Alternatively, you have another option. I could ablate it, which, in many centers, is the standard of care. After ablating, even if I eradicate the dysplasia, you are still going to need follow-up endoscopes every 6 months, and then every year, the same way we would if you had not had ablation."

So, many of my patients say, "Then what's the point?". They hear about potential chest pain and potential stricture formation, with ablation, and so they may opt-out. That's okay, unless, or until, they develop high-grade dysplasia at some time in the future, which may never happen. So, I have that discussion with the patient.

Then, there are other patients who I push for ablation. I had a patient whose brother died at a young age with esophageal cancer. I recommended that since he had low-grade dysplasia, he needed to be ablated. I had another patient who had low-grade dysplasia who was getting chemotherapy for myeloma, and the concern was that the chemotherapy could cause some accelerated high-grade dysplasia development or carcinoma development, and the patient opted for ablation. Then, there are some other patients who are absolutely terrified, and they want ablation. Even though we are going to keep scoping them as though they never had ablation, they want it because it'll give them some peace of mind.

If I'm dealing with a patient who previously had high-grade dysplasia which we eradicated but now they return on follow-up surveillance with some low-grade dysplasia on one or two biopsies, we recommend ablation. Assuming that your pathologist's findings are confirmed, once they have had an element of high-grade dysplasia, I will definitely treat the patient who returns with low-grade dysplasia.

The majority of my patients who are found to have low-grade dysplasia de novo decide that since they're going to be endoscoped every 6 months for at least a year, and then every year after that, despite ablating or no ablating, they decide that they might as well just hold off on ablation.

Eventually, we may see some national guidelines come out with firm recommendations that once you eradicate the Barrett's esophagus in low-grade dysplasia, you can now get a little bit laid back and push the endoscopies out to once every 3 years. If that recommendation comes out, we may want to do more ablations.

The patient chooses to have an ablation.

How do you perform your ablations at MCW?

We no longer use photodynamic therapy to ablate Barrett's esophagus. Currently, the most common technique used for eradication is radiofrequency ablation and that is what we use. The probes come in various shapes and sizes. We have a probe that ablates 360° covering large areas, another one with 90-degree ablation, a longer 90-degree ablator, and 90-degree Ultra. The 360-degree probe has to be passed over a guide wire outside the endoscope, whereas the 90-degree probes are mounted on the endoscope like a cap. Then, there is a probe that can be introduced through the accessory channel of the endoscope. We also have cryoablation catheters that we generally reserve for patients who fail RFA ablation, although this approach can also be used upfront.

Is this generally a pretty benign procedure?

Patients can feel significant chest pain and odynophagia following ablative therapy, especially after using the 360-degree probes and ablating a long segment of Barrett's esophagus. Patients can also develop ulcers and strictures, especially if ablation is applied over overlapping areas that otherwise should be avoided. Rare perforations have occurred.

Do all patients respond to ablation or are some resistant? If so, what do you do in cases that are resistant to ablation?

A few patients are resistant, which seems to occur in patients who have reflux that is not adequately controlled, generally associated with a large hiatal hernia. No matter how much PPI you give them, you cannot control their reflux. So, I will encourage those patients to get a laparoscopic repair of their hernia. Of course, we first try a very strict anti-reflux regimen including weight loss, smoking cessation, and exercise. In others who fail RFA, some practitioners start using cryoablation.

Case 3 A 57-year-old man with a BMI of 32 is referred with a finding of a nodule in the background of Barrett's esophagus. The patient was first diagnosed with Barrett's esophagus 3 years earlier, and at that time, there was no dysplasia present. He has been receiving pantoprazole since then. Now, on his first follow-up EGD, he is found to have C4M6 Barrett's esophagus with a 3-mm nodule present. He is sent to you for a second opinion.

When you see a small nodule will you biopsy it, or do an ablation, or EMR?

If somewhere in the Barrett's esophagus segment, there is a nodule, then one should do an EMR. There are two reasons to avoid simply doing a biopsy. First, there could be something deeper that is more sinister, where your biopsy may come back showing high-grade dysplasia, but deeper down there is carcinoma. Second, your biopsy may cause some submucosal fibrosis and that may create difficulties with the endoscopic mucosal resection. If there is a bump or a nodule, we always do

EMR rather than ablation. As compared to EUS, histopathology of the resected tissue will also give better depth of invasion and margin involvement if it is adenocarcinoma.

Will you ablate the surrounding Barrett's esophagus at the same time?

This can be done, but we generally avoid it for fear of perforation, especially if using balloon ablation and cryogas. We usually wait for the histopathology results and plan accordingly. Generally, waiting for 8 weeks after EMR/ESD is recommended.

How do you evaluate the remainder of the field of Barrett's esophagus?

Once I see a nodule, I will do 4-quadrant biopsies every 1 cm. I want to see if there is any multifocal dysplasia or even carcinoma. You can have carcinoma that may be completely flat and miss it if you don't do biopsies. Always use NBI (or other such imaging on other company endoscopes) and magnification in all patients with Barrett's at each examination. There are several other enhanced imaging modalities available such as confocal microscopy [7] and OCT (see WATS-3D below).

What would you do if the biopsies of the remaining Barrett's esophagus show no dysplasia, would you do ablation?

If the nodule shows high-grade dysplasia or carcinoma in situ, I would want to eradicate the remaining Barrett's esophagus, even if the remaining Barrett's esophagus has no dysplasia on biopsy. If there is one site that declared itself, I expect that the entire field of Barrett's esophagus is probably unstable and hence would favor eradication.

Are there new techniques available for screening and diagnosing Barrett's esophagus in the community?

There are new techniques being studied, but not widely available, they are not being done here at MCW. Endoscopy continues to be the mainstay for the diagnosis of Barrett's esophagus (BE). However, this strategy is not cost-effective and carries a potential risk of harm from the procedure. Because of this, there is much interest in the development of tools and testing modalities which are less invasive and more cost-effective for screening and diagnosing BE with substantial progress over the last decade. Of these, the modality that has the most data available is the use of tethered cell collection devices in combination with biomarker testing. Devices such as the Cytosponge™ with trefoil factor family protein 3 (TFF3) immunohistochemical staining, EsophaCap™ with a methylated DNA marker panel, and EsoCheck™ also with a methylated DNA marker panel have shown good accuracy in diagnosing BE [7]. Of these, the most studied has been the Cytosponge™ with TFF3 immunohistochemical staining, with one study showing up to a 90% sensitivity and 94% specificity when compared to endoscopy in patients with a BE segment of 2 cm or greater [8].

Given the progress in the development of these devices, the most recent guidelines have included using a swallowable, non-endoscopic capsule sponge device combined with a biomarker as an acceptable alternative to endoscopy for BE screening [1]. However, these devices have not become widely adopted in the USA as of this moment.

Another promising technology is the use of a wide-area transepithelial sampling with computer-assisted three-dimensional (WATS-3D) analyses [3, 7]. This technology provides advanced sampling by using an abrasive brush to sample deeper layers and larger surface areas of the esophagus. These specimens are then analyzed by a computer software which identifies abnormal cells. Studies have shown that WATS3D may increase the yield of dysplasia detection with a recent meta-analysis [9] showing that WATS3D increased the absolute yield of dysplastic BE by 7.2% (95% Cl 3.9–11.5) over conventional forceps biopsies. Currently, one of our society guidelines (AGA) supports its use as an adjunctive technique to sample the suspected or established BE [7].

References

1. Shaheen NJ, Falk GW, Iyer PG, Souza RF, Yadlapati RH, Sauer BG, Wani S. Diagnosis and management of Barrett's esophagus: an updated ACG guideline. Am J Gastroenterol. 2022;117(4):559.
2. Sharma P, Shaheen NJ, Katzka D, Bergman JJ. AGA clinical practice update on endoscopic treatment of Barrett's esophagus with dysplasia and/or early cancer: expert review. Gastroenterology. 2020;158(3):760–9.
3. Qumseya B, Sultan S, Bain P, Jamil L, Jacobson B, Anandasabapathy S, Agrawal D, Buxbaum JL, Fishman DS, Gurudu SR, Jue TL. ASGE guideline on screening and surveillance of Barrett's esophagus. Gastrointest Endosc. 2019;90(3):335–59.
4. Manner H, Rabenstein T, Pech O, Braun K, May A, Pohl J, Behrens A, Vieth M, Ell C. Ablation of residual Barrett's epithelium after endoscopic resection: a randomized long-term follow-up study of argon plasma coagulation vs. surveillance (APE study). Endoscopy. 2014;46(01):6–12.
5. Kolb JM, Shah S, Chahine A, Chang K, Samarasena JB. Hybrid argon plasma coagulation for Barrett's esophagus. VideoGIE. 2021;6(8):339–41.
6. Canto MI, Shaheen NJ, Almario JA, Voltaggio L, Montgomery E, Lightdale CJ. Multifocal nitrous oxide cryoballoon ablation with or without EMR for treatment of neoplastic Barrett's esophagus (with video). Gastrointest Endosc. 2018;88(3):438–46.
7. Muthusamy VR, Wani S, Gyawali CP, Komanduri S, Conference CB. AGA clinical practice update on new technology and innovation for surveillance and screening in Barrett's esophagus: expert review. Clin Gastroenterol Hepatol. 2022;20(12):2696–706.
8. Kadri SR, Lao-Sirieix P, O'Donovan M, Debiram I, Das M, Blazeby JM, Emery J, Boussioutas A, Morris H, Walter FM, Pharoah P. Acceptability and accuracy of a non-endoscopic screening test for Barrett's oesophagus in primary care: cohort study. BMJ. 2010;341:c4372.
9. Codipilly DC, Chandar AK, Wang KK, Katzka DA, Goldblum JR, Thota PN, Falk GW, Chak A, Iyer PG. Wide-area transepithelial sampling for dysplasia detection in Barrett's esophagus: a systematic review and meta-analysis. Gastrointest Endosc. 2022;95(1):51–9.

Chapter 10
PEG Tubes

William Berger

Case 1 We have a 75-year-old man who had a PEG placed following a stroke a month earlier. He is sent back to the office because he has continuous drainage from the PEG site.

Many gastroenterologists find this a common complication. How do you deal with it?

First of all, what sort of drainage are you dealing with? In some patients, it's only clear liquid which may be gastric fluid, which can be very irritating. Other patients have feedings come out around the tube, and still others have a lot of mucus or even purulent discharge.

The most common sort of drainage is tube feedings. To have tube feedings draining out the stoma, there must be something causing an abnormal pressure differential. Because if you remember back to the work of William Beaumont, he studied a French trapper named Alexis St. Martin, who had been shot in the abdomen and had a large unhealed fistula between his skin and his stomach. Beaumont was able to look into the trapper's stomach and observe what goes on in the stomach during digestion. The hole was so big that Beaumont could actually peer into it, and he could place various things into the stomach and watch how the stomach reacted. The point of the story is that the trapper could eat regular food, and it didn't come pouring out onto his shirt because the pressure inside the stomach is typically negative relative to the outside. So, if the pressure inside the stomach is negative, we should

W. Berger (✉)
Division of Gastroenterology & Hepatology, Medical College of Wisconsin,
Milwaukee, WI, USA
e-mail: wberger@mcw.edu

not see any leak through the G tube site. So then, why do we have any leak? Why would we have a higher pressure in the stomach than the atmospheric pressure outside, which is what causes liquid to leak out?

One possibility is that you just have dramatic overfeeding. Another could be that the patient has gastroparesis, and the stomach fills up but doesn't empty properly. In fact, any kind of gastric motility disorder, outlet obstruction, or anything else causing increased pressure in the stomach will cause more leakage.

A third, which I see not infrequently, is a PEG tube placed in the antrum. During gastric peristalsis, antral contractions start on the incisura and push toward the pylorus generating high pressures. When the tube is in the antrum, these high pressures can force fluid out around the tube because the tract becomes the path of least resistance. The proximal stomach is for capacitance—that's where the adaptive relaxation and accommodation occur. The antrum—beyond the incisura—is functionally a different organ as far as acid secretion, peristalsis, and the like.

Now, why do some patients have increased gastric acid leakage? The acid leakage usually is because they're hyper-secretors. For these patients, you place them on a PPI, and frequently, the problem goes away. Not only does it alleviate the causticity of the discharge, but also the volume of it.

If you have purulent drainage, it usually means you have an infection. Sometimes, it just looks like mucus, but quite often it's an infection in the abdominal wall. Sometimes it's obvious just looking at it, but other times you get an ultrasound or CT, and you may even find a small abscess there. With the infection, you occasionally have to take the G tube out, leave it for a few days, and then put another G tube in at a different location.

What do you think leads to these infections?

By taking a PEG tube and dragging it down the patient's throat, you're taking a foreign body, coating it in saliva, and sticking it in a fresh wound. So, it's not surprising that we see some immediate infections.

Delayed infections, months or years later? I don't know what causes them, but usually there's some kind of nidus, and it's not just a local cellulitis. Usually, there's an abscess. Usually, even if you give them antibiotics, it may clear up for a while, but it comes right back because the foreign body is still there. So, I usually take the G tube out, let it heal, and settle down at least a few days, with or without antibiotics, and then, put another G tube in at another site.

Sometimes, there's no infection, but you'll see marked irritation on the skin surrounding the G tube probably related to the caustic damage from gastric acid. I treat this like a bad diaper rash with absorbent pads and zinc oxide. PPIs should help as well.

What if we have a G tube that's in the body of the stomach, not the antrum, there's no gastroparesis, and you have ongoing drainage that's either clear or slightly mucoid. There's some local irritation around the surrounding skin from leakage. What are some strategies to deal with this?

In all these cases of G tube dysfunction, you want to identify any physiological conditions that are correctable. If you find them and correct them, there is a pretty high success rate. In this case, there's no obvious underlying condition, and then, you have to do a systematic approach. By aspirating gastric contents through the PEG tube we can quantify gastric residuals. If that is increased, solve that problem first.

Next is usually the PPIs, which at least make it somewhat less caustic and sometimes cut down the volume of drainage. In the worst cases we will place an ostomy bag around the stoma if the leakage is severe. These unfortunate patients have to hook themselves up for feedings and then drain the excess fluid that comes out.

We always want to make sure that we are not dealing with a buried bumper. In those cases, they're pumping in the food, and it comes right back out around the stoma. So, one of the things I almost always do is scope the patient to see what the site looks like, make sure the bumper is intact and not buried, and make sure the tube is not located in the antrum. If you go down and the tube is in a normal position, there's not a big gastric pool, the pylorus is wide open, yet they still seem to leak, and you have two options. Either try replacing, repositioning the G tube in a new location, or simply apply symptomatic control of the leakage.

Have you ever dealt with this problem by leaving the tube out for a number of hours and let the hole close up by itself so the opening is smaller?

That presumes that resistance to flow around the tube is the problem. Following that logic, we see people placing bigger and bigger tubes in an attempt to plug the hole. So, if you start out with a 20 Fr tube, the hole may loosen, so it is now 22 Fr diameter. Then, if you place a 22 Fr tube in to plug it up, it'll become a 24 Fr hole, and it just gets progressively wider. It loosens itself up as you go. Wanting to just plug it up to take care of the problem is destined to fail. It may give you a temporary sense of control, but the underlying problem is the pressure differential, and trying to increase the resistance so that it won't leak while you still have the underlying pressure differential is at best a temporizing measure.

It makes you feel better, so you can send them back to the nursing home, but the only way they don't come back is if they get sick of dealing with you and send them to someone else.

On a similar note, we occasionally get consulted about patients who have had a surgical J tube placed with a lot of bile leakage. The feedings don't come back, but bile leakage can be massive and caustic to the skin. It turns out that it is almost always because somebody put a balloon tube in the jejunum and it's causing a partial downstream obstruction for fluid coming from upstream. Peristalsis is generating internal pressure, while clamping down on the balloon blocking the lumen just as the bile bolus is being pushed from upstream. This just makes the J tube stoma the path of least resistance. So, what you do is just get rid of the balloon and secure the jejunostomy tube externally by suturing it in place.

Do you ever consult wound care nurses?

Often, one of their tricks is to place the ostomy bag over the tube, as I alluded to previously. It's messy and it's inconvenient, but it will work. That's a worst-case, last-resort scenario. The wound care nurses are basically going to deal with what comes out, and they're going to assume it's going to continue to come out because they are ostomies. That's what these nurses work with. Otherwise, like I said, you just need to try to figure out what's coming out and why it's coming out.

Do you ever use antibiotics or antibiotic ointments?

If it is at all purulent, the ointments aren't really going to help, it has to be systemic, and you can usually get that with pills, occasionally you have to resort to IV antibiotics. Quite often because the foreign body is still there, and that's what's really acting as the nidus of infection, I usually end up taking the tube out. Of course, I have a pretty low threshold for doing that. I will put down an NJ tube or something else to take care of them for 3, 4, and 5 days until that stoma cools down and closes up and then replace the tube somewhere else.

In some cases, where PEG tubes have been in place for a long time and then are removed because the patient no longer needs them, the tract fails to close. How do you deal with this?

Again, consider the underlying cause. Typically, it is because the tube has been in so long that the tract—that was originally lined with granulation tissue, which seals up pretty quickly—has become epithelialized. Usually for those, I try using a silver nitrate stick inside the tract to try to ablate the squamous tissue and try to create some granulation tissue. Then, you take a four by four and fold it corner to corner until you have this little pyramid, stick that in there, and cover it over tightly with tape. That'll keep it from leaking. I won't send them to surgery to close the fistula until they've tried a few sessions of that over a couple of weeks. Denuding the epithelium in the tract can be painful, so if you are going to be aggressive, first injecting lidocaine around the stoma can be kind.

Clogged NG, NJ, and PEG tubes are a common problem. Do you have strategies to deal with these?

One thing to be aware of is that crushed pills can clog a tube. Sometimes, liquid medicines are used for this reason. However, you need to know that a lot of the medicines that come in liquid form are sweetened, because it is assumed that they're for children. They'll often use a sugar-free sweetener, usually sorbitol. By the time you get three or four medicine doses of sorbitol a day, you have a real diarrhea problem. What people don't appreciate is that there are other ways to avoid crushed meds other than using liquid meds. You can just crush them very finely, or you can disolve them with water.

Some of the more common causes for a clogged J tube include administering meds like Carafate (which ironically is meant to be delivered to the stomach) or potassium pills (also ironic, as this used to only come in liquid form). These will both clog up a J tube quickly.

We will occasionally use Viokase (pancreatic enzyme) and bicarbonate to unclog tubes. G tubes are fairly short and wide enough that they usually don't clog. There are devices you can twirl down a G tube to unclog it. So, it turns out that it's the J tubes that are the biggest problem. I usually just start out with coke because it's cheap, it's easy, and it's immediately available. The carbonic acid in coke will clean your car battery terminals and also clean out G tubes and J tubes reasonably well.

The biggest reason for clogging a lot of the J tubes out there is both NJ tubes and G-J tubes are side holes. What happens is they'll have a little tiny hole at the end. That gets clogged up immediately, but feeds and meds can still come out the side holes. Then, more stuff packs up and the most distal side hole gets plugged. Then, one by one, all the other side holes clog up.

So, I use a J tube of polyvinyl chloride (PVC) with a blunt cut end and no side holes. The blunt end may be more difficult to get past the pylorus. If you can maneuver the blunt end into the jejunum, you can just use a 3- to 5-ml syringe, shoot some water through, and the clog will shoot right out. Some folks, who don't understand basic hydraulics will put on a big ol' 60cc syringe, but you get your most hydraulic force using a small barrel syringe.

Case 2 *A 56-year-old man had a PEG placed for bulbar palsy 2 years earlier. The original tube had been replaced with a MIC PEG replacement a year ago, which itself has been replaced several times for occlusions. Now, he is found to have vomiting after feeding and is found to have evidence for gastroparesis.*

How would you manage this?

I would exchange the PEG tube for a G-J tube. I find them very easy to do, although for some reason, most people seem to think it's too complex or difficult, but yes, it sounds like the patient needs it. I tracked 179 J tubes and found that about half of those were for aspiration and about a quarter were for gastroparesis. PEG-J seemed to work pretty well for both.

Now, many patients with gastroparesis have poorly controlled diabetes. Poor control causes the gastroparesis, and the gastroparesis leads to retention or dumping, resulting in poor control. I recall a study I think out of Iowa from the late nineties which studied patients with a glycohemoglobin of at least 14, who had been hospitalized twice in the last year for inability to tolerate feeds and been on TPN at least once. They put those folks on PEG-J tube feedings and then used a continuous pump, 24 h a day, and administered ultralente insulin to bring their glucose under control. Within 2–3 months, those people were able to come off J tube feedings and eat normally. After 2 years of follow-up, none of them ended up back in the hospital and their glycohemoglobin stayed under 11. Okay, so in many cases, we can make a huge difference in gastroparesis by controlling the underlying problem.

Can you describe the method(s) you like to use to place a G-J tube?

I like to start out with a large bore G tube and that's one of the reasons that we have the 24 French PEG set. We scope through the G tube using a 4.2-mm ultra-thin gastroscope that will fit through a 24 Fr tube but not the routine 20 Fr PEG tube. Go through the G tube with the thin endoscope, past the pylorus, past the ligament of Treitz, and pass a wire down the endoscope well into the jejunum. Then, we withdraw the scope over the wire and use the wire to place the J tube into the jejunum.

Although it may seem that this requires special equipment, most GI laboratories have an ultra-thin "neonatal" scope (also useful for trans-nasal endoscopy). The larger PEG tube can easily be ordered, even up to 28 Fr. Other benefits to this technique are that no medication is needed, airway issues are avoided, and it is fast. This can also be done at the time of initial PEG placement, if you already know that a G tube alone will be inadequate.

Case 3 *A 65-year-old man is found to have laryngeal cancer. He is started on radiation treatment, and his oral intake decreases substantially. A PEG is desired.*

Would you do the routine sort of PEG in someone with laryngeal cancer? What do you think about concerns of potentially seeding tumor doing this, do you think they are overblown?

The literature has been a little all over the place with that. The frequency of seeding is fairly low, and estimates have ranged from 0.6% to 5% of cases. It's important to differentiate between seeding and metastasis. Seeding means that you took laryngeal cancer cells and implanted the cells at the PEG site, while metastasis means that the tumor has developed the ability to spread throughout the body on its own. These have very different prognostic significance.

The thing is that if seeding is going to occur, it usually doesn't show up for 6–12 months. Many of the people who have seeding are those who are going to die within a year or two anyway. However, if you have a more viable patient, seeding can usually be taken care of with focal radiation therapy or resection, so it's usually manageable.

In reality, this is an uncommon complication, but I try to teach the fellows the Russell (introducer) PEG insertion technique, which does not involve pulling the PEG tube down the throat. This technique can also be beneficial in patients with narrowing of the esophagus, where you are not sure if you can get your bumper to go through or if you have a patient with narrowing high up in the larynx and you worry that you might obstruct the airway if you drag a bumper through. In cases like this, the Russell technique can also come in handy. This is the technique the radiologists use. In fact, we use the same kit with T-fasteners and dilators with a peel-away sheath that IR uses.

This said, I certainly don't criticize gastroenterologists who place PEGs through the routine Ponsky technique even in patients with active ENT or esophageal cancers.

Case 4 *A patient is malnourished and has poor oral intake, and a swallowing exam shows that he aspirates. As part of his workup for weight loss, an abdominal CAT scan is done and is essentially negative. The decision is made to place a PEG. Reviewing the CT scan, however, it appears there is not a good window for you to do PEG placement.*

Do you trust the CT interpretation, or do you find that when you attempt PEG placement in someone like this you are often successful in spite of the CT interpretation?

I really don't place too much reliance on the CT because you're going to inflate the stomach with air, and who knows what you'll find. The CT is showing a tiny little collapsed balloon of stomach that's up underneath the ribs, where it should be when it's empty, but when you inflate it, either with the endoscope or when a radiologist pumps air in with an NG tube, then it becomes a football, and you may have easy access.

So, it's never bad to have a CAT scan. I've had cases where a CAT has been done, and we find that the patient had an umbilical hernia repair with a big chunk of mesh in the way. It's good to know about the mesh, because you can't put your PEG tube through the mesh. If you ever hear the word mesh in a surgical repair, you definitely want to get a CT or an ultrasound before doing a PEG so that you can map it out and mark where the mesh is on the abdominal wall. And then you can try to be at least 2 cm away from it when you put your PEG in.

The other thing that's interesting from a radiologic perspective is that if you have a patient with an upper abdominal midline incision, and you're afraid that the colon may be adhered by scar tissue, there is a technique to make sure the colon is not in the way of your planned PEG placement. The patient drinks about a half cup of barium mixed with a half cup of water the day before and then does the PEG under fluoroscopy. By that time, barium will be distributed through the colon pretty evenly, so imaging can help me find a window, massage the colon out of the way, or confirm that there is no window.

Case 5 *A patient with advanced type 1 diabetes has refractory gastroparesis. The desire is to be able to provide enteral feeds, while at the same time performing a "venting gastrostomy."*

How would you do this?

I would place a 28F PEG tube and put a Y connector on before putting the J tube in. It's a little bulky, but it works pretty well. Then, I usually use a bile collection bag. On the bottom of that bag is a valve that you can easily open for venting and drainage.

Also, on occasion, we've had patients with apparent duodenal obstruction sent for venting gastrostomies where we have been able to place a venting G tube and a feeding G-J tube because we were able to get our endoscope past the obstruction and feed a wire and allow for a feeding jejunostomy. One caveat is if there is a lot of drainage of gastric fluid and/or bile, this needs to be reduced as much as possible. A PPI can help with gastric secretions, but bile may need to be re-infused through the J tube. If not, significant potassium and bicarbonate loss can occur.

Case 6 *A 65-year-old woman is sent to have PEG placement. At the time of the procedure, you do not see good trans-illumination within the stomach. There is a good finger indentation, however.*

Would you proceed with this case?

I have aborted in many of these cases, but there are others where you don't see a good light, but there might be a good explanation for this, like they weigh 400 pounds. Sometimes I'll go ahead and try it using the safe-track technique (see below).

Case 7 *A PEG is placed in an 82-year-old woman. Placement was somewhat challenging but was eventually successful. She goes for a CT scan 2 weeks later to help evaluate some abdominal pain, and the CT scan shows the PEG tube traversing the liver and going into the stomach. It is not causing any bleeding.*

How would you manage this? Have you had, or seen other practitioners have, complications of PEG placement where another organ was entered? Do you have any advice on how to avoid these complications?

This problem should be avoidable using the safe-track technique. That's where you get some fluid in your syringe, and you place a nice long needle on it. Then, you advance the needle along your proposed tract aspirating as you go in. Keep an eye on the inside of the stomach with your scope to see where the needle's going to come in.

Just as the needle becomes visible in the stomach, the person who is looking at the screen will say "Needle" and the person putting the needle in and watching the syringe should say "Air," when bubbles suddenly aspirate into the syringe. (Note: The person watching the syringe should not be trying to watch the screen and the person who's watching the screen should not be trying to glance at the syringe.) Then, if you get the audible from both people simultaneously—in stereo—you know that you're in the stomach and you didn't hit the colon or anything else. If you get back air but don't see the needle in the stomach, it may be passing through the colon. If you're not seeing the needle in the stomach but you get a big flashback of red blood, you're probably going through the liver.

However, in this case they've already gone through the liver, unaware they had done so, and had no major clinical problems. Going through the liver is actually not that uncommon. Jeffrey Ponsky actually reported a case where they intentionally went through the liver to place a PEG in a kid with a huge liver that covered the whole belly, and there was no problem.

There have been two times that I've encountered this scenario, and in neither case, was there a problem. Just remember that with PEGs through the liver the problems are when it comes time to replace the tube.

The tract needs to be really mature—at least a few months. Then, the tube must be removed atraumatically. This means endoscopically snared and pulled back up the esophagus. If you were to try "traction removal" as the tube was designed for, you could stimulate significant bleeding. This is if you are lucky enough to know your tract is through the liver.

However, if you try to replace a tube in a tract without knowing it is through the liver, you could end up with the tip of the tube in the liver parenchyma. Tube feedings making their way into the hepatic vein is uncool. There is even a case report of someone testing their tube placement with an air flush, which immediately became a fatal air embolism.

When you replace a PEG tube do you do it endoscopically, or blindly? And do you always do a gastrografin study to make sure it's in the right place?

The original tube is designed to be removed by traction, without endoscopic guidance, and we have not seen significant complications when we simply pulled them out.

We usually don't get a gastrografin study to confirm the location inside the stomach. What I do is just go ahead and feed that replacement tube in about 9 cm through the tract, with an uninflated balloon and put suction on it. If I get back some gastric fluid, bile, or mucus, then I know I'm in the correct place. Then, blow up the balloon, cinch it up a bit, and send them home.

If I can aspirate, that's my preferred method, I think that using gastrografin in every case is a bit of overkill, but you want to be really careful with your replacement tubes to make sure that you aspirate some good gastric fluid. I had one where the tract was not solid, although 14 months old. It had somehow been placed through the posterior wall of the stomach, interposing the omentum in the tract. The replacement tube initially landed in the peritoneal cavity between the abdominal wall and the stomach. However, when we tried to aspirate, we weren't getting good gastric juice back, and we knew not to start feedings.

The other thing you should do if you're trying to aspirate fluid and you get nothing back is to inject some water into the tube and then see if you can suck that back. If you're in the peritoneal cavity and you put 60 ML of water in, you won't get that return because it's not going to sit there. If that's the case, then we'll definitely get an X-ray to check on the position. So, if you can put fluid in and suck fluid out, then you're in the stomach.

The first thing to remember is that the first replacement is the most dangerous. It's not pulling out the original PEG tube that is the tricky part, it's putting that first replacement tube in. It depends on how long the original tube has been in. Your task may be more daunting if the original tube has only been in for a month or two. In that case, you could potentially rupture the tract with the pullout. If it's less than 2 weeks, obviously this requires an emergency room visit, because you won't have a mature tract. On the other hand, if it's been a year and a half, 2 years, that tract is as solid as it's going to be.

It turns out that in Europe it is mandated to change the primary PEG tube once a year, but also to change any balloon tubes every 3 months. To replace, PEG tubes involves taking a patient from the nursing home, putting them in an ambulance, transporting them to the emergency room, having somebody take out the old tube, and put the new tube in. If mandated to do that four times a year, it would be easier and cheaper to just replace the primary tube endoscopically.

That's what they usually do in Europe, just replace the primary tube. So, you have a Ponsky tube in there with a bumper, no balloon. We can usually get at least 2 years out of a Ponsky primary tube.

When you place a new PEG do you put gauze under the bumper?

Initially, I do, on day 1. That way, any discharge or bleeding will collect in the gauze, but when we loosen the tube the next day, they take the gauze out and leave it out. Usually, the stoma is dry and there's no need to have gauze there.

We're concerned that if we leave the gauze there and the patient goes back to the nursing home, it won't get changed and you increase the risk of infection long term.

How tight do you make the PEG bumper, and how much do you loosen it the next day?

We used to make it very tight to prevent pneumoperitoneum, but since we started using CO_2 instead of air during our PEG placements, we have much less problem with pneumoperitoneum. So, we usually leave 0.5 cm of play at placement. The trauma surgeons seem to clinch their bumpers in real tight and they are more likely to get a buried bumper or an ulcer underneath the internal bolster, just from pressure necrosis which can happen within a few days.

When you place a PEG, the thing is that you're going through perpendicularly oriented layers of muscle in the gastric wall and the abdominal wall. So, when your needle goes through those layers, it just spreads them apart and you get a pretty good seal. There was a paper by Ponsky, again, back in the eighties, where he investigated how tight you needed to cinch up the bumper. He put 10 PEG tubes in 10 dogs. The first one he put in and cinched it up nice and tight. The second one, he put a centimeter loose, and the next dog was 2 cm loose and then 3 cm and so forth. He got all the way up pushing 10 cm of tube into the abdomen. All 10 dogs did fine. There were no leaks anywhere.

Now, I'm not leaving it that loose. I want it so that several days later there is at least 0.5–1.0 cm of play. Now, right after the procedure I might leave 0.5 cm of play but when we examine the patient the next day the bumper may be tight, no play, because the abdominal wall had increased in thickness due to either edema from the injury or hematoma.

The other thing that's interesting is that you do have a difference in your abdominal wall thickness between when you're laying down and sitting up. So, somebody lying down may have 0.5–1.0 cm play, but when they sit up, there may be no play at all. So, if it's really cinched down, then the amount of time they spend sitting up may be the amount of time that they're getting pressure necrosis.

It's one of those things to be aware of. You can't make it too loose; you can definitely make it too tight.

Will you place a PEG in someone on DOACs or Plavix?

I try to get the patient to hold those, simply because you're likely to get bleeding from either the mucosa or the skin edge. If they can't and they need the tube, I go ahead anyway. If you get mucosal bleeding, usually that stops. That's one of the times that I might tighten up the internal bolster because that'll hold pressure on it and then loosen it the next day. Bleeding at the incision site, worst-case scenario, you go in there with some silver nitrate and you burn it to make it stop, but I like to see the bleeding stop before I send them back upstairs.

I will hold the DOACs for a couple of days, I will hold warfarin until the INR is 1.5. I don't hold the antiplatelet meds, but if the patient can't hold the anticoagulation because of an acute post-stroke or some other reason, I just do what needs to be done.

Case 8 *You are attempting to place a PEG but the light shows up in an undesirable location—either too high—at the xiphoid, or too low, or too much to the left or right.*

Will you proceed in these situations? What is the risk involved? Is there some way of minimizing the risk?

If I have to, although usually you'll find that if you get the stomach well inflated then you will have multiple potential sites. Inside the stomach, I would like to be 2 cm proximal to the incisura on the anterior wall of the stomach. On the outside, I try to stay off of the midline because the Linea alba doesn't make for a good tract, going through the tendon. I also try to stay 2 cm off the rib margin because that can be really uncomfortable. For those patients, it hurts every time they take a breath because the tube is rubbing against their lower rib.

As I mentioned before, the safe-track technique can help reassure you, but I also make sure to use tiny finger circles at candidate sites, not just finger pokes, which can be misleading.

Case 9 A 37-year-old man who suffered severe brain anoxia following a self-hanging attempt *has a PEG tube placed. Two weeks later, he involuntarily yanks the tube out.*

How would you manage this situation?

You generally don't see gastric perforations in people who've yanked out their PEG tubes too early. It seals up, as long as you don't put a lot of stuff in the stomach.

I'd keep him NPO on NG suction for 24 h and then feed him via the NG tube on days 2 and 3 and then go ahead and place another PEG.

You generally end up placing a totally new PEG rather than using the old tract.

When the tube comes out, the muscle fibers typically fall back and seal pretty well. It may be that the tract is already established, within even a few days, but if you go back in and you try to put a needle through where the old tract was, it rarely comes out where the inside tract was in the stomach. So, you generally end up placing a new PEG in a totally new location.

A case reported in the Milwaukee Journal-Sentinel told of a local nursing home patient who returned from the hospital with a fresh PEG tube, which he pulled out on transit to the nursing home. The charge nurse, having replaced PEG tubes before, dutifully put in a new tube and fed through it. Unsurprisingly, feeds went into the peritoneal cavity, the patient got septic, and he died. Our post-procedure orders clearly state that if a PEG tube comes out under any circumstances in the first 2 weeks, bring the patient to the emergency room.

How do you manage the buried bumper?

Usually, if there's still a tract that communicates with the inside of the stomach, I can put a wire down the tube and assuming the wire makes its way into the stomach, and I grab the wire and pull the tube out over it. Then, I just place another PEG tube over the same wire by a regular Ponsky technique and make sure the tube length and play are appropriate and that the external bolster is not over-tight.

When you talk about using a wire to place your J tubes do you always try to use fluoroscopy? What techniques do you use when fluoro is not available?

I use fluoro when I can, but it's not always available. When you don't have access to fluoro, the way you control the wire is critical, but working with the fellows I always hold the wire. You have to keep the wire from coiling in the stomach. The person holding the wire has to keep his hand completely steady, because the wire moving forward, even a few inches as you're feeding the tube in will cause the tube to coil up in the stomach. Then, once it's coiled, even if you're holding the wire firm after that, then it just pulls the wire back and continues coiling up in the stomach.

Because I'm tall, I can just hold it up, arm length, really high, and then try to keep the wire as straight as possible between my hand and the patient's nose (NJ) or G tube (PEG-J) and don't let the wire move. One thing that can be very helpful for the PEG-J is to loosen the external GT bumper to allow the GT to be fed into the stomach ~10 cm toward the pylorus before feeding the PEG-J tube in. Then, there's only a short distance between the tube tip and the pylorus, so the tube is less likely to coil in the stomach.

Finally, try to avoid any big loop in the wire in the stomach during scope withdrawal, and decompress the stomach of as much gas as possible as you withdraw your scope.

Chapter 11
Autoimmune Metaplastic Atrophic Gastritis

Francis Edeani

Case 1 *A 48-year-old diabetic male patient is referred to you by his primary care physician for chronic osmotic diarrhea, anemia, and a sore tongue. Laboratory evaluation reveals macrocytic anemia, and a vitamin B12 level returns low. The diagnosis of pernicious anemia is entertained.*

How would you confirm this diagnosis?

I would order intrinsic factor antibodies and anti-parietal cell antibodies. If intrinsic factor antibodies return positive, these are highly specific for PA. However, they are not that sensitive. Antibodies to parietal cells are more sensitive (80%) but not that specific. In addition, I order a gastrin level. In advanced PA, there is hypochlorhydria or achlorhydria with a resultant hypergastrinemia.

The patient's intrinsic factor and anti-parietal cell antibodies both return positive, and gastrin level is elevated at 540.

How would you further evaluate this patient?

In patients with pernicious anemia, I would do endoscopy with gastric mapping. I suspect the patient has autoimmune metaplastic atrophic gastritis (AMAG). I want to confirm the presence of gastric atrophy, evaluate the extent of inflammation, and look for any changes of metaplasia or dysplasia.

Which portions of the stomach tend to be involved in AMAG?

AMAG tends to involve the fundus and body of the stomach, generally sparing the antrum. Autoimmune destruction of oxyntic mucosa leads to a decrease in acid, pepsin, and intrinsic factor. The antrum is not involved and so antral G cells

F. Edeani (✉)
Division of Gastroenterology and Hepatology, Department of Internal Medicine, GI, Medical College of Wisconsin, Milwaukee, WI, USA
e-mail: fedeani@mcw.edu

© The Author(s), under exclusive license to Springer Nature Switzerland AG 2023
W. H. Sobin et al. (eds.), *Managing Complex Cases in Gastroenterology*,
https://doi.org/10.1007/978-3-031-48949-5_11

proliferate, stimulated by hypochlorhydria and resulting in hypergastrinemia. The hypergastrinemia also leads to ECL proliferation, which may stimulate growth of carcinoids.

Endoscopically what do you tend to see in AMAG?

You tend to see loss of gastric rugae in the gastric body and fundus, and because of thinning of gastric mucosa, submucosal vessels may stand out. Uneven destruction of oxyntic mucosa may lead to pseudopolyps—representing residual oxyntic mucosa that has not been destroyed.

Are patients with AMAG at a higher risk of developing gastric cancer?

Yes, they are at a heightened risk for gastric carcinoids and gastric adenocarcinoma. The gastric carcinoids result from the ECL proliferation that results from hypergastrinemia. The gastric adenocarcinoma is a result of inflammation leading to metaplasia eventually resulting in dysplasia that over time may evolve into adenocarcinoma. There are various types of metaplasia that may occur—pseudopyloric metaplasia, incomplete intestinal metaplasia, or complete intestinal metaplasia.

Because of the increased risk of gastric malignancy how often would you repeat surveillance endoscopy?

Every 3 years and more often if there is a family history of gastric malignancy.

This patient is diabetic. Is there an increased incidence of other "autoimmune diseases in AMAG?"

Yes, about 1/3 of AMAG patients have autoimmune thyroid disease and 10% have diabetes.

Case 2 A 55-year-old Caucasian man is evaluated and referred to gastroenterology for endoscopic evaluation of occult blood loss anemia. An EGD is performed, which shows erythema and edema in the gastric mucosa of the antrum. Biopsies revealed atrophic gastritis, and Warthin silver stain reveals H. pylori organisms.

What is the association between HP and atrophic gastritis?

The most common association is environmental metaplastic atrophic gastritis (EMAG). EMAG differs from AMAG in that antibodies for IF and parietal cells are generally not present, and gastrin levels are normal. HP is the most common cause of EMAG, but HP has also been linked as a possible trigger in some cases of AMAG.

EMAG differs from AMAG in other ways as well. Atrophic gastritis can be present anywhere in the stomach in EMAG and actually is most common in the antrum (which is usually spared in AMAG). Normal gastrin levels mean that ECL hyperplasia and carcinoid tumors are uncommon.

EMAG may progress to dysplasia and there is an increased incidence of gastric adenocarcinoma just as with AMAG. Indeed, HP is the most common etiologic factor associated with gastric adenocarcinoma.

Can you prevent the development of gastric adenocarcinoma by eradicating HP in cases of EMAG?

It is clear that treating HP will not prevent all cases of adenocarcinoma. Once dysplasia has occurred, the disease has usually progressed too far. Indeed, once extensive intestinal metaplasia has occurred many cases may already be too far gone. However, it is felt that if you treat EMAG prior to development of extensive metaplasia most cancers may be prevented.

Do all polypoid lesions have to be removed in AMAG and EMAG?

No, many polyp-like lesions are actually pseudopolyps, normal viable oxyntic mucosa that remains adjacent to areas of oxyntic destruction, but all polypoid lesions should be biopsied to make sure there is no dysplasia or cancer.

You mention gastric mapping. What technique do you recommend?

I would get at least two biopsies from both the antrum and the body, biopsying both lesser and greater curvature, and one from the incisura. In addition, any suspicious or polypoid lesions should be biopsied. If polypoid lesions are biopsied, you should also biopsy flat areas adjacent to the polyps.

It is crucial to label the biopsies from the antrum and body specifically. There is a form of metaplasia where mucosa in the body of the stomach can be replaced by antral-type mucosa, termed pseudopyloric metaplasia. The only way to make this distinction histologically is to label the biopsies from the corpus separately.

Chapter 12
Subepithelial Lesions and NETs

Phillip Chisholm

Case 1 A 68-year-old man has an EGD performed for chronic heartburn. He is found to have mild grade A esophagitis accounting for his symptoms, but incidentally noted is a lesion indenting the gastric fundus, about 1.5 cm in size. The overlying mucosa appears normal.

How would you determine the location of this lesion and its malignant potential?

Lesions that are present under the mucosal layer of the stomach may be intramural or extramural. These are usually found incidentally at the time of endoscopy-like in this case.

Extramural lesions could include surrounding organs, or blood vessels, pancreatic pseudocysts, or liver cysts. Intramural lesions could be tumors or intramural vessels.

Determining the etiology of the lesions can be done with tunneled biopsies—where using a jumbo biopsy forceps multiple biopsies are done, one on top of the next. More often we evaluate them with EUS. EUS allows a determination of the location of the lesion, what layer it's located in, and allows for FNA to arrive at histology.

Many of these lesions are submucosal, and one of the most common gastric submucosal lesions is the GIST. On EUS, these lesions are hypoechoic, usually in the fourth layer, rarely in the second. GISTs are most commonly found in the stomach (40–60%), next most frequently in the small intestine (20–30%), and less common in the colon and rectum (15%), and <1% are found in the esophagus. On histology, GISTs are spindle cell tumors that stain positive for C-kit+ (CD117) and CD34.

P. Chisholm (✉)
Hep Division/Department of Medicine—GI, Medical College of Wisconsin, Milwaukee, WI, USA
e-mail: pchisholm@mcw.edu

© The Author(s), under exclusive license to Springer Nature Switzerland AG 2023
W. H. Sobin et al. (eds.), *Managing Complex Cases in Gastroenterology*,
https://doi.org/10.1007/978-3-031-48949-5_12

The differential of submucosal gastric lesions includes leiomyomas. These are also usually located in the fourth layer on EUS, occasionally the second. These are differentiated from GISTs by histology, which reveals smooth muscle actin and stains are negative for spindle cells and C-kit.

A third submucosal lesion is the lipoma. These are most common in the colon, but can be present anywhere in the GI tract. The overlying mucosa appears normal but is occasionally yellow. When using biopsy forceps to push on the lesion, there is the characteristic pillow or tent sign.

The patient has an EUS with FNA, and histology is consistent with a GIST.

How would you manage this lesion?

For gastric GISTs <1 cm in size, observation alone is recommended. For lesions >2 cm, it is felt that surgical resection is necessary. This lesion is 1.5 cm in size, and careful follow-up observation is warranted unless the patient wants to proceed with surgery.

Case 2 A 59-year-old man was found, on screening colonoscopy, to have a small subepithelial lesion in the rectum removed with snare cautery that revealed a well-differentiated neuroendocrine tumor. It was completely excised, and there was no lymphovascular invasion. The quantity of Ki67 was <1%. It was felt to be a rectal carcinoid.

What is the significance of finding a neuroendocrine tumor in the GI tract?

Neuroendocrine tumors of the gut are generally termed carcinoid tumors. Neuroendocrine tumors in the pancreas are pancreatic islet cell tumors or PNETs. Some neuroendocrine tumors may be functioning, secreting hormones, while others are non-functioning. Functioning tumors include VIPomas, gastrinomas, insulinomas, and glucagonomas. These are usually PNETs. Small bowel carcinoids may be functional, releasing serotonin and other vasoactive amines.

The patient described above has a small rectal carcinoid. Not expecting this to be functional we wouldn't bother with hormonal testing. Endoscopic resection is generally curative.

Case 3 A 63-year-old man without a significant past medical history is admitted to the hospital with melena and acute anemia. An EGD is performed, which reveals a 2.5 cm ulcerated lesion in the gastric body. The remainder of the examination is unremarkable. Biopsies obtained from the lesion reveal a gastric neuroendocrine tumor, a carcinoid. A gastrin level returned 25. It was felt that the patient probably had a type 3 carcinoid.

What is the implication of this finding? Is this usually as innocent as the rectal carcinoid described earlier?

Gastric carcinoids have been divided into three types. Type 1 is generally innocuous and represents a growth of enterochromaffin-like cells (ECL) as a reaction to hypergastrinemia. These patients have atrophic gastritis, often with associated pernicious anemia. The elevated gastrin is an appropriate reaction to hypochlorhydria or achlorhydria. This has also rarely been described in patients on chronic PPI therapy. Type 1 gastric carcinoids have a very low malignant potential.

Type 2 gastric carcinoids are also a reaction to hypergastrinemia and also grow from ECL cells. They are often multifocal. In type 2 carcinoids, the tumors arise from hypergastrinemia from ZE syndrome. These carcinoids are usually benign, but there needs to be further searching to locate another biologically active NET of the pancreas or chest, which is secreting gastrin. These tumors may be malignant.

Type 3 gastric carcinoids also develop from ECL cells. However, the growth of these cells is not stimulated by hypergastrinemia. These carcinoids tend to have a high malignancy risk with poor prognosis. These cases require surgical resection and lymphadenectomy.

Case 4 *A 51-year-old woman with a history of hypothyroidism presents with symptoms of epigastric discomfort and fatigue. She has no heartburn and denies nausea, vomiting, or weight loss. Her sister died from gastric adenocarcinoma at age 48. Laboratory studies show a Hbg of 11, ferritin of 6, iron of 18, and vitamin B12 of 100. Upper endoscopy reveals atrophic mucosa with a 3-mm polyp in the fundus that is removed. Histology reveals a monomorphic collection of neuroendocrine cells.*

How would you interpret this case?

This patient almost certainly has pernicious anemia with associated gastric atrophy with hypochlorhydria or achlorhydria and intrinsic factor deficiency. These patients tend to have a rebound hypergastrinemia that stimulates growth of the ECL cells. In addition, the achlorhydria is associated with decreased iron absorption and a mixed anemia, both IDA and megaloblastic type (the latter due to low vitamin B12). This fits the criteria for a type 1 gastric carcinoid, which tends to run a very benign course.

What further testing should be done in a patient with suspected gastric carcinoid?

Further testing might include checking a gastric pH, as well as biopsies for HP. A fasting gastrin level should be checked off of PPI. In patients with elevated gastrin suspected of having Zollinger-Ellison syndrome, a secretin test should be performed. In normal controls, secretin should cause a decrease in serum gastrin. In Z-E syndrome, there is an inappropriate rise in serum gastrin. Some of these patients will also benefit from a CT chest and abdomen along with somatostatin scintigraphy—either dotate or octreotide PET scan.

What about small bowel carcinoids?

Small bowel carcinoids account for a large number, about 40% of small bowel malignancies. They are most common in the ileum. Small bowel carcinoids tend to be slow-growing tumors, but they cause an intense desmoplastic reaction that might lead to small bowel obstruction. In addition, some of these lesions are functioning, releasing serotonin and other biologically active amines. These can cause a carcinoid syndrome that includes diarrhea, flushing, and hypotension. Usually, carcinoid syndrome from small bowel carcinoids occurs in patients who have liver metastases. It is diagnosed by an elevation of 5 HIAA.

Chapter 13
Viewpoints on Managing Common Clinical GI Disorders from a Practitioner with Over 50 Years of "Real-World" Experience

Helmut Ammon

Constipation

Case 1 *A 35-year-old woman is having problems with chronic constipation. She would prefer to use a natural product because she doesn't like the idea of taking drugs.*

Our first choice is Metamucil, which works in over 30%, maybe 50% of our patients. We start out telling the patient to take one packet of Metamucil in a glass of water, with a meal, preferably breakfast. If taken before a meal, patients tend to fill up too quickly. Usually, one packet a day is sufficient; rarely, a patient needs a second packet with lunch or dinner. We tell the patient that their constipation is a result of not having enough water in their stool and that Metamucil mixed in water takes care of that problem along with providing bulk.

The patient tries the Metamucil but stops it because she gets too gassy, even if she cuts back to half a packet a day.

She agrees to try some drug. What do you like to use here?

Everyone these days seems to prescribe Miralax, which works well, but another agent to keep in mind, which has been used over the decades, is milk of magnesia (MOM). It's not the most fashionable drug these days, but it works quite predictably, is quite cheap, and can be used on a chronic basis, as long as the patient doesn't have renal insufficiency. We start with one tablespoon a day, but if needed you can go to one tablespoon two or three times a day, with meals, with plenty of fluid [1].

H. Ammon (✉)
Division of GI and Hepatology/Department of Medicine, Medical College of Wisconsin, Milwaukee, WI, USA
e-mail: hammon@mcw.edu

The important thing to remember in treating constipation is not to overdo things and create severe diarrhea, where the patient gets tempted to take Lomotil or Imodium. You want to be consistent, and not get into a pattern of blasting them out and then going in the opposite direction, and then having to go back and forth. You want to get them on a regular regimen they can adhere to where they take the same dose of medicine every day and have an adequate bowel movement on an ongoing basis.

When you start patients on treatment for constipation, they shouldn't expect to experience a bowel movement the very next day, it takes time to prime the pump. They needn't worry if it takes a couple of days for them to start going, there is nothing wrong with that.

How do you feel about the use of Surfak or Colace?

These meds are surfactants, they are detergents, and they all inhibit electrolyte and water absorption and stimulate secretion. Generally, they are quite effective, but you can get the same effect by using olive oil. These triglycerides are broken down, and their fatty acids act as detergents. Some people use linseed oil, and in the old days, they used castor oil. Ricinoleic acid, the fatty acid in castor oil, is poorly absorbable, which makes it effective [2]. We tell patients to take one or two tablespoons of olive oil and put it on their salad, or cook with it, and get the same laxative effect.

How about the use of senna or bisacodyl (Dulcolax)?

Senna is considered safe [3]. Its long-term use can cause melanosis coli. Bisacodyl can cause significant mucosal injury [4, 5]. For this reason, we don't like to use it on a chronic basis. Dulcolax suppositories have been known to cause rectal ulcers due to their local effects.

How do you feel about the use of anorectal manometry?

We usually reserve this for patients who don't get relief from their constipation with our medications. Our patients appreciate the fact that we are trying to come up with a scientific explanation for their symptoms, using anorectal manometry. Unfortunately, when you diagnose dyssynergic defecation, it turns out that many patients are not good candidates for biofeedback. In the end, there are relatively few patients who will benefit from anorectal manometry.

Acute Diarrhea

Case 2 *A 38-year-old man who you have seen previously calls with the complaint of new-onset diarrhea of 5-day duration without any clear-cut precipitating factors.*

In a case like this is it necessary to do any testing? How would you manage the patient? Is Pepto-Bismol useful?

Most patients with this problem have self-limited viral, or less often, bacterial diarrhea that will resolve with no treatment, so there is no indication for stool cultures. We simply tell patients to stay well hydrated, occasionally recommending

Gatorade. We do not prescribe Pepto-Bismol. It would be hard to appreciate whether Pepto was of any benefit, since the diarrhea will generally resolve in a few days, with or without treatment.

IBS-D

Case 3 *A 28-year-old woman is having diarrhea and cramps over the past 6 months. Her primary care doctor orders laboratories, including a celiac panel and stools, including stool for calprotectin, and all tests return negative. He prescribes a low FODMAP diet but she gets no relief. She is referred to you for a second opinion.*

How would you proceed?

I assume you are trying to describe a patient with functional complaints. In reality, you end up with a colonoscopy to exclude organic disease first. The main tool here is the history. Why in the world did this 28-year-old woman develop these symptoms at this time? What happened in her life to precipitate this change? We ask the patient to tell us her story because oftentimes the answer is in the telling. When there is a strong psychological underpinning, we may refer her to a psychologist or psychiatrist. Most gastroenterologists are not trained to take a detailed psychological history.

In terms of management, we often try Metamucil first, and it absorbs excess water and provides bulk, which may be beneficial. Imodium can certainly be used. An antispasmodic occasionally works. Peppermint oil is an over-the-counter antispasmodic that is inexpensive. Some patients will respond to dicyclomine or hyoscyamine. It is important to reassure the patient of the benign nature of her symptoms, which can produce anxiety. Oftentimes medication is not necessary, and we adhere to what Marvin Schuster once said, "Don't medicalize IBS, don't make it into a disease, it's part of the human condition."

What about using cholestyramine in IBS-D or post-cholecystectomy diarrhea?

For cholestyramine to work, there must be some bile acid malabsorption. According to Camilleri, 25–50% of patients with IBS-D have bile acid malabsorption, and it is not so clear whether they all will respond to cholestyramine, but it may be worth a trial [6, 7]. However, it's a different story if the patient has had a cholecystectomy, in which case there may be bile acid malabsorption, which can cause diarrhea and cramps, simulating IBS-D. These patients will frequently respond to cholestyramine.

Cholestyramine works best when given with meals. The bile acid pool is largest in the morning, so giving it with breakfast has the largest benefit. Cholestyramine binds bile acids as they get dumped into the small intestine in response to a meal. Patients with post-cholecystectomy diarrhea respond well to cholestyramine, but oftentimes this is a self-limited disease that corrects over time. Before embarking on long-term treatment, a therapeutic trial with cholestyramine 4 g with each meal and at bedtime for 72 h will tell. If the diarrhea is not controlled, it is not caused by bile acids. Most patients get away with taking it with breakfast or with breakfast and lunch. Since cholestyramine can bind medications as well, the patient needs to be instructed to take all medications at least 1 h apart from cholestyramine. Patients taking cholestyramine on a chronic basis are at risk of developing deficiencies in fat-soluble vitamins and need to be monitored accordingly.

Gastroparesis (We Are Presenting Several Scenarios Here for Comparison)

Cases 4–6 *The first patient is a 35-year-old woman who complains of chronic fullness and nausea but has no history of diabetes. She experiences significant weight loss of about 15 pounds over 2 months. She claims to avoid eating because it exacerbates her nausea. An EGD is performed and is negative except for mild gastric retention of semi-solid food. A gastric emptying scan at 4 h showed 30% retention (normal < 10%).*

The second patient is a 50-year-old obese woman with type 2 diabetes of 5-year duration who gives a history of persistent nausea and vomiting. Her hemoglobin A1C is 7. EGD and a gastric emptying scan are consistent with gastroparesis.

The third patient is a 55-year-old diabetic patient with poorly controlled diabetes and a HbA1C of 11. She suffers from peripheral neuropathy in her toes and retinopathy.

In the first case, history is very important. What happened to this 35-year-old woman to create these symptoms at this point in her life? Was there some precipitating cause, any depression or other factor? When patients are nauseated, they usually have delayed gastric emptying but what came first, the nausea or the gastroparesis?

The most worrisome thing in this history is the fifteen-pound weight loss. Has she had a full work-up for weight loss? Might she have an eating disorder? Take a calorie count to document whether there has been decreased caloric intake.

In the second case, we question the correlation between diabetes and gastroparesis seeing how the diabetes is only of 5-year duration and there is no peripheral or autonomic neuropathy.

In the third case, it is clear that diabetes is an important factor. In dealing with patients with gastroparesis and diabetes that is poorly controlled the first thing you need to do is to get the diabetes under better control. However, an interesting pearl about diabetic gastroparesis is that the symptoms may fluctuate. There are times when symptoms are worse and times when they are better. Sometimes the symptoms correlate with diabetes control, and sometimes they don't.

In treating gastroparesis, we generally try a prokinetic agent first, and it is usually metoclopramide. If the metoclopramide is helping, we will continue it for 4–6 weeks, we avoid using it any longer. The longer the patient takes metoclopramide the risk of tardive dyskinesia gets much higher and the efficacy of the drug diminishes, because of tachyphylaxis. So, we usually use a 4 to 6-week cutoff. You don't want to get complications from your therapy.

GERD

Case 7 *A 35-year-old man with chronic heartburn takes PPIs and his symptoms keep recurring whenever he tries to stop the medicine. Occasionally, he gets breakthrough symptoms despite once daily PPI. An EGD is performed off of PPIs, which returns negative.*

Do you have a favorite PPI? Is there one that is superior? How long will you maintain a patient on PPIs? What do you make of the fact that the PPI is working inconsistently?

Our favorite PPI is the PPI that works for that patient (unfortunately we're often stuck with the one the insurance company will pay for). Not all PPIs work the same in all patients, some will respond better to one PPI than another. We generally try omeprazole first and go from there.

If a patient is getting a suboptimal result from his PPI, the first thing to do is to make sure he is taking it properly, a half hour before the meal. If they are not responding to several different PPIs, it is possible they are a fast PPI metabolizer, in which case they may do better with rabeprazole [8].

We believe in maintaining PPIs as long as they are needed, we are not that concerned about long-term side effects from PPIs, which seem questionable. We feel it's more important to keep the patient out of the hands of the surgeons for as long as possible. If patients need to remain on PPIs indefinitely, we are comfortable with that.

Microscopic Colitis

Case 8 *A 67-year-old woman presents with chronic diarrhea. A screening colonoscopy 2 years ago was negative. The patient has been on statins for 20 years.*

The patient had a negative colonoscopy. How would you evaluate her now?

In this age range, microscopic colitis is a distinct possibility. A negative colonoscopy (without biopsy) 2 years ago does not rule that out. So, performing a colonoscopy with biopsy is indicated.

The colonoscopy is grossly normal but biopsies show microscopic colitis.

How would you proceed?

Our first choice is usually budesonide.

How long will you continue budesonide?

If budesonide works, the condition often improves, and you can taper off the medicine. If you stop the medicine and symptoms return, they usually don't recur immediately, so the patient usually experiences a hiatus in drug therapy. If there is a clear relapse, we restart budesonide and try to taper the dose to 6 mg or 3 mg. In most cases, long-term therapy is not needed, but if it is necessary, we are generally comfortable with long-term treatment with 3 mg and to some extent, 6 mg.

Fecal Incontinence

Case 9 *An 83-year-old woman presents with the complaint of occasional fecal incontinence. She is aware of the urge to defecate, but when these "incidents" occur she can't "hold it in" long enough. This happens about once a week, and during these episodes, she actually defecates into her pants. There is nothing to suggest that she has constipation with overflow incontinence. On your rectal examination, she has some anal tone, but it is diminished. Her last colonoscopy was 5 years ago and was negative except for diverticulosis. Her only meds are anti-hypertensives and statins.*

What are your considerations in managing this patient?

In a woman with anal incontinence, an obstetric history is important. Were there vaginal deliveries, and if so, how many? Were there any lacerations at the time of the deliveries? We want to know if there is a rectocele or cystocele. So, if there was a significant obstetric history, we definitely want the patient to get a good pelvic examination.

What is the stool pattern? If the stool is soft or watery or even of normal consistency, we might try Imodium first. If the patient has hard balls of stool we probably would not. Metamucil can also be helpful in some of these patients.

We also want to know when the incidents occur in relation to the time of day, the time of meals, and the type of food eaten. If a connection can be established, a behavior may be able to be changed.

The question of whether to proceed with defecography in an 83 years old, if a rectocele is highly likely, is debatable. If the patient is not a good surgical candidate, it is not worth putting her through the examination, and in elderly patients, you don't want to be overly aggressive.

Diverticulitis

Case 10 *A 35-year-old man comes in with a history of two episodes of diverticulitis in the last 9 months. CAT scan documented sigmoid diverticulitis in both cases. Both episodes were treated with outpatient antibiotics.*

How would you manage this patient?

The unusual thing in this case is the patient's young age. We haven't been told whether he has diffuse diverticulosis, or diverticulosis that is limited to the sigmoid, which may alter our management.

In this case it was limited to the sigmoid.

The fact that the patient has had two episodes of diverticulitis in 9 months at such a young age makes it very likely that he will have more episodes in the future. We would put him on a high-fiber diet, and Metamucil. We would have a low threshold to refer him to a surgeon if there was another episode of diverticulitis in the future. At this age, the likelihood of recurrence is high, and he is a good surgical risk, but you need to know your surgeon, and a colon resection for diverticulitis is not always a walk in the park.

References

1. Loening-Baucke V, Pashankar DS. A randomized, prospective, comparison study of polyethylene glycol 3350 without electrolytes and milk of magnesia for children with constipation and fecal incontinence. Pediatrics. 2006;118(2):528–35.
2. Ammon HV, Thomas PJ, Phillips SF. Effects of oleic and ricinoleic acids on net jejunal water and electrolyte movement. Perfusion studies in man. J Clin Invest. 1974;53(2):374–9.
3. Godding E. Laxatives and the special role of Senna. Pharmacology. 1988;36:230–6.
4. Saunders DR, Sillery J, Rachmilewitz D, Rubin CE, Tytgat GN. Effect of bisacodyl on the structure and function of rodent and human intestine. Gastroenterology. 1977;72(5 Pt 1):849–56.
5. Saunders DR, Haggitt RC, Kimmey MB, Silverstein FE. Morphological consequences of bisacodyl on normal human rectal mucosa: effect of a prostaglandin E1 analog on mucosal injury. Gastrointest Endosc. 1990;36(2):101–4.
6. Camilleri M. Bile acid diarrhea: prevalence, pathogenesis, and therapy. Gut Liver. 2015;9:332–9.
7. Camilleri M, Vijayvargiya P. The role of bile acids in chronic diarrhea. Am J Gastroenterol. 2020;115(10):1596–603.
8. Sachs G, Shin JM, Howden CW. Review article: the clinical pharmacology of proton pump inhibitors. Aliment Pharmacol Ther. 2006;23(Suppl. 2):2–8.

Chapter 14
Small Intestinal Bacterial Overgrowth

Benson Massey

Case 1 *A 64-year-old woman presents with abdominal distension, flatus, diarrhea, weight loss, and anemia. She has malodorous, fatty, foul-smelling stools several times a day. She has systemic sclerosis with significant GI tract involvement. In addition, she has had recurrent bouts of small bowel obstruction, which have led to repeated explorations and resultant adhesive disease. In addition, she's had exploratory laparotomies for profound pneumoperitoneum and pneumatosis in the bowel, but no perforation or ischemia has been identified. On presentation, she has anemia with low vitamin B_{12}, hypoalbuminemia, low vitamin D, and elevated INR.*

Do you think this patient has SIBO?

Yes, I think it's very likely that the patient has many manifestations of SIBO syndrome [1] and has many factors that would predispose to having SIBO. In SIBO, you have an abnormal accumulation of primarily anaerobic bacteria in the small bowel, in sufficient quantities to disrupt normal intestinal digestion, absorption, and transit, leading to various clinical manifestations.

What are the consequences of this anaerobic proliferation? One is consumption of vitamin B_{12} by the bacteria within the gut. They use this as part of their metabolism. Interestingly, however, while bacterial metabolism markedly reduces vitamin B_{12} it often generates folate. So, patients with SIBO will often have a very high serum folate, along with a low vitamin B_{12}. In addition, not only does bacterial metabolism in SIBO lead to B_{12} deficiency, but it also causes breakdown of carbohydrates and proteins so that they're no longer available for human nutrition. In addition, bacterial action will cause bile acid hydrolysis. As a result, we don't have

B. Massey (✉)
Division of Gastroenterology and Hepatology, Department of Medicine, Medical College of Wisconsin, Milwaukee, WI, USA
e-mail: bmassey@mcw.edu

© The Author(s), under exclusive license to Springer Nature Switzerland AG 2023
W. H. Sobin et al. (eds.), *Managing Complex Cases in Gastroenterology*,
https://doi.org/10.1007/978-3-031-48949-5_14

81

bile acids to help micellize fats. Therefore, fat, protein, and carbohydrate deficiencies are encountered. Bacterial overgrowth also leads to damage to the intestinal lining, resulting in reduced disaccharide levels. The divalent sugars are not absorbed and empty into the colon to be fermented by bacteria, resulting in an increase in the luminal osmolality, giving us an osmotic, laxative-type diarrhea.

Furthermore, because of bacterial enterocyte damage, particularly in the distal small bowel, we can have a reduction of the enterohepatic circulation of bile acids. Therefore, more bile acids will leak into the colon, which stimulates further fluid secretion, yet another reason to have diarrhea.

As a consequence of this anaerobic proliferation, many patients have diarrhea, some have steatorrhea and weight loss, and in severe cases, we can see severe protein-calorie malnutrition, with low serum albumin and edema. As a result of vitamin B_{12} losses, we can see manifestations of pernicious anemia and peripheral neuropathies.

After being seen in the ER, the patient gets a KUB that demonstrates massively dilated loops of bowel, but she also has air under the diaphragm and there is pneumatosis intestinalis. CAT scan shows no other signs of perforation, ischemia, or inflammation.

Now, in this case, the patient has pneumoperitoneum and pneumatosis without obvious ischemia, perforation, or obstruction. Can this be due to bacterial overgrowth?

Yes, with all the tremendous fermentation that's going on, these patients often complain of bloating and excessive flatus. In extreme cases, the increased gas from bacterial fermentation can lead to pneumatosis intestinalis and, rarely, even profound pneumoperitoneum.

What are the mechanisms that predispose a patient to develop SIBO?

The most common is impaired clearance through the gut. We see this in patients with intestinal strictures, patients who've developed adhesions, chronic partial small bowel obstruction, and patients with multiple small bowel diverticula. These can all act as areas of stasis that become a nidus for bacterial proliferation. In addition, some patients have coloenteric fistulas that lead to a direct backflow of bacteria into the small intestine.

The next most common etiology for delayed clearance would be impaired motility. This woman has systemic sclerosis, which is a classic disorder associated with delayed motility. This can also be seen in chronic intestinal pseudo-obstruction and certain neurodegenerative disorders, such as multiple sclerosis. Certainly, we always have to remember drugs, particularly narcotics.

Another etiology for SIBO is impaired bacterial killing. One example of this is the patient with profound achlorhydria, as is seen in autoimmune gastritis. This can also happen in certain bypass situations where the stomach has been mostly excluded.

Yet another mechanism is when there's excess substrate for bacterial growth, because, normally, nutrients are being cleared (absorbed) from the small bowel, but if you have chronic pancreatitis, or if you have a reduction of lipase and amylase for any reason, you may have nutrients sitting around longer in the small intestine, encouraging the development of bacterial overgrowth.

We can also see bacterial overgrowth with immune deficiencies such as common variable immunodeficiency.

The patient underwent a glucose breath test where glucose was administered and breath samples were collected for hydrogen and methane over a course of 3 h. Normally, the fasting values for hydrogen after glucose administration are less than 10. This patient started out with an extraordinarily high baseline of 238 and subsequently had whopping elevations after administration of glucose. The diagnosis of SIBO was confidently confirmed.

How do you treat your patients with SIBO?

There are no controlled studies on this, but I will start with the cheapest antibiotic that the patient hasn't already been exposed to. I keep them on this until they develop resistance, which will eventually happen. Hopefully, you can get 6 months, maybe a year, out of the antibiotic, but at some point, it's going to fail, and then, you have to switch to another agent, and then, after that one fails, switch to yet another one.

In the past, I'd use agents such as metronidazole or fluoroquinolones, but it's been clear for years now that there are potential toxicities with long-term use of these, such as peripheral neuropathy and tendon rupture, and so, I avoid their long-term use.

I will say that in my experience, rifaximin, usually in the dose of around 1200 milligrams a day, is actually quite helpful, but the problem is that it does not have an FDA-approved indication for treating SIBO, so we're using it off-label, and it's very expensive. It's very hard to get it covered by insurance even after appeal.

The patient receives three courses of different antibiotics and responds for months at a time. Now, she is no longer responding after trials of various antibiotics.

What do you do for the patient who initially responded to several rounds of antibiotics but now nothing is working?

First, I would confirm that the SIBO condition is still active. I would do an updated breath test on the current therapy, and if it's abnormal, I would get a duodenal aspirate for quantitative culture and sensitivity. Using this, we can try to find out what the dominant organism or organisms are and what antibiotics they are susceptible to. We can also make sure the patient hasn't developed yeast overgrowth from all these antibiotics, but in severe end-stage cases, you may need to resort to an elemental diet or TPN.

Case 2 This is a 24-year-old law student who's been having intermittent abdominal cramps, occasional rectal urgency, and some diarrhea. She has a frequent sense of bloating and passing gas after meals.

She's working all day to get her law degree, neglecting a lot of healthy lifestyles, eating a highly processed takeout diet, and has gained 10 pounds since the start of the semester.

Because of her GI symptoms, she started searching online and read about SIBO. She took a home lactulose breath test where she collected breath samples after consuming some lactulose and sent these off to the commercial laboratory. Her early hydrogen readings were all less than 10 until 60–75 min out where they went up to the 30–45 range. She did feel slightly bloated at that time. This was reported out as a positive breath test for SIBO, and she was instructed to contact her physician for antibiotic treatment.

She has no other past medical history and is not taking any medications. When you examine her, she has an elevated BMI; otherwise, her examination is normal and her laboratory studies are normal.

Do you agree that this patient has SIBO?

I think it is dubious. If you're considering the diagnosis of SIBO in a patient, you have to consider what predisposing conditions might be leading up to it. In the absence of those predisposing conditions, the diagnosis is unlikely [1], and clearly, many of the symptoms that may be attributed to SIBO, including diarrhea and flatus, are much more commonly seen in various functional disorders such as functional bloating, IBS-D, and IBS-C.

Then, we have to realize that the testing for SIBO really is imperfect. There is no gold standard that's agreed on. So, with imperfect testing, if you're not careful about who you choose to investigate for SIBO, you will have a lot of false positives.

However, let's step back a minute and talk about breath testing, which is the main way people try to diagnose SIBO in this day and age. There are some generally agreed-upon principles about breath testing. One is that human metabolism does not produce hydrogen or methane. They are a product of bacterial metabolism, and when hydrogen or methane are produced, they diffuse into the circulation at whatever site they're being produced, be it mouth, small intestine, large intestine, or bladder, and then, they're transported to the lungs, and these gasses are expelled during exhalation. These can be detected with very sensitive gas analyzers. So, if you see hydrogen and methane in someone's breath, it tells you that bacterial fermentation is going on somewhere in their body. It does not tell you where this is occurring or just what is being fermented.

By itself, the production of hydrogen or methane does not confirm that a disorder like SIBO is present. Why is that? First of all, we have to realize that fermentation in the gut is a normal process that depends on what you eat and where the bacteria are located. Levels of bacteria are low in the stomach and proximal small bowel and orders of magnitude higher in the colon than in the small bowel, even in someone who has small bowel bacterial overgrowth. Therefore, when you give a patient a carbohydrate test substance and detect a rise in hydrogen or methane production in the breath, you have to be certain that the production is not occurring in the colon before you diagnose the patient as having SIBO.

The problem with using lactulose for breath testing is that once this undigestable (by humans) carbohydrate reaches the colon, bacteria there will metabolize this and generate gas that can be detected in the breath. Most people using this test make the assumption that SIBO must be present if hydrogen or methane concentrations in breath specimens rise significantly (10–20 ppm) before 90 min. This is based on an assumption that the orocecal transit time is 90 min or longer. However, in a landmark study of diarrhea-predominant IBS patients when the lactulose was given with a radioactive tracer, so that the location of the lactulose bolus could be determined when the breath hydrogen levels increased, it was found that in 79% of the "abnormal (hydrogen rose before 90 min)" tests, the rise in hydrogen actually occurred after the bolus had already reached the colon. Indeed, the mean orocecal transit time in these cases was 41 min, well under 90 min. This is consistent with prior work showing that functional diarrhea patients have a more rapid orocecal transit time. Therefore, using lactulose breath testing without concurrently measuring the orocecal transit time leads to a tremendous rate of false-positive tests [1]. The only reasonably reliable test result with lactulose is a negative one.

How about glucose breath testing, which was the gold standard for breath testing? The working assumption for a glucose breath test is that all glucose is completely absorbed within the small intestine. Therefore, if you see a rise in hydrogen or methane, after giving glucose, this has to be due to bacteria in the small bowel metabolizing glucose. This is a reasonable assumption so long as you can be certain that the patient does not have rapid gastric emptying, rapid small bowel transit, or small bowel mucosal disease. Any of these three factors could lead to incomplete small bowel absorption of glucose, resulting in colonic fermentation of that glucose, and hence a false-positive glucose breath test.

At MCW, we have the ability to perform glucose breath testing with concurrent scintigraphy, and so, we can monitor where the head of the bolus is when we start detecting bacterial fermentation. We only make the diagnosis of SIBO if the gas levels rise before the bolus reaches the cecum.

It turns out that about half the time when we see abnormal glucose breath tests, they're actually falsely positive from rapid transit. In our studies, the overall average orocecal transit time was 75 min. So, the studies that argue that any time you see a rise of hydrogen before 90 min SIBO must be present are erroneous.

If you look at people who've had major upper GI tract surgery, such as a gastric bypass, the vast majority of these have an abnormal breath test, but in most cases, it's abnormal due to rapid transit. However, even without such surgery, about one in nine abnormal breath tests were falsely positive, which is better than with lactulose, but still points out a high rate of false-positive testing if one were to use glucose alone without a concurrent measure of orocecal transit time.

Clearly, defining SIBO based on breath tests is problematic. What about performing quantitative bacterial cultures from small bowel aspirates obtained during endoscopy? This approach is very expensive and invasive. It's going to cost several thousand dollars by the time you count in the endoscopy and the culture processing in the microbiology laboratory. Furthermore, there is a concern that obtaining samples from only the duodenum will not detect bacterial overgrowth located more distally. Finally, there is uncertainty about what concentration of bacteria represents a true problem with overgrowth. While previous work has suggested that patients with symptomatic SIBO have concentrations of $>10^5$/ml, a recent study in healthy subjects on a high-fiber diet can have bacteria concentrations this high. Furthermore, treating patients for SIBO based on a finding of this relatively low concentration in duodenal aspirates has not been shown to result in better clinical outcomes.

Ultimately, the problem we are facing today is one of indiscriminate testing in patients with nonspecific symptoms who have no predisposing conditions or findings that would lead one to suspect the presence of SIBO (i.e., low pretest probability). In this setting, I would expect the pretest probability of having SIBO is at best 1%, but for the point of argument let's say it is as high as 10%. If we perform in this patient group a glucose breath test, which has a sensitivity and specificity of about 80%, then among those with a positive result about 4% (a third, at the higher pretest prevalence) will actually have SIBO.

So, if you start doing more indiscriminate testing, you're going to diagnose a lot more people with SIBO who don't really have SIBO. Therefore, I think we have to come up with a more rational approach to testing here. First of all, I think we have to increase the pretest probability, and to do that, we have to start limiting testing to patients who have abnormalities that are associated with SIBO. Patients with anemia, particularly vitamin B_{12} deficiency-related anemia, and those with steatorrhea, or low albumin. Those people who have conditions that are known to predispose to SIBO, such as chronic small bowel pseudo-obstruction, common variable immunodeficiency, or systemic sclerosis, are reasonable candidates (if actually symptomatic). We can't just keep testing people with nonspecific symptoms, and we also need to have a reliable testing protocol. We can't use lactulose breath testing unless it's combined with scintigraphy to measure orocecal transit. You also need to be sure that patients are on the appropriate pretest (no FODMAPs) diet before breath testing. Because constipated patients can release preformed colonic gas during breath testing, this needs to be treated before performing breath testing. Breath test findings cannot be interpreted accurately in patients with major foregut surgery without a concurrent measure of transit time. If a patient with no good *a priori* indication nevertheless tests positive on glucose breath testing, consider repeating the test with a concurrent measure of orocecal transit time. Otherwise, if one truly thinks the test result is accurate, then one is obligated to investigate further to try to find the underlying reason the patient has developed SIBO, to see if that can't be corrected, rather than just treating the test result with antibiotics.

Reference

1. Massey BT, Wald A. Small intestinal bacterial overgrowth syndrome: a guide for the appropriate use of breath testing. Digest Dis Sci. 2021;66(2):338–47.

Chapter 15
Unusual Causes of Abdominal Pain and Controversies in Diagnosis

W. Harley Sobin and Patrick Sanvanson

In the selections below, we briefly examine a number of controversies in the diagnosis of abdominal pain, along with a review of some of the rarer etiologies of abdominal pain. They are not meant to be an exhaustive examination of the topics, but, rather, a brief review of diagnoses to consider in the patient with an elusive presentation, a checklist of zebras to keep in mind.

Case 1 *A 35-year-old woman presents with chronic abdominal pain. The pain has been present off and on over the past 2 years. The pain is located in the mid-abdomen. It is worse when she is stressed. It does not radiate. Bowel movements are normal, and stool for H pylori was negative. A trial of PPIs for a month was not helpful. Her CBC, CMP, and lipase were all normal. An abdominal ultrasound was normal. She had an esophagogastroduodenoscopy (EGD) by a different gastroenterologist that was negative. You tell the patient that there is no sign of serious pathology and you explain the functional nature of her symptoms. She does not buy into your explanation; instead, she is upset that nothing has been found and requests a CT scan.*

How beneficial is a CT scan in evaluating chronic abdominal pain?

In a young patient like this, with negative laboratory results, a CT scan is unlikely to add much useful information. CT scans are vastly over-utilized in the diagnosis of chronic abdominal pain. They are costly, expose the patient to radiation, and have

W. H. Sobin (✉)
Division of Gastroenterology and Hepatology, Medical College of Wisconsin, Milwaukee, WI, USA
e-mail: hsobin@mcw.edu

P. Sanvanson
Division of Gastroenterology and Hepatology, Department of Medicine, Medical College of Wisconsin, Milwaukee, WI, USA
e-mail: psanvans@mcw.edu

© The Author(s), under exclusive license to Springer Nature
Switzerland AG 2023
W. H. Sobin et al. (eds.), *Managing Complex Cases in Gastroenterology*,
https://doi.org/10.1007/978-3-031-48949-5_15

a high incidence of insignificant incidentalomas. Unless there are findings on physical or basic laboratory data to suggest organic disease, CT scans have a low likelihood of providing data that will alter management.

Incidental findings increase healthcare costs for limited benefit for the patient. There is a certain allure to CT scans that drive patients to ask for them and doctors to order them, when there are no findings of organic disease on initial examinations to explain symptomatology [1–3]. However, if there is nothing to suggest organic disease, we should try to resist that temptation.

After explaining your reasons to decline ordering the test, the patient becomes argumentative. She talks about the stress in her life and says that it will relieve her stress to have the CT scan.

It is very problematic to order a CT scan simply to allay a patient's fear if you fully believe the CT scan will be negative and will more likely cause harm than benefit. After explaining your arguments, after explaining the nature of functional symptoms, the majority of patients will be happy to learn that they do not have serious organic pathology. They will be happy to drop the issue and go on with their lives, but we have all experienced a few challenging patients who make demands and try to coerce us [4].

This patient alludes to all the stress in her life, and patients with increased stress are more likely to have functional GI pain syndromes and disorders of gut-brain interaction [5]. Many of these patients may benefit from psychotherapy. There is a high frequency of anxiety and somatization in those patients who have disabling IBS symptoms.

In all cases, it is essential to have a strong doctor-patient relationship and spend the time necessary to explain the nature of DGBI. Some patients will definitely benefit from the use of central neuromodulators that can work on abdominal pain and anxiety and depression. In a case like this, communication and strategies to address the stress are much more likely to help the patient than ordering a CT scan [6].

The patient, rather than going to see a mental health specialist, makes an appointment with her OB-GYN doctor, who reluctantly orders the CT scan. The CT scan fails to show anything in the upper or mid-abdomen to explain her symptoms but does show some thickening in the area of the cecum. The reading reports that this could be due to under-distension and presence of stool, but cannot rule out a cecal mass.

How likely is it that the patient has colon cancer?

Unfortunately, this finding, a thickening of the colon wall, is notoriously nonspecific. A routine contrast CT scan (as opposed to CT colonography or PET scan showing intrinsic colon disease) has a very high number of false-positive results, due to stool, lack of adequate distension, or other artifacts. In one study [7], only 13% of patients with cecal thickening on CT scan had pathology on follow-up colonoscopy. This is an example of one of the hazards of ordering a CT, the incidentaloma, which probably occurs in about 5% of all cases.

Case 2 *A 45-year-old slightly obese woman presents with intermittent RUQ pain.*
On the examination, she has very minor RUQ tenderness. Laboratories, including
LFTs, are normal. An US (ultrasound) is normal. She wants to have her gallbladder
removed.

Would you send her to a surgeon to take out her gallbladder?

While the ultrasound is good for ruling out cholelithiasis, it is not as good at ruling out microlithiasis and does not evaluate biliary dyskinesia. On the one hand, there are patients who have a normal ultrasound whose pain is due to gallbladder disease, but, on the other, we do not like to send a patient to surgery without some objective abnormality on imaging or laboratory.

Therefore, if the patient's symptoms sound typical of cholecystitis, but the US is normal, we like to order scintigraphy with a CCK-HIDA scan. If there is non-filling of the gallbladder, or if the ejection fraction after injection of CCK is significantly <38%, this suggests biliary dyskinesia and an increased incidence of microlithiasis and/or chronic cholecystitis [8]. In these cases, if there are no other findings to explain their symptoms, we will send patients for surgical evaluation, knowing that we can't guarantee a cholecystectomy will resolve the problem in all of them. Many patients will get symptomatic improvement after surgery, but a few will not, and therefore, an abnormal CCK-HIDA scan has to be evaluated with some healthy skepticism [9].

Case 3 *A 35-year-old woman complains of mid-abdominal pain. The pain is fairly*
chronic but worsened by meals. She has chronic constipation, only moving her bow-
els every 2–3 days. You examine her and hear a bruit over her abdomen. Because of
this, you send her for a CT scan that reveals median arcuate ligament narrowing of
the celiac axis.

How likely is it that this is causing the pain?

Both superior mesenteric artery compression (SMA syndrome) and median arcuate ligament compression (MALS) on CT scan have been objects of controversy. There are patients who have these radiographic findings who are asymptomatic [10], and a number of patients have had surgical repairs that did not result in improvement [11]. There are certainly a number of patients with SMA syndrome and MALS who have improved with surgery, but in other cases the X-ray findings end up being a red herring [12].

It is important to rule out other etiologies for abdominal pain. Only then, if the history is consistent with a vascular cause of pain, should angiographic studies be performed to measure the flow velocity across the vessel and document whether there is significant stenosis. Not everyone with the radiologic finding has significant clinical disease. It is important to inform the patient that although these may be the correct diagnoses, frequently patients will go for surgery/revascularization depending on the diagnosis, and the symptoms may not completely resolve.

Some factors suggesting a good result with celiac decompression for MALS include postprandial pain, age between 40 and 60, and weight loss of more than 20 lbs. [13]. Factors that suggest a poorer outcome include alcohol, and drug use and a history of significant psychiatric disorder [13, 14].

Case 4 A 35-year-old woman comes in for a second opinion. She complains of persistent abdominal pain located on the right side of her abdomen. The pain has been there for a year but has been getting more intense recently. When you push on her abdomen, she complains of extreme pain, but the abdomen is very soft and there is no guarding. Her vitals are normal, and her heart rate is 70, even when she complains of severe pain. Her basic laboratory panel is normal. She has had an US and EGD elsewhere, which were normal. Your impression is that her pain is probably functional.

It is very difficult to manage patients with chronic abdominal pain who have no apparent organic abnormalities. Do you have any special insight into treating these patients?

Many of the patients we see with complaints of chronic abdominal pain will not have an organic reason. Generally, when they do, it can be elicited with a basic history, physical examination, and simple laboratory panel. Not every patient complaining of pain warrants an EGD, colonoscopy, and CT scan.

How do we approach these patients who lack any organic findings? Some of them fit established criteria for well-defined disorders of gut-brain interaction such as irritable bowel syndrome (IBS), functional dyspepsia (FD), and centrally mediated abdominal pain syndrome (CAPS), which, although not associated with organic findings, are accepted as diagnostic entities with a well-defined treatment algorithm. Not all of these patients come to medical attention, but the ones who do, and the ones who are more resistant to treatment, tend to have higher levels of psychological distress [15].

Many of these patients have complaints that are vastly exaggerated relative to their physical findings. These patients tend to perseverate over symptoms, catastrophize, and, in many ways, end up inflating the severity of a symptom that would normally seem innocuous. It is a form of visceral hypersensitivity [16].

Some patients get secondary gain from their role as a patient, getting attention from doctors, family, and friends that reinforces the behavior. If we recognize that a patient has symptoms that are way out of proportion to the physical and laboratory findings, we can often anticipate that these factors are at play.

The patient described above most likely has a disorder of gut-brain interaction (DGBI, used to be called functional GI disorder-FGID). In DGBI patients, painful stimuli are exaggerated rather than inhibited. Many patients who do not respond to primary treatment regimens have this sort of misalignment. It is essential to explain to patients that this is a positive diagnosis, so that they don't go around thinking that no one can come up with an answer for their symptoms. There are specific treatments for these disorders, and it is important to communicate this insight to the patient [5]. There are more insights into management of DGBI in other chapters, later in this text.

Case 5 *A 46-year-old man comes to you with the complaint of abdominal pain. The patient had an episode of pancreatitis 1 year ago and was placed on narcotic pain medications as an inpatient, which were continued as an outpatient. He has not seen a gastroenterologist since discharge from the hospital. He has reportedly quit drinking, although he keeps smoking, but still complains of abdominal pain and keeps asking his primary care doctor to renew his narcotics. His doctor recently told him that he would not refill the narcotics unless he saw a gastroenterologist who recommended they be continued. The patient is complaining of severe, constant pain. His vitals are stable. On examination, the only thing of note is that his abdomen feels full, probably from retained stool, but his abdomen is soft and lacks involuntary guarding, although he complains of diffuse tenderness.*

Will you continue narcotic pain medications in a patient like this?

While narcotic pain medications may benefit patients with acute pancreatitis in the short term, their efficacy wears off quickly and these drugs need to be stopped as early as possible. One concern is addiction, the second is tolerance, with patients requesting ever higher doses, the third is side effects such as opioid-induced constipation, and the fourth is the most remarkable, that after a while, continued use of narcotics actually increases the level of pain, causing hyperalgesia [17].

You need to explain to the patient that you think the drugs are actually contributing to the pain. They need to start tapering the dose of narcotics while getting onto alternative analgesics such as gabapentin or duloxetine. The gastroenterologist may need to enlist help from a pain specialist. Unfortunately, patients tend to resist this explanation, but it is a necessary first step.

Case 6 *A 64-year-old woman complains of intermittent diarrhea and abdominal cramps that have been ongoing for 3 months. She avoids eating to avoid diarrhea and has lost 10 lbs. as a result. She had her last screening colonoscopy at age 60, and it was negative. Her 35-year-old daughter was recently diagnosed with IBS, and she questions whether that is her diagnosis as well. Her CBC, iron studies, and chemistries were all normal.*

How would you manage a patient like this?

In a 35-year-old with a history of chronic diarrhea and pain, IBS-D is often the explanation, but in a patient who is over the age of 50, with no history of functional GI illness, IBS is infrequent. In this case, there is a good chance that what sounds like IBS-D is actually microscopic colitis [18], and a repeat colonoscopy with random biopsies is indicated.

What if a patient in this age range presented with upper abdominal pain and ulcer-like symptoms, but had a negative EGD and US. Would you think this is likely functional dyspepsia (FD)?

No, once again it is much less common for a disorder of gut-brain interaction (DGBI) like FD to first present at 64 years, and, in this age range, organic pathology needs to be ruled out [19]. An EGD would be recommended, and, if that is negative, a triple-phase CT scan to rule out pancreatic malignancy or other organic pathology may be warranted in the appropriate patient.

Case 7 A 78-year-old man comes into the ER with a history of moderately severe pain in his mid-abdomen. He had several similar episodes of pain over the prior 4 months, but this one was more severe and lasted about 3 h before remitting. His CBC, lactate, and chemistries were normal. A CT scan showed diffuse atherosclerosis involving mesenteric vessels. The small bowel and colon appeared normal.

Is this likely acute bowel ischemia?

The finding of diffuse atherosclerosis will be present in a large number of individuals in this age range who are totally asymptomatic. The absence of acute bowel wall edema makes it less likely; this is acute ischemic colitis, or acute mesenteric insufficiency. Making a diagnosis of chronic mesenteric ischemia is more difficult. It is generally necessary to rule out other causes of pain, which might require upper endoscopy, ultrasound, or dedicated cross-sectional imaging.

When would you proceed to revascularization?

If this patient, with documented mesenteric atherosclerosis, has recurrent episodes of pain that are suggestive of ischemia, and the work-up shows no other etiology for the pain, we would refer the patient to a vascular surgeon for consultation.

Case 8 A 37-year-old woman has intermittent RUQ pain after eating fatty foods. The pain is very similar to the symptoms she had prior to cholecystectomy 1 year earlier. She had cholelithiasis, but her symptoms weren't much better after cholecystectomy and still occur intermittently. She is referred to you for the evaluation for sphincter of Oddi dysfunction (SOD).

What is your approach to patients with potential SOD disorder?

In this setting, it is essential to know what her liver enzymes are during the episodes of pain. We would also get a magnetic resonance cholangiopancreatography (MRCP) to rule out a retained common duct stone. Assuming there is no stone, we would consider the diagnosis of an SOD disorder only if there is an appropriate bump of liver function tests (LFTs) during the episode that might suggest intermittent spasm or obstruction. The finding of elevated LFTs and dilation of the bile duct must be present to consider this diagnosis. In the past, we used to consider endoscopic retrograde cholangiopancreatography (ERCP) and manometry based on the symptoms alone. This approach was associated with a high frequency of complications [20]. Now, if we have the requisite elevation of laboratories and bile duct dilation, we would go directly to ERCP and sphincterotomy without manometry.

Case 9 A 46-year-old woman is seen with the complaint of chronic suprapubic pain. She has a history of constipation for which she started taking laxatives. Although her constipation improved, her suprapubic pain did not. In addition, she is troubled with low back pain. She is pre-menopausal, and the suprapubic pain is worse during her menstrual periods. Her gynecologist ordered a pelvic ultrasound that was negative. She had a negative screening colonoscopy 1 year ago. The possibility of endometriosis is entertained.

How do you proceed with investigating possible endometriosis?

Diagnosis of endometriosis is challenging, and basic tests may return negative. A history of dyspareunia, dysmenorrhea, low back pain, abnormal uterine bleeding, and bowel or bladder abnormalities are common symptoms [21]. Pelvic ultrasound and examination by a gynecologist with special interest/training in diagnosing and managing patients with endometriosis are essential since this is frequently a difficult diagnosis to make. Gynecologists will occasionally obtain pelvic MRIs for additional information. A GI work-up to exclude other gastrointestinal pathology may be warranted. The ultimate diagnosis of endometriosis is made by laparoscopy.

Is a diagnostic and therapeutic medical trial ever appropriate before performing laparoscopy?

In patients with typical but less severe symptoms, a trial of oral contraceptive pills (OCPs) may be given. Pain relief with OCPs supports the diagnosis. But if symptoms are more severe, or patients do not respond to OCPs, laparoscopy may be performed prior to starting GnRH agonists or antagonists.

Case 10 A 27-year-old woman comes in complaining of chronic abdominal pain. He says the pain is steady, unrelated to meals, occasionally worse when he defecates, particularly if he is straining. His appetite is good, and he denies nausea or weight loss. On examination, his abdomen is soft, and bowel sounds are normal, but he has localized abdominal wall tenderness. When you ask him to tense his abdominal muscles and raise his head (while supine), the tenderness seems to worsen. Basic laboratories are all normal.

Is it possible to get chronic abdominal pain from the abdominal wall?

Yes, some patients develop chronic abdominal wall pain [22]. The Carnett maneuver, described above, is important in making the diagnosis [23]. In some cases, patients may have an anterior cutaneous nerve entrapment syndrome. We have tried lidocaine patches in a few, generally with limited success, but, in the patient with more severe pain, we will contact the anesthesiologists in the pain clinic to consider a local injection [24, 25]. For patients who don't respond to injection, abdominal wall neurectomies have been successful [26].

Another cause of abdominal wall pain is a Spigelian hernia, an uncommon hernia that may present with pain alone in some individuals. If we are considering this diagnosis, a good ultrasound can confirm it, and we will generally get an experienced surgeon to weigh in.

Case 11 A 57-year-old man presents with LLQ pain of 4-h duration. After evaluation in the ER, he is found to be afebrile but has mild leukocytosis of 14,000. Diverticulitis is suspected, but the CT scan reveals a round fat-attenuating structure with associated inflammation on the lateral wall of the rectosigmoid consistent with epiploic appendagitis.

Epiploic appendagitis is a self-limited entity that presents just like diverticulitis, but does not require antibiotics. In uncomplicated cases, it can be managed with NSAIDs. Rather than a mini-perforation of a diverticulum as we see in diverticulitis, this involves inflammation/ischemia of the appendages of the bowel mesentery. The presentation oftentimes is suggestive of diverticulitis or appendicitis but requires a CT scan for diagnosis. We emphasize the self-limiting nature and symptoms that average about 10 days. However, if conservative treatments fail and symptoms persist/worsen, rarely patients may need surgery [27, 28].

Case 12 A 27-year-old woman presents to the ER with the complaint of abdominal pain, nausea, and *vomiting and also pain and tingling in her hands and legs. She has had three other ER visits for abdominal pain and has had an EGD, CT scan x 2, and US, all of which were negative. She is having her menstrual period. On the examination, she seems agitated and mildly confused. Pulse is 115, and BP is 150/110. Her abdomen is moderately tender and distended with increased tympany and high-pitched bowel sounds. A KUB showed an ileus with no free air. Because of her altered mental status, a drug screen was sent off and returned negative for cocaine or other drugs. Because of her multiple ER visits with negative findings in the face of abdominal pain, now accompanied by symptoms suggesting CNS abnormality, a urine porphobilinogen (PBG) was sent off. Result is 12 mg/24 h (normal < 4 mg/24 h.).*

How would you manage this patient?

The finding of elevated urine PBG is specific for porphyria, and this patient's clinical course is consistent with porphyria [29]. Since she is symptomatic and her urine PBG is significantly elevated, treatment should be administered with IV hemin (Panhematin). While waiting for hemin to be made available, IV glucose loading should be initiated [30]. Hemin should be administered once daily for 4 days or longer.

For patients with repeated episodes of acute intermittent porphyria (AIP), there is a drug, givosiran, which interferes with the gene that is induced during an AIP attack, thereby preventing attacks or decreasing their intensity. This drug needs to be administered subcutaneously on a monthly basis.

Case 13 A 67-year-old man presents with a complaint of chronic abdominal pain gradually worsening over the past month. He has a past history of cholecystectomy when he was 30 years old and also required surgery for small bowel obstruction when he was 35 years old. On examination, there is mid-abdominal fullness and a possible mass. You order a CT scan that reveals a 5-cm mass in the mesentery and a fat ring sign. There is calcification within the mass and surrounding lymph nodes. The differential diagnosis is most likely sclerosing mesenteritis (or panniculitis), or less likely neoplasm.

How would you proceed?

Laparoscopy and tissue biopsy are required.

The surgical findings and biopsy are consistent with sclerosing mesenteritis.

How would you manage the patient?

Treatment for sclerosing mesenteritis involves a course of steroids and long-term therapy with tamoxifen. Tamoxifen acts as an anti-fibrotic agent. Prednisone is administered for 3 months and then, if there is symptomatic improvement, tapered over 3 months. Tamoxifen is continued indefinitely [31, 32].

Case 14 *A 36-year-old man presents for an office consultation with a history of recurrent episodes of abdominal pain and nausea. His past history includes migraine headaches. When you ask him whether the abdominal pain coincides with the migraine headaches, he says, "I think it does. I hadn't thought of that. I don't get abdominal pain with every migraine but, yes, when I get the pain, it is often shortly after the start of a migraine."*

He is feeling well when seen. His examination is unremarkable, and baseline laboratories are normal.

How do you make a diagnosis of abdominal migraine?

Patients usually have a history of migraine headaches. The abdominal pain may or may not coincide with the migraines. Episodes of pain are described as "paroxysmal," coming on suddenly and then often lasting for 15–20 min. Patients often have nausea and vomiting along with headaches that may accompany the pain. The abdominal pain is usually relieved with migraine medications. Meds used for prophylaxis of migraines may prevent episodes of abdominal pain [33]. There is no specific test to diagnose abdominal migraine. As with many of the other uncommon etiologies for abdominal pain, the diagnosis requires ruling out other organic causes for the GI symptoms. If abdominal migraine is suspected, a clinical trial of sumatriptan should be given. If the patient responds, but has repeated episodes of abdominal pain, medications used to prevent migraine headaches can be offered. Beta blockers, calcium channel blockers, valproic acid, and topiramate have all been used prophylactically.

Case 15 *A 55-year-old woman with rheumatoid arthritis (RA) presents to the ER with a 2-h history of excruciating abdominal pain. On examination, there is marked tenderness and rebound. Non-contrast CT scan reveals free air and inflammatory change around the stomach suggestive of perforated ulcer. The patient was on methotrexate for her RA and was taking naproxen on a regular basis over the past 3 months for increased joint pains. When questioned, she denied having chronic abdominal pain, although she experienced some mild nausea or "indigestion" for the past week. The patient is sent to surgery, and a perforated gastric ulcer is identified and oversewn.*

Isn't it extraordinary for a peptic ulcer to lead to perforation without warning signs of abdominal pain leading up to that?

There is a high frequency of peptic ulcers in patients with RA taking NSAIDs. In one study [34], 26% of patients taking naproxen for 3 months developed peptic ulcers. Only 7% had abdominal pain.

The finding of asymptomatic peptic ulcers is not limited to patients with rheumatologic disorders. In one Chinese study, largely asymptomatic patients were having EGDs to screen for gastric cancer [35]. In that study, 11% had peptic ulcer disease (PUD) and 2/3 of ulcer patients were asymptomatic. Current smoking and obesity were associated with increased incidence of asymptomatic ulcers. Smaller ulcers and healing ulcers were less likely to cause symptoms.

It is not unusual for peptic ulcers to first present with a complication. In about 25% of PUD patients, the first manifestation is perforation or bleeding. Of patients with bleeding ulcers, somewhere between 43% and 87% are asymptomatic.

It has been argued that NSAID use may increase the likelihood of asymptomatic PUD due to its analgesic effects. However, more recent studies show that most NSAID-associated gastric ulcers are symptomatic [36].

Age also factors in when determining the incidence of asymptomatic ulcers. Only 7% of patients under 50 years old were without abdominal pain, while 29% of patients over 60 were without pain [37].

Case 16 *A 70-year-old woman is brought into the ER by her daughter with a temp of 100 and new-onset confusion. She is on prednisone 5 mg daily for temporal arteritis. There was no prior history of abdominal pain. On examination, she has minimal tenderness in the epigastric area and RUQ. She has a WBC of 10,000 with 5% bands. An US suggests cholecystitis. A CT scan is ordered that suggests phlegmonous cholecystitis but is otherwise negative.*

Isn't it unusual to see a patient with cholecystitis presenting with altered mental status and minimal abdominal pain?

Older patients who present to the ER with abdominal pathology are generally more likely to present with advanced-stage disease. Elderly patients are more likely to have vague symptoms, nonspecific physical findings, and may lack laboratory abnormalities. Elderly patients with cholecystitis lacked the classic pain patterns in 84% and had no pain at all in 5%. They were more likely to have an absence of leukocytosis (41%) and fever (56%) and are much more likely to require surgery on presentation [38].

The most common finding in elderly patients presenting to the ER with acute abdominal pain was acute cholecystitis. In younger patients, the most common etiologies were nonspecific abdominal pain followed by appendicitis.

When elderly patients do present with appendicitis, they can have unusual presentations. Only 23% had fever, and many more elderly patients were found to have diffuse tenderness, distension, and rigidity because they waited longer before presenting to the ER [39, 40].

Another cause of intra-abdominal emergency in the elderly is an abdominal aortic aneurysm (AAA). Many significant AAAs may be asymptomatic and may not be diagnosed until there is rupture [41, 42]. Of course, in elderly patients presenting with abdominal pain, vascular insufficiency always has to be considered. The classic story is the elderly patient with severe pain that seems out of proportion with the physical findings [43].

Besides ischemic bowel, AAA, and cholecystitis, other causes of abdominal pain that are more common in the elderly include acute pancreatitis and diverticulitis. They are also more likely to have intra-abdominal cancer.

Another factor that may lead to decreased symptoms and physical findings in the elderly is the increased use of medications such as beta blockers and steroids that may mask normal alterations in vital signs.

References

1. Mwinyogle AA, Bhatt A, Ogbuagu OU, Dhillon N, Sill A, Kowdley GC. Use of CT scans for abdominal pain in the ED: factors in choice. Am Surg. 2020;86(4):324–33.
2. Kanzaria HK, Hoffman JR, Probst MA, Caloyeras JP, Berry SH, Brook RH. Emergency physician perceptions of medically unnecessary advanced diagnostic imaging. Acad Emerg Med. 2015;22(4):390–8.
3. de Burlet KJ, MacKay M, Larsen P, Dennett ER. Appropriateness of CT scans for patients with non-traumatic acute abdominal pain. Br J Radiol. 2018;91(1088):20180158.
4. Roberts LW, Dyer AR. Caring for "difficult" patients. Focus. 2003;1(4):453–8.
5. Drossman DA. David sun lecture: helping your patient by helping yourself—how to improve the patient–physician relationship by optimizing communication skills. Off J Am Coll Gastroenterol|ACG. 2013;108(4):521–8.
6. Drossman DA. Do psychosocial factors define symptom severity and patient status in irritable bowel syndrome? Am J Med. 1999;107(5):41–50.
7. Cai Q, Baumgarten DA, Affronti JP, Waring JP. Incidental findings of thickening luminal gastrointestinal organs on computed tomography: an absolute indication for endoscopy. Am J Gastroenterol. 2003;98(8):1734–7.
8. Sharma BC, Agarwal DK, Dhiman RK, Baijal SS, Choudhuri G, Saraswat VA. Bile lithogenicity and gallbladder emptying in patients with microlithiasis: effect of bile acid therapy. Gastroenterology. 1998;115(1):124–8.
9. Gudsoorkar VS, Oglat A, Jain A, Raza A, Quigley EM. Systematic review with meta-analysis: cholecystectomy for biliary dyskinesia—what can the gallbladder ejection fraction tell us? Aliment Pharmacol Ther. 2019;49(6):654–63.
10. Park CM, Chung JW, Kim HB, Shin SJ, Park JH. Celiac axis stenosis: incidence and etiologies in asymptomatic individuals. Korean J Radiol. 2001;2(1):8–13.
11. Ylinen P, Kinnunen J, Höckerstedt K. Superior mesenteric artery syndrome. A follow-up study of 16 operated patients. J Clin Gastroenterol. 1989;11(4):386–91.
12. Cohen LB, Field SP, Sachar DB. The superior mesenteric artery syndrome. The disease that isn't, or is it? J Clin Gastroenterol. 1985;7(2):113–6.
13. Reilly LM, Ammar AD, Stoney RJ, Ehrenfeld WK. Late results following operative repair for celiac artery compression syndrome. J Vasc Surg. 1985;2(1):79–91.
14. Skelly CL, Stiles-Shields C, Mak GZ, Speaker CR, Lorenz J, Anitescu M, Dickerson DM, Boyd H, O'Brien S, Drossos T. The impact of psychiatric comorbidities on patient-reported surgical outcomes in adults treated for the median arcuate ligament syndrome. J Vasc Surg. 2018;68(5):1414–21.
15. Keefer L, Drossman DA, Guthrie E, Simrén M, Tillisch K, Olden K, Whorwell PJ. Centrally mediated disorders of gastrointestinal pain. Gastroenterology. 2016;150(6):1408–19.
16. Mayer EA, Gebhart GF. Basic and clinical aspects of visceral hyperalgesia. Gastroenterology. 1994;107(1):271–93.
17. Drossman D, Szigethy E. The narcotic bowel syndrome: a recent update. Am J Gastroenterol Suppl. 2014;2(1):22–30.
18. Nguyen GC, Smalley WE, Vege SS, Carrasco-Labra A, Flamm SL, Gerson L, Hirano I, Rubenstein JH, Singh S, Stollman N, Sultan S. American Gastroenterological Association Institute guideline on the medical management of microscopic colitis. Gastroenterology. 2016;150(1):242–6.
19. Moayyedi PM, Lacy BE, Andrews CN, Enns RA, Howden CW, Vakil N. ACG and CAG clinical guideline: management of dyspepsia. Off J Am Coll Gastroenterol|ACG. 2017;112(7):988–1013.
20. Cotton PB, Pauls Q, Keith J, Thornhill A, Drossman D, Williams A, Durkalski-Mauldin V. The EPISOD study: long-term outcomes. Gastrointest Endosc. 2018;87(1):205–10.
21. Ballard KD, Seaman HE, De Vries CS, Wright JT. Can symptomatology help in the diagnosis of endometriosis? Findings from a national case–control study—part 1. BJOG Int J Obstet Gynaecol. 2008;115(11):1382–91.

22. Srinivasan R, Greenbaum DS. Chronic abdominal wall pain: a frequently overlooked problem: practical approach to diagnosis and management. Am J Gastroenterol. 2002;97(4):824–30.
23. Takada T, Ikusaka M, Ohira Y, Noda K, Tsukamoto T. Diagnostic usefulness of Carnett's test in psychogenic abdominal pain. Intern Med. 2011;50(3):213–7.
24. Alnahhas MF, Oxentenko SC, Locke GR, Hansel S, Schleck CD, Zinsmeister AR, Farrugia G, Grover M. Outcomes of ultrasound-guided trigger point injection for abdominal wall pain. Dig Dis Sci. 2016;61:572–7.
25. Boelens OB, Scheltinga MR, Houterman S, Roumen RM. Management of anterior cutaneous nerve entrapment syndrome in a cohort of 139 patients. Ann Surg. 2011;254(6):1054–8.
26. van Assen T, Brouns JA, Scheltinga MR, Roumen RM. Incidence of abdominal pain due to the anterior cutaneous nerve entrapment syndrome in an emergency department. Scand J Trauma Resusc Emerg Med. 2015;23(1):1–6.
27. Sand M, Gelos M, Bechara FG, Sand D, Wiese TH, Steinstraesser L, Mann B. Epiploic appendagitis–clinical characteristics of an uncommon surgical diagnosis. BMC Surg. 2007;7(1):1–7.
28. Akubudike JT, Egigba OF, Kobalava B. Epiploic appendagitis: a commonly overlooked differential of acute abdominal pain. Cureus. 2021;13(1):e12807.
29. Herrick AL, McColl KE. Acute intermittent porphyria. Best Pract Res Clin Gastroenterol. 2005;19(2):235–49.
30. Ortega AJ, Cherukuri S, Kalas MA, Lee B, Guzman J, Robles A, Zuckerman MJ, Al-Bayati I. A perfect storm: abdominal pain and ileus explained by acute intermittent porphyria caused by prehospitalization and intrahospitalization factors. J Investig Med High Impact Case Rep. 2022;10(2):3247096221109206.
31. Danford CJ, Lin SC, Wolf JL. Sclerosing mesenteritis. Off J Am Coll GastroenterolACG. 2019;114(6):867–73.
32. Anderson KE, Bloomer JR, Bonkovsky HL, Kushner JP, Pierach CA, Pimstone NR, Desnick RJ. Recommendations for the diagnosis and treatment of the acute porphyrias. Ann Intern Med. 2005;142(6):439–50.
33. Roberts JE, deShazo RD. Abdominal migraine, another cause of abdominal pain in adults. Am J Med. 2012;125(11):1135–9.
34. Hawkey CJ, Laine L, Simon T, Quan H, Shingo S, Evans J. Incidence of gastroduodenal ulcers in patients with rheumatoid arthritis after 12 weeks of rofecoxib, naproxen, or placebo: a multicentre, randomised, double blind study. Gut. 2003;52(6):820–6.
35. Lu CL, Chang SS, Wang SS, Chang FY, Lee SD. Silent peptic ulcer disease: frequency, factors leading to "silence," and implications regarding the pathogenesis of visceral symptoms. Gastrointest Endosc. 2004;60(1):34–8.
36. Kim HM, Cho JH, Choi JY, Chun SW, Kim YJ, Cho HG, Song SY, Han KJ. NSAID is inversely associated with asymptomatic gastric ulcer: local health examination data from the Korean National Health Insurance Corporation. Scand J Gastroenterol. 2013;48(12):1371–6.
37. Hilton D, Iman N, Burke GJ, Moore A, O'Mara G, Signorini D, Lyons D, Banerjee AK, Clinch D. Absence of abdominal pain in older persons with endoscopic ulcers: a prospective study. Am J Gastroenterol. 2001;96(2):380–4.
38. Parker LJ, Vukov LF, Wollan PC. Emergency department evaluation of geriatric patients with acute cholecystitis. Acad Emerg Med. 1997;4(1):51–5.
39. Elangovan S. Clinical and laboratory findings in acute appendicitis in the elderly. J Am Board Fam Pract. 1996;9(2):75–8.
40. Kraemer M, Franke C, Ohmann C, Yang Q, Acute Abdominal Pain Study Group. Acute appendicitis in late adulthood: incidence, presentation, and outcome. Results of a prospective multicenter acute abdominal pain study and a review of the literature. Langenbeck's. Arch Surg. 2000;385:470–81.
41. Fielding JW, Black J, Ashton F, Slaney G, Campbell DJ. Diagnosis and management of 528 abdominal aortic aneurysms. Br Med J (Clin Res Ed). 1981;283(6287):355–9.

42. Marston WA, Ahlquist R, Johnson G Jr, Meyer AA. Misdiagnosis of ruptured abdominal aortic aneurysms. J Vasc Surg. 1992;16(1):17–22.
43. Bala M, Kashuk J, Moore EE, Kluger Y, Biffl W, Gomes CA, Ben-Ishay O, Rubinstein C, Balogh ZJ, Civil I, Coccolini F. Acute mesenteric ischemia: guidelines of the world Society of Emergency Surgery. World J Emerg Surg. 2017;12(1):1–1.

Chapter 16
Vascular Disorders of the Intestine

Jim Nelson

Case 1: Acute Mesenteric Insufficiency (AMI) *A 64-year-old male smoker is recovering from a recent MI in a rehab center. One evening, he develops acute abdominal pain and is brought into the ER. There is moderate abdominal tenderness on the examination. WBC 15,000. Elevated lactate and D-dimer. Creatinine is 1.6. KUB reveals thumbprinting.*

There is a suspicion of intestinal ischemia here. There is mild renal insufficiency. Is a contrast CT required for diagnosis? Can an MRA be used instead?

That's one of the gray areas and really depends on how significant the renal insufficiency is. Generally speaking, a mild degree of chronic kidney disease is not a major contraindication to using CT in these circumstances. There are many reasons why a CTA is the preferred study. The sensitivity and specificity of a CTA are much better compared to an MRA [1]. In addition, CTAs don't take nearly as long to complete. So, if the patient has difficulty lying down for a long time, is in a significant amount of pain, or can't hold their breath for any period of time, it makes MRA much more difficult and less useful. In addition, the MRA often lacks some of the resolution that the CTA has in terms of documenting stenosis. The MRA may overestimate the degree of occlusion and may not visualize the IMA sufficiently, although the IMA isn't usually a clinically significant vessel in acute mesenteric ischemia. So, for all these reasons CTA is the preferred imaging study. In this case, a CTA is reasonably safe and appropriate to properly evaluate for AMI.

A CTA is performed that reveals an embolus in the SMA confirming the diagnosis of AMI.

J. Nelson (✉)
Department of Medicine, Division of Gastroenterology and Hepatology, Medical College of Wisconsin, Milwaukee, WI, USA
e-mail: jnelson@mcw.edu

© The Author(s), under exclusive license to Springer Nature Switzerland AG 2023
W. H. Sobin et al. (eds.), *Managing Complex Cases in Gastroenterology*,
https://doi.org/10.1007/978-3-031-48949-5_16

101

Is there a predilection for emboli to occlude the SMA?

Yes, there is a predilection for emboli to occlude the SMA, which relates to the anatomy of the SMA [2, 3]. Many, if not most of these cases of AMI, are embolic in etiology. The SMA, being a large caliber vessel, allows emboli to more easily pass into it. Also, compared to the 90-degree takeoff of the celiac artery, the takeoff of the SMA is a less acute angle. Emboli, therefore, generally bypass the celiac artery takeoff and pass into the SMA much more readily. So, for those reasons there is a predilection for emboli to occlude the SMA.

How long do you have in AMI before you need to intervene?

Several studies indicate that if there's 100% occlusion of the SMA, you have approximately 6 h before bowel infarction will occur. If you have a 75% occlusion, you have about 12 h before you would need to intervene before infarction occurs [3]. While this may seem like time is on your side when attempting to make a diagnosis of AMI, it's not and any delays increase mortality and can complicate surgery. Bottom line: "AMI is a medical emergency."

How would you manage this?

Any patient that has acute mesenteric ischemia, whether it's embolic or thrombotic, should receive systemic heparinization [1]. Therefore, the initial approach, when there is a concern for AMI, should be to immediately start full anticoagulation with IV heparin. They should be NPO and placed on broad-spectrum antibiotics to cover bacteremia secondary to bacterial translocation and the potential for sepsis. Definitive treatment is ultimately going to require revascularization, either radiologic or surgical.

When do you decide to use surgery as opposed to interventional radiology?

Decisions regarding revascularization require consultation with both vascular surgery along with interventional radiology [4]. If a patient is showing signs of peritonitis or advanced ischemic changes/infarction such as worsening abdominal pain, fever, or leukocytosis, surgical intervention is indicated. Otherwise, radiologic intervention, specifically embolectomy or angioplasty/stenting, is the preferred initial approach.

Do you know how useful the finding of thumbprinting on KUB is? Is it sensitive, specific?

It's not very sensitive and you don't see it very often, but when you do it usually indicates severe ischemia or infarction. Therefore, plain X-rays of the abdomen are generally not very helpful in the diagnosis or management of AMI.

The patient has a mesenteric angiogram and thrombectomy but afterward develops hypotension with a BP 90/60.

Is there any role for pressors in a hypotensive patient with mesenteric ischemia?

Yes, but with care. If you do decide that a patient needs pressor support, you should, in general, avoid alpha-adrenergic pressors, such as vasopressin, as they can cause vasoconstriction of the splanchnic arteries and worsen the ischemia. While low-dose vasopressin might be safe to use, more often dobutamine or dopamine are used since they don't cause vasoconstriction of the splanchnic arteries [2].

A follow-up X-ray shows jejunal distension with wall thickening, pneumatosis, and air in the portal vein.

How would you manage this?

These are worrisome signs of bowel infarction. The patient needs surgical intervention for possible resection of the infarcted bowel. A second look operation is many times done during the same hospitalization to evaluate and remove any remaining, non-viable bowel. Short bowel syndrome is an unfortunate outcome of large resections.

The patient goes to surgery and a section of necrotic small bowel of 100 cm is removed distal jejunum and proximal ileum.

Is this the most common etiology for short bowel syndrome?

Yes, the main cause of short bowel syndrome is surgical resection for ischemia. Crohn's disease is the second most common cause. Recurrent chronic obstruction from adhesive disease from prior surgeries is another etiology.

Following resection, the patient has a slow but consistent recovery.

Case 2: Mesenteric Vein Thrombosis (MVT) *A 73-year-old man with a history of metastatic renal cell carcinoma presents to the ER with a history of acute onset of mid-abdominal pain. There is moderate abdominal tenderness and decreased bowel sounds. Laboratories reveal leukocytosis and mild metabolic acidosis. A CT scan reveals thrombosis of the SMV and portal vein with edema and dilation of small bowel loops. The impression is that this patient has acute mesenteric vein thrombosis. A surgical consult is called, but the decision is made to treat with anticoagulation.*

Should you do a thrombophilia work-up in all of these patients?

Statistically, the majority of patients who develop mesenteric venous thrombosis have a primary hypercoagulable disorder as the cause. A smaller percentage have a malignancy causing a secondary hypercoagulable state. So, in this case, although he has a malignancy, it's not unreasonable to do a limited hypercoagulable work-up.

The patient is found to have factor V Leyden deficiency.

Is it sufficient to treat with anticoagulation? Is surgery ever indicated? If so, when?

Anticoagulation is the primary therapy [1]. If they don't improve or if the patient progresses to peritonitis and presumed infarction, surgery would be necessary.

Is there usually a different clinical presentation in acute SMV thrombosis vs acute SMA thrombosis?

SMV thrombosis is more common in males, while SMA thrombosis is more common in females. Many patients with SMV thrombosis have a history compatible with or have a diagnosis of chronic mesenteric ischemia. They often have a history of postprandial abdominal pain and weight loss.

In comparison with SMA thrombosis which presents acutely, patients with SMV thrombosis have a more insidious course with chronic or subacute symptoms. SMA thrombosis tends to present with more acute, severe pain, while SMV thrombosis typically presents with a dull pain that develops over days to weeks.

Which veins tend to be involved in acute MVT? How does this lead to organ damage, does gangrene occur?

Most of the time it's the SMV, which leads to damage of the distal small bowel [2]. Rarely is it the IMV. The pathophysiology is like any form of venous outflow obstruction. The bowel wall gets edematous causing increased intramural pressure resulting in a reduction in arterial flow through the bowel wall. If the reduction in submucosal arterial blood flow is severe, bowel infarction can occur.

How successful is anticoagulation?

Very successful. Anticoagulation almost eliminates in-hospital mortality in these patients. Overall mortality is less than 5% in patients who have been treated quickly and adequately anticoagulated. Most of these patients will need to remain on long-term anticoagulation since their thrombotic risk continues indefinitely.

Case 3: Chronic Mesenteric Ischemia A 75-year-old man presents with a 1-month history of abdominal pain and weight loss. The pain is periumbilical and tends to occur about a half hour after meals. The patient also experiences mild nausea after meals. To prevent nausea and abdominal pain, he has been avoiding eating and lost 15 lbs. over the past month. The abdominal examination is benign without a bruit. The CBC, chem panel, and liver enzymes are all normal. EGD is negative. US abdomen is normal. CT abdomen and pelvis reveal a normal-appearing pancreas, but there is extensive atherosclerosis of the mesenteric vessels. There is no suggestion of acute ischemia. Bowel loops appear normal. Because of these findings in the setting of abdominal pain and weight loss, the diagnosis of possible CMI is raised.

Is there any way to make a clear-cut positive diagnosis of CMI or do you have to exclude other causes first and then chronic ischemia becomes a diagnosis of exclusion if the CTA or angio are consistent?

In most cases, it's hard to come to a definite diagnosis of CMI. Only a small percentage of patients have the classic clinical trial of abdominal pain, weight loss, and abdominal bruit. In general, you first want to rule out other potential causes of postprandial pain, like biliary tract disease, that can mimic the same clinical presentation as CMI. Once other causes of postprandial abdominal pain and weight loss have been excluded, and a CTA shows significant stenosis in at least 2 of the 3 mesenteric arteries, then there is a high likelihood of CMI.

What percentage of patients in this age range will have vascular abnormalities simulating CMI, and yet be asymptomatic?

About 60% of older patients have radiologic findings of mesenteric vascular disease in one or two vessels but are asymptomatic. Another 15–20% will have atherosclerotic disease in all three vessels and are asymptomatic.

What is the role, if any, of duplex Doppler?

I think a lot of people would gravitate to this test first to screen for CMI but a CTA should be done to confirm the diagnosis. Duplex Doppler is more of a physiologic test that is highly sensitive and specific at detecting abnormally high mesenteric arterial velocities suggesting CMI [1]. A peak systolic velocity > 275 cm/sec in the SMA suggests significant stenosis [2].

If you've convinced yourself this is CMI, how do you manage it?

The first approach usually involves radiologic revascularization, specifically angioplasty and stenting.

The patient is evaluated by IR and surgery, and the decision is made to perform endovascular revascularization. Following this, the patient's pain resolves and he gains back the weight lost over the next 2 months.

Case 4: Nonocclusive Mesenteric Ischemia (NOMI) *A 72-year-old man with a history of CHF and the recent diagnosis of chronic cholecystitis is scheduled to have an elective cholecystectomy. When presenting to the pre-op area of the hospital, he was noted to be hypotensive BP-90/50. IV fluids were started, but the patient started complaining of increased pain across his abdomen, different from his usual gallbladder pain. An urgent CT was performed, which revealed small bowel edema with probable pneumatosis. There were scattered plaques in the abdominal aorta and mesenteric vasculature but no occlusive disease. There was also a spasm of the arterial cascade emanating from the SMA. Because there was concern for bowel ischemia, urgent laparoscopy was performed. A section of dusky appearing distal jejunum was identified and resected. Adequate pulsations to the rest of the bowel were ascertained. There was no evidence of thrombosis or embolism to any blood vessels. The post-op impression was nonocclusive mesenteric ischemia.*

What are the risk factors for NOMI? Which patients are most at risk?

This patient was hypotensive on presentation possibly due to evolving sepsis from cholecystitis. Most often these are critically ill patients in ICUs who have some form of hemodynamic instability [3], whether it's septic shock, hemorrhagic shock, or cardiogenic shock [2, 4]. Be alert to a critically ill ICU patient with hypotension who develops abdominal pain, distension, or signs of a GI bleed as NOMI would be a concern.

Was surgery mandatory? Can you make a case for pre-op vasodilators?

Yes, especially with the finding of possible pneumatosis on CT. Other findings concerning severe bowel ischemia are fever, leukocytosis, and an elevated lactate level. If NOMI is suspected, vasodilator treatment should be promptly initiated [4]. Vasodilators, like PGE1 or papaverine, infused directly into the SMA or IV are options. Equally important and what is still primary therapy is treating the underlying cause of the hemodynamic instability.

Could the diagnosis be ascertained by CTA alone with confidence?

Yes, the classic finding is the irregularity of the vascular arcade suggesting spasm [3]. There may also be hypo-enhancement of the intestinal wall. Many of these patients also have some degree of atherosclerotic narrowing of their SMA without occlusion. The degree of narrowing, however, is generally not sufficient to explain the severity of ischemia and symptoms.

Case 5: Colon Ischemia (CI) *A 65-year-old man presents to the ER with a history of rectal bleeding. He has no past history of cardiovascular disease, hypertension, etc. He does have occasional constipation. His last screening colonoscopy 2 years earlier was negative except for mild diverticulosis.*

He is on no meds. He was fine until that afternoon when he felt a sudden weakness, sweating, and nausea causing him to sit down and compose himself. Shortly after the episode, he developed abdominal cramping, following which he had two or three bowel movements that were loose and mixed with blood. In the ER, he was normotensive, his HR was 90 and regular, and he was afebrile. On the abdominal examination, there was minimal abdominal tenderness and no rebound, and bowel sounds were normal without a bruit. His laboratories showed a Hgb of 12 and a

WBC of 13,000. There was no metabolic acidosis, but a CRP was 30. A CT scan was obtained and showed colitis involving the splenic flexure. CI is suspected. Overall, the patient appears quite stable.

How would you manage this patient, other than starting IV fluids? Would you start antibiotics? Would you do a colonoscopy?

In general, you don't need to start antibiotics if the patient appears stable and doesn't have any worrisome clinical findings, such as a high white count, fever, significant abdominal tenderness, or more evidence of significant damage on CT. Current ACG guidelines indicate you should consider starting antibiotics in patients with moderate or severe disease, which is based primarily on colonoscopy findings. Findings of severe CI include deep ulcerations and cyanosis of the mucosa. If these abnormalities are found on colonoscopy, then antibiotics should be started.

The vast majority of these patients have mild disease and do well with supportive care alone. As to whether you perform a colonoscopy on a patient that has suggestive findings such as segmental colitis in the watershed regions on CT depends on whether there are concerns for other causes of segmental colitis such as Crohn's disease. A colonoscopy can be helpful in differentiating between CI and other causes. A finding that is pathognomonic for CI [5] is longitudinal ulcerations, the so-called stripe sign, which extend down the long axis of the colon. It's generally safe to do a colonoscopy as long as you don't advance the scope past the area of injury.

Colonoscopy is performed to the splenic flexure where there is a region of typical ischemic colitis noted with longitudinal ulcers, dusky mucosa, and bluish blebs. Because these findings are consistent with severe CI, the patient was started on IV antibiotics.

CI seems to occur in a number of patients who have no risk factors. Comments?

Because most cases of CI occur in the 60–80-year age group, they often have undiagnosed atherosclerotic mesenteric vascular disease, especially if they have other risk factors such as a history of hypercholerolemia, hypertension, coronary artery disease, or peripheral vascular disease.

Another risk factor is constipation which the patient reported. Yes, based on several studies, constipation is a risk factor for ischemic colitis [5, 6]. The reason that constipation is a risk factor, along with other causes of bowel distension such as colonoscopy [7] or prepping for a colonoscopy, is that distension can lead to compression of submucosal vessels resulting in ischemia.

There are some medicines that have been associated with precipitating ischemic colitis [5, 2] including nasal decongestants, methamphetamines, digoxin, cocaine, Tamiflu, rizatriptan, diuretics, alosetron, estrogens, and clozapine.

Some patients have microvascular thrombotic disease or a previously undiagnosed hypercoagulable state, but still most patients with CI have small or large vessel atherosclerotic vascular disease.

The patient's clinical course is unremarkable and he goes home after a few days' hospitalization.

The outcome in most of these CI cases is almost uniformly excellent in my experience. Has that been your experience as well?

Yes, usually it takes longer for patients with more severe damage to improve, often several days, as in the example case, but the majority who have mild disease improve in 2–3 days.

Do you do any follow-up colonoscopy?

No, not routinely. If there is a concern, for instance, for a neoplasm based on a history of constipation or IBD, then a follow-up colonoscopy would be appropriate.

It seems to me that a number of these patients present with nausea or weakness prior to developing abdominal pain, diarrhea, or rectal bleeding, just like this patient. Any comments?

It may be due to a vagal response to some degree of pain or they're simply not eating or drinking enough fluids due to a mild ileus that potentially may develop preceding the ischemic event.

Case 6: Median Arcuate Ligament Syndrome (MALS) A 53-year-old woman with a history of epigastric pain and postprandial nausea and early satiety presents with 20 lb. weight loss. There is no history of smoking or cardiovascular risk factors. She is placed on a PPI without relief. She has an EGD that is normal and a gastric emptying scan that reveals mild delay. A gastroparesis diet does not help much. A CT scan is negative except for mild small bowel dilation that is no longer present on CTE. She visits the ED after an episode of more severe pain where she is found to have mild abdominal tenderness, an abdominal bruit, slightly elevated lipase and lactate. A CT scan is ordered and suggests MALS.

Is MALS a real entity? Do some of these patients have functional symptoms, and do they really require surgery?

The European Society of Vascular Surgery guidelines consider this to be one of the most common causes of mesenteric ischemia that is not associated with atherosclerosis or thrombosis. In other words, they consider it a real entity.

One of my patients who had surgery for MALS did well for about a year, but then started having recurrent abdominal pain likely due to untreated depression. I realize now that part of her disease process was probably untreated depression. There are studies showing that patients who have untreated psychiatric problems frequently have poorer outcomes after surgical treatment of MALS [8]. While this was a mixed result for my patient, MALS surgery should still be considered after a thorough evaluation ruling out other causes and first treating associated conditions such as depression.

How does duplex Doppler US help you?

A duplex Doppler US has good sensitivity (80%) and even better specificity (95%) when used to screen for MALS. There are specific velocity patterns that are seen in MALS including a change in pulse velocity with respiration. A dynamic MRA or preoperative angiography is also sometimes done to see if there is compression of the celiac artery during the respiratory cycle.

Why are you interested in a dynamic MRA? Why is there a change during the respiratory cycle?

A hallmark of MALS is expiratory compression of the celiac artery by the ligament of the diaphragm crux with an increase in flow velocity that can be found on Doppler US. Most of the time it is related to an anatomic variation in the location of takeoff of the celiac artery that is higher than normal.

How would you manage this patient?

I would refer the patient to a vascular surgeon who has experience treating patients with MALS.

Pre-op angiogram shows narrowing of the celiac with expiration. Surgery is performed, releasing the ligament and decreasing vascular resistance. The patient remains asymptomatic 1 year after surgery.

References

1. Clair DC, Beach JM. Mesenteric Ischemia. N Engl J Med. 2016;374:959–68.
2. Ahmed M. Ischemic bowel disease in 2021. World J Gastroenterol. 2021;27(29):4746–62.
3. Gnanapandthan K, Feuerstadt P. Review article: mesenteric ischemia. Curr Gastroenterol Rep. 2020;22:17.
4. Blaser AR, et al. A clinical approach to acute mesenteric ischemia. Curr Opin Crit Care. 2021;27:183–92.
5. YuShuang X, et al. Diagnostic methods and drug therapies in patients with ischemic colitis. Int J Color Dis. 2020;36:47–56.
6. Fitzgerald JF, Hernandez LO III. Ischemic colitis. Clin Colon Rectal Surg. 2015;28:93–8.
7. Sadalla S, et al. Colonoscopy-related colonic ischemia. World J Gastroenterol. 2021;27(42):7299–310.
8. Goodall R, et al. Median arcuate ligament syndrome. J Vasc Surg. 2020;70:2170–6.

Chapter 17
Polypectomy

Zachary Smith and Matt Mohorek

Cold vs. Hot Snare for Flat Polyps

Case 1 *A 52-year-old male comes in for his first screening colonoscopy and is found to have a 1.2-cm flat polyp in the sigmoid colon.*

How do you decide whether to use cold snare polypectomy or hot snare?

I will start by saying that I frequently favor cold snare over hot snare polypectomy, but anyone doing a polypectomy should evaluate three things. The first is the anatomic location of the polyp, the second is the polyp morphology, and the third is whether to do en bloc vs. piecemeal resection.

In this case, most gastroenterologists would resect the polyp en bloc using hot snare polypectomy. While hot snare polypectomy is more likely to lead to delayed bleeding, in this case, we're dealing with a polyp in the left colon and we know that polyps in the left colon are less likely to have delayed bleeding compared to polyps in the right colon [1]. The second thing is that if you take a 12-mm polyp out with a cold snare, the chance of complete en bloc resection is far less compared to taking that polyp out with a hot snare. So, for those reasons hot snare polypectomy may be favorable in this situation.

Unfortunately, we don't have good data to evaluate polyp recurrence rates in comparing cold snare piecemeal polypectomy with hot snare en bloc polypectomy. Now intuitively, one would think that en bloc resection is going to have less of a

Z. Smith (✉)
Division of GI and Hepatology, Department of Medicine, Medical College of Wisconsin, Milwaukee, WI, USA
e-mail: zsmith@mcw.edu

M. Mohorek
Department of Gastroenterology, GI Associates, Wauwatosa, WI, USA
e-mail: matthewm@wigia.com

chance of recurrence compared to piecemeal and hot is going to have less chance of recurrence compared to cold. Per the guidelines, if you have a single 10 mm + adenoma removed en bloc, that's a 3-year interval for repeat colonoscopy, whereas if you take it piecemeal, you might feel less comfortable waiting 3 years.

So, there are a lot of things to consider in this case, but I think, putting together all of the available data, hot snare polypectomy is still probably the preferred modality in this case.

Let's say you are referred a patient with a large, laterally spreading granular tumor. You favor cold snare polypectomies. Do you have a size limit beyond which you will not use cold snare?

No, I do most of my EMRs cold and I have taken out polyps that occupy >50% of the circumference of the right colon cold. What cold snare EMR has done is that it has changed the conversation and allowed us to have very safe options for removing large polyps in high-risk patients. We are frequently referred patients who were scoped by community gastroenterologists after being found to be anemic, and large polyps were discovered. Some of them are in their eighties, on Eliquis, and they're poor surgical candidates. The referring doctor is uncertain how to manage the situation. Whereas previously I might have been reluctant to offer one of these high-risk patients conventional (hot snare) EMR due to the inherent risk of delayed bleeding, etc., I am now much more willing to proceed, using cold snare EMR. It expands the patient pool where we are able to offer therapy with polypectomy while maintaining a risk/benefit ratio that is still favorable. After all, it's hard to assess whether a 7 cm laterally spreading granular tumor without high-grade dysplasia will turn into colon cancer during a patient's lifetime. It's much more satisfying if we can safely remove the polyp.

With hot snare EMR it is advised to ablate the margins of the resection site. Do you ablate the margins when you do a cold snare polypectomy?

No, I don't. The technique is still in its infancy where we don't have a lot of data on the optimal way to do things. Conventional, hot EMR has been around for decades, and we just found out in 2019 that ablating the edge of the polyp is a good way to minimize recurrence [2]. I don't know if we are going to have cold EMR ablation data for quite a while so my practice personally is to do more of a wide-field resection where you are taking several millimeters on the circumference of normal-looking mucosa.

When you are doing this, you are thinking of a couple of things. First, the safety profile of cold EMR is favorable, but it is also much more cost-effective. We were able to show this in a cost-effectiveness study published in *Endoscopy [3]*. The main determinant of cost-effectiveness for cold EMR is the lack of need for prophylactic clipping. On the sensitivity analysis, when you are looking at various factors determining cost-effectiveness, including the cost of clips, cost related to polyp recurrence, and cost related to complications such as bleeding or perforation, it turns out that the number one determinant of cost-effectiveness is the cost of clips and the reason is that Medicare and most commercial insurances don't reimburse the cost of endoscopic clips. So, if you take out a 6-cm polyp and you use 8 clips and each clip is $200, that is a significant cost to the patient.

Therefore, consistent with this, when I perform a large polyp EMR cold, I try to keep my device usage as low as possible. If you are going to ablate the edges of a polyp that would require opening up some other device, either a hot snare (using the tip for ablation) or an APC catheter. Until we have evidence that it helps tremendously, it is not my practice to ablate the edges when using cold EMR technique.

Can you discuss the different types of snares on the market and the advantages and disadvantages of each type?

There are a host of snare sizes, shapes, and designs. One can get very overwhelmed with the available options. My suggestion is to get comfortable with at most five and know how to use those. There are a lot of snare options, such as duck-billed snares and rotatable snares, and in my opinion, a lot of this is overly nuanced and not clinically useful. So, I think that if you have a cold snare that you are comfortable with, and a couple of hot snares of various sizes, you can do most anything. Certainly, be willing to try new snares, but folks are going to be most successful by knowing their own arsenal and what they are most comfortable with.

Now, for cold snares specifically, there are a handful of dedicated cold snares out on the market. Boston Scientific and STERIS are probably the two most well-known. Boston makes the Captivator cold, which is a 10-mm oval snare. Steris makes the Exacto, which is a 9-mm hexagonal snare. Both of these function similarly. There are some other companies that have dedicated cold snares with various shapes and sizes. Diversatek has both a 10-mm and 15-mm cold snare that is rotatable.

What you want with a cold snare is something that is going to capture tissue and cut reliably. Without the use of diathermy, you need to rely on the mechanical force of the snare to get through tissue. There are some technical nuances to that as well, but what you don't want to do is use a snare designed for hot polypectomy for cold snare EMR. The manufacturers of hot snares don't put a premium on using mechanical force to cut through the polyp without heat, and so it is going to be much more challenging to do cold EMR with those devices.

Anticoagulation After Polypectomy

Case 2 *A 65-year-old woman who is on apixaban for atrial fibrillation (held for 2 days prior to colonoscopy) is found to have a 1.5-cm sessile polyp in the right colon.*

Would you prefer to use cold snare or hot snare to remove this, why?

Personally, if anybody is on an antithrombotic, I am using a cold snare. Post-polypectomy and post-EMR bleeding can be morbid, and over 50% of the time, it will require a second colonoscopy, so there is a significant cost associated with that complication. Back in the days when I was doing more frequent conventional EMR, I would instruct patients to avoid traveling for 2 weeks because if they are going to have a delayed bleed, they need to be where good health care is accessible. We're seeing very low bleeding rates with cold EMR, the delayed bleeding risk is negligible. Therefore, I almost always place the patient back on their antithrombotic agent on post-procedure day 1, unless there is an extenuating circumstance, I have never had a delayed bleed and am well over 200 cold EMRs currently. The impetus for delayed bleeding is diathermy-induced ulcers, and with cold, we just don't have that.

After resection would you routinely place clips to close the polypectomy site?

Cold EMR does not require clips. I think that this is a tough pill for people to swallow sometimes. You take a big polyp out from the right colon and then leave it unclipped, which can be a little unnerving for people. I think in all of the cold EMRs I have done, I have placed two clips total and they were for vessels that were persistently bleeding. The bottom line is that the observational data available suggest that clips are not needed with cold EMR [4, 5].

Now for hot EMR the clinical trial data obviously suggest otherwise. The most robust data for this are from LPS, a study published in Gastro in 2019 where they randomized polyps larger than 2 cm to clips vs. no clips following hot EMR [1]. In patients who had right-sided polyps proximal to the splenic flexure, the bleeding risk in the clip arm was reduced by about two-thirds from 9% to 3%. The caveat to this is that not every defect can be closed completely. In the LPS trial, only about two-thirds of defects were able to be closed with clips, either because they were too big, or in a difficult location. So, current evidence tells us that if you take out a large polyp in the right colon using hot EMR you should attempt to close the defect with clips.

How long would you hold apixaban afterward?

My anecdotal evidence suggests that if the polyp was removed with cold EMR, anticoagulation can be restarted on day one after polypectomy. Every once in a while, I will wait a little bit longer if I have a gut feeling that a patient is at low risk for a cardio-embolic event but higher risk for bleeding. I may wait an extra day, but otherwise I will restart the next day.

Would any of the above three answers differ if the patient was on clopidogrel instead of apixaban?

Not based on my experience. Remember, most people on antiplatelet therapy are receiving it for prophylaxis of cardiovascular stent thrombosis or stroke prophylaxis. Major cardiovascular and cerebrovascular events are a larger threat to these patients' lives, and therefore, the importance of promptly restarting anticoagulation far outweighs the risk of having a delayed bleed from cold EMR. So, I would absolutely resume these medications on day one.

Do you hold anticoagulation or antiplatelet agents prior to an elective screening colonoscopy?

I do, and the reason is that you never know what you are going to find. Personally, I don't do a lot of screening colonoscopies, but because I do EMR and I am comfortable doing higher-risk endoscopic maneuvers on an index colonoscopy, I want the patient to be prepared for possible EMR. For example, if I find a 5-cm polyp on a screening colonoscopy I would remove it right there rather than bringing the patient back. With that being said, there are data from the Annals of Internal Medicine that looked at cold snare vs. hot snare in patients on antiplatelet therapy and cold snare was significantly safer. So, we can do cold snare polypectomy on anticoagulation/antiplatelet agents, and I would not hesitate to do that if the need arose, but generally, we don't find many situations where a patient is too sick to hold anticoagulation/antiplatelet therapy for an appropriate length of time but is still appropriate for screening colonoscopy. Having said that, if I'm called in to assist on a case where I encounter an 8 mm sessile polyp in a patient on anticoagulation I would have no hesitation to remove it with a cold snare.

EMR

Case 3 *A 68-year-old man comes in for his first screening colonoscopy with his community gastroenterologist and is found to have a 3-cm flat adenomatous appearing polyp in the transverse colon.*

If a gastroenterologist in the community finds a large flat polyp on an index colonoscopy, should he generally remove it then, or come out and discuss it with the patient after the procedure and set it up for another day? Or, for that matter, should he refer it to someone who specializes in EMR?

This entirely revolves around the skill set of the endoscopist. This is a recurring theme and something that I am very passionate about. For me personally, as someone who is a high-volume EMR provider and comfortable with techniques that minimize the risk profile of EMR, I would have no hesitation taking this out at the time of the index procedure. That being said, there are some medical-legal things to consider. For example, if you are very cursory with your consent process and you have not specifically talked about high-risk interventions, it is very justifiable to bring the patient back.

However, the thing that I can't stress enough is that if someone finds a large polyp on colonoscopy and they don't do a lot of EMR, the last thing you want to do is to start taking out the polyp and not finish the job. Doing an incomplete polypectomy causes a lot of submucosal fibrosis, which makes any attempt at salvage resection markedly more challenging. So, if you start resecting and then determine the polyp is in a difficult spot, or it's bigger than you thought it was, or it starts bleeding and you decide to just stop, and refer it out, or attempt it another day, realize that you're jeopardizing the success of the polyp resection. A good way to increase the chance of a patient needing surgery for a benign polyp is to do an incomplete EMR before referring the patient to an expert center. So, if you look at the polyp and you can't tell yourself with 100% certainty that you can remove it, then you should not attempt it. So, for your standard community practice general GI doc who sees a gambit of GI pathology and is not a high-volume EMR person I would not resect this for the reasons I have mentioned above.

Do you feel like there is any role for EMR in an ambulatory endoscopy center not attached to a hospital?

The reason not to do an EMR in an ASC, everything else being equal, is lack of resources in case something goes wrong. If I run into trouble at an ASC, an emergency surgery consultation is just not available. Part of the reason that the rate of surgery for benign polyps continues to rise (at least through 2014 according to observational data) is that a lot of people are averse to using EMR technique, but if people can get more comfortable with cold EMR technique, understand the technique, understand that it is adequate, and fully grasp that the risk profile is markedly reduced, I think many more of these polyps will be removed by gastroenterologists, rather than being referred to surgeons. I think that doing a cold EMR at an ASC becomes much more justifiable because the likelihood of a complication, where you need an emergency surgery consultation, is so negligible. Having an immediate perforation from a cold EMR is a reportable case event, and the ones that have been reported are near surgical anastomoses or in patients who have some sort of predisposition. In a patient who has a native colon, no inflammatory bowel disease, or other risk factors, the chance of a perforation on a cold EMR is basically zero. So, I think that it is completely justifiable to use cold EMR techniques at an ASC.

What do you like to use to inject to lift polyps? Will you ever use saline for lifting?

Typically, I do still lift polyps and will use one of the commercially available viscous solutions. However, emerging observational data from Michael Bourke's group and others suggest that lifting for large cold resections may not be necessary [5, 6]. However, I think the verdict is still out on that. LPS-2, which we are involved in, is a 2×2 randomized trial comparing hot and cold EMR as well as commercially available viscous injectate vs. saline and methylene blue. So, there should be some comparative data on solutions from this trial. A lot of the data on injection solutions have looked at durability of lift, completeness of resection, resection time, and polyp recurrence, so establishing meaningful endpoints is important. Sometimes these solutions can be cost-prohibitive for smaller centers. In those circumstances, saline or hydroxyethyl starch and methylene blue is an appropriate alternative. For me personally, with EMR, unless I am doing an underwater EMR technique, I am still injecting a submucosal agent.

This is your partner's case and he is doing a submucosal injection and is finding that this relatively flat polyp is flattening out further with the injection making it difficult to get a snare around the polyp and calls you in for advice.

How do you avoid this problem with your injection?

One benefit of the commercially available injectates is that for the most part they don't tend to spread laterally as much as saline does. With that said, flatness of injection can happen for a couple of reasons. First, it can be a technique problem and there are ways to potentially combat this. They include:

Inject Slowly. If the injectate seems to be spreading laterally and not lifting, stop and consider re-inserting the needle in a different place.

Direct the tip of the colonoscope upward to create tension away from the colon wall while injecting.

If using saline and not using a viscous solution (commercial or otherwise), consider changing.

Second, there are other situations, like ulcerative colitis, where you might get lateral spread of the injectate. Even if these patients have quiescent colitis, they have had some submucosal fibrosis over time and this interferes with lifting.

There are some endoscopic techniques to try to get the snare to capture, even when the polyp remains flat and doesn't lift. Some of those are more advanced techniques that I do not recommend unless one is trained. One example is to do a mucosal incision as if you were doing an endoscopic submucosal dissection around the polyp and then create a little notch around the mucosa where the snare is able to latch on and grab the tissue. This is commonly referred to as precut EMR.

Sometimes, just changing your snare to a thinner wire snare is enough to combat this problem. Sometimes approaching the polyp from a different angle will help.

Is there anything to do once flattening has occurred?

Mucosal incision is one suggestion. Another suggestion is to convert to an underwater technique. Here, you take air out of the colon and then you immerse the colon with water using your pedal. Water immersion has a buoyant effect on the submucosa. This was first described by Ken Binmoeller in San Francisco when he was doing endoscopic ultrasound. He noticed that when water was instilled while looking at submucosal lesions, there was expansion of the submucosa and he parlayed that into the world of endoscopic resection. Underwater EMR gives you a lot of benefits, it allows you to work in a collapsed space, and tissue is much easier to grab in a collapsed space. It allows you to work very close to a polyp, giving you a magnified view of everything. So, in this situation I would probably quickly convert to an underwater technique.

Do you always inject into the polyp? Do you ever inject just adjacent to it?

It depends on the size and location of the polyp. I will inject into the polyp if it is 2 cm. or less, especially with sessile serrated polyps, just to get one uniform injection. If it's a big polyp or in a saddle distribution (meaning over a fold), I will typically start by injecting on the oral side of the polyp and then work toward the anal side. I won't try to inject a whole 5 cm polyp at once, I will inject the part that I am going to cut out first and then I will re-inject and take the rest of the polyp. This seems to keep things plump when you are doing the cutting and doesn't allow injectate to diffuse out while you are working on the other side of the polyp.

What is your technique for removing large polyps using a cold snare technique?

The most important things are the same regardless of cold vs. hot technique. You want the scope to be straight, reduced, and have the polyp at the 5:00 to 7:00 region. I always lock my wheels. I want scope stability as much as possible.

The main difference is that cold snares are smaller and so typically you are taking less tissue out per bite. When I am teaching people, I compare it to mowing your lawn. You start on the edge near your sidewalk and you are then going to have some overlap every time you go back and forth. So, you put your snare down, you make a cut, it doesn't matter how big your first cut is, and then your second cut is going to lay on the edge of the resection defect of your first cut and is going to grab mucosa.

So, if you are working left to right, the left side of the snare is going to sit in the submucosa where you made your first cut, the right is going to scoop tissue on the right, you are going to bring it together, and move down the line. When the back side is done from left to right you move a little toward the anal side and overlap a little with the resected zone on the oral side and repeat the process until you are done.

When you remove bigger polyps, you are going to see some lumps and bumps of adenoma that don't come up with the cold snare and you can go back and take those with snare or avulsion techniques. For the most part, it is a systematic process and it goes a lot faster than people think it will.

When you're removing a large flat polyp in the cecum would you manage it differently to avoid complications?

Probably not. While cecal polyps can hide in funny places, like behind the ileo-cecal valve or juxtaposed to the appendiceal orifice, making things more challenging, for the most part my technique is going to remain the same whether the polyp is located in the cecum, ascending colon, or transverse colon.

What are the polyps that you will send to the surgeon?

Usually, surgeons send me polyps. It is common for patients to be referred to surgery for "unresectable" polyps by general community gastroenterologists. We now know that surgery is associated with higher morbidity and mortality, higher rates of procedure intervention, higher cost, and longer hospital stays than endoscopic resection. For the vast majority of people, surgery is not the best option.

Some gastroenterologists don't understand the full implications of surgical intervention required to address the lesions detected. Take for example a case where two large "unresectable" polyps are detected in the ascending colon and splenic flexure. What they need to think about is that the surgery that is required to address this would require a subtotal colectomy and that has a major impact on the patient's quality of life. There are data from Stanford and Australia that both suggest that in patients who are referred to surgery for large, "unresectable" polyps, referral to an expert endoscopist or a high-volume EMR center can avoid surgery 90% of the time.

Having said that, there are a few instances where I will send the patient to a surgeon. The first is recalcitrant polyps. What I mean by this is if we remove a large polyp and bring the patient back 6 months later to take another look there is a significant recurrence of polyp. We then resect the polyp regrowth. Then, on follow-up, 6-12 months later there's significant recurrence and you realize that you are not able to completely resect it. These situations are more common in patients who have significant fibrosis, either because they had a previous, limited EMR attempt prior to seeing me, or they have some other condition that predisposes them to submucosal fibrosis like ulcerative colitis.

The second instance is when I am referred to a polyp that is presumed to be benign but it turns out there is invasive cancer on the resection specimen. Occasionally, this is apparent on initial inspection using careful optical observation with electronic chromoendoscopy, near-focus imaging, and you see clear evidence of deep submucosal invasion. You do targeted biopsies, it proves cancer. Those patients go to surgery, or, the polyp may look benign, but once you start taking it out, it becomes obvious that there is cancer by the way it is behaving. Either it's not lifting well, there is a lot of tissue that is matted to the submucosa, or it is bleeding more than you would expect. All of those are indicators that there is invasive cancer. In those circumstances, they go to surgery as well.

Most of the time, if I am referred to a polyp that has not been intervened on, I am successful in removing the polyp and keeping the patient out of the operating room. It is usually these few extenuating circumstances that could lead to an operation. The vast majority of time, if someone else doesn't partially remove the polyp we are usually able to durably resect and cure those lesions.

What are the endoscopic features that most strongly suggest deep submucosal invasion?

I would encourage people to become familiar with a pit pattern classification such as Kudo. I think the simplest one for me is the NICE classification. It is a narrow-band classification validated on the Olympus platform. It is a way to distinguish hyperplastic and serrated lesions from traditional adenomas and from submucosal invasive cancer. It is a very simple classification, and I think you just have to look very carefully. If you are using a 190-series adult scope, do near-focus imaging. Sometimes, imaging something underwater is another way to get a nice perspective of the pit pattern.

I do very careful optical examination before I remove a polyp, because if there is submucosal cancer my approach is very different. Another important finding on the optical examination is surface ulceration. The finding of surface ulceration, visible on regular high-definition white light imaging, goes hand in hand with NICE type III pit pattern classification. If something looks ulcerated on the surface, the chance of submucosal cancer is high regardless of the size.

I just had a case where a patient was referred by a community gastroenterologist for EMR of an 11 mm polyp in the cecum with high-grade dysplasia. Although the polyp was not that large it had surface ulceration and I explained that I was concerned about possible invasive cancer, based solely on the surface ulceration. I did the EMR. The polyp lifted great, we did an en bloc resection, the base of the polyp looked pretty reasonable, clipped it, and the pathology came back as margin-positive invasive adenocarcinoma. He ended up with a hemicolectomy anyway.

Another indicator of malignancy is any lesion that is near circumferential. The chance is high that there is an invasive cancer somewhere in that lesion. Then, if something is just bleeding or oozing more than it should, that is usually a good indication that you might be dealing with cancer.

What about the use of the Paris classification to suggest the likelihood of deep submucosal invasion?

In the Paris classification, lesions that have a central depression, either IIc or II a + c lesions (something that is raised on the edge and depressed in the middle), can harbor cancer. These are usually accompanied by surface ulceration. Lesions that have a 1-s component (which is what we call a dominant nodule) tend to harbor high-grade dysplasia, not necessarily cancer per se. I always look for those areas specifically to ensure that I'm concentrating on getting those sections out. So, as far as the benign Paris lesions, those are the two that would indicate potential cancer.

Pedunculated Polyp

Case 4 *A 55-year-old man is found to have to have a large (about 1.8 cm) pedun-culated polyp on a thick stalk.*

Is there any role for cold snare polypectomy of a pedunculated polyp?

I would say no, it's just going to turn into a bloody mess if you are able to tran-sect it. If you are unable to transect it, which is the most likely scenario because you are cutting through a huge stalk and big vessel, then you are just getting yourself in trouble. These polyps invariably require hot snare.

I will take out pedunculated polyps less than 1 cm in size in the left colon with cold snare, especially if I already have a cold snare out and have already been using it. They will bleed a little bit more in the short turn, but they will thrombose and stop quickly.

Do you like to pre-treat the stalk in patients with a thick stalk? If so, what do you like to use?

I will if it is a big polyp and I am having difficulty getting a snare around it. If you inject standard epinephrine into the stalk of the polyp that will diminish the flow from the feeding vessel(s) and result in an ischemia-induced reduction in size. The polyp will shrink in real time and that may make enough of a difference to change something from not capturable to capturable. Stalk, injecting into the stalk.

If I can get a snare around a polyp comfortably, I'm usually not pre-treating the stalk. When I'm removing a polyp on a thick stalk, I know beforehand that I will probably clip the stalk afterward. I prefer to clip it following polypectomy, rather than before, because if a stalk starts bleeding post-polypectomy and you clip it and it stops, then you know your clip is in the right place and you can feel good about it.

Some people will place standard endoscopic clips at the stalk base prior to pol-ypectomy. I have avoided doing that because the stalks are frequently thicker than the standard 11 mm clips and you can't be sure that you are effectively tamponading the vessel. Now that there are larger, 18 mm clips, and there may be more of a role for them, but so far that is not my practice.

If I encounter a very high-risk polyp with a thick stalk and I am tempted to clip prior to polypectomy, I prefer to use a detachable snare. A lot of people are uncom-fortable with the deployment of a detachable snare because the deployment systems can be a little tricky. When you cinch down on a detachable snare, you run the risk of cold-ligating the stalk causing heavy bleeding if you aren't careful or you deploy it and it isn't tight enough, which makes it ineffective. So, there is a very systematic way to open the snare, get it around the polyp, and get the cinch down to the point where you know that there is tamponade of the vessel that is indicated by color change of the polyp as you tighten the loop.

In those cases, where you opt to use hot snare discuss the various cautery settings that are available and how you decide on the particular ones in a par-ticular setting.

There has always been a blue-pedal-yellow-pedal debate (on the ERBE). I have always been on team yellow, but there was a pretty well-done randomized control trial looking at this exact question, yellow vs. blue pedal for complex polypectomy, and found no difference in resection success and complications [7], so it looks like you can probably do either in those circumstances. Some people feel that the blue pedal has more cautery associated with it so maybe your bleeding risk is going to be less. Any source of blended current (if you are using an ERBE or similar device) is going to have some cautery current built-in with the cutting current. There is usually some tissue impedance that directly feeds back to the generator that allows it to alter the settings as it cuts through. So, I still use the yellow pedal for pretty much everything (ENDOCUT Q for ERBE systems). Then it's just personal preference on cut duration, cut interval, and effect. I think whatever you are comfortable with is what you should stick with.

Your partner is performing the polypectomy and has not pre-treated the stalk. There is heavy bleeding at the stalk immediately following polypectomy.

How do you like to manage this?

You can do a handful of things. I think mechanical tamponade is the best approach. If you want to inject epinephrine to slow things down so you can better see where the bleeding is coming from that is also completely appropriate. But standard endoscopic clips are fine in this scenario, and I think that while heavy bleeding does impair visualization, I always tell the fellows that bleeding is a good thing because once it is treated and the bleeding stops you know that your clips are in a good position.

Post-Polypectomy Bleeding

Case 5 Your partner performs a cold snare polypectomy on a 48-year-old patient in good health. The polyp was described as 6 mm in size, located in the sigmoid colon. That Friday night you get a call from the patient that he has had two bloody bowel movements since the colonoscopy that morning, about 4 h apart.

How would you advise this patient?

Anytime the patient calls, regardless of how the polyp was taken out, you want to clearly assess their symptoms. Are they lightheaded? If so, is this postural?

If a polyp was taken out in the left colon, it was under 1 cm in size, and removed cold, the chance of having a bleed that requires intervention is well below 1%. What I mean by that is not the proportion who have cold snare polypectomy, but the proportion of those who call you with bleeding after a cold snare of a diminutive polyp in the left colon. So, reassurance is the most common thing, but besides that, I want to make sure we are keeping an eye on things, the patient knows when to go to the emergency department, etc.

The next morning the patient is still having bloody bowel movements and you decide to perform a repeat colonoscopy that weekend. There is ongoing bleeding from the polypectomy site. How would you treat it?

I would clip it.

There is frequently mild oozing of blood at the time of cold snare polypectomy. How do you decide whether the bleeding will stop spontaneously? When does the bleeding appear excessive?

It is very unusual for something to bleed persistently at the completion of a procedure. Most things have slowed down to a trickle or have stopped completely, even after a big EMR. Every once in a while, you can hit a big vessel with a cold snare so if something doesn't look like it is slowing down and you have given it 5 min or so, nobody is going to fault you for putting a clip or two on there, but this is rarely needed with cold polypectomy.

Do you ever see delayed bleeds after a cold snare polypectomy starting up days after the event?

It is very uncommon. Again, we think the impetus for delayed bleeding is diathermy and ulcer formation so it just rarely happens.

Slightly different scenario is the polyp is now 1.5 cm in size and was located in the descending colon and removed with hot snare. The bleeding starts up 7 days post-procedure and is quite brisk. You admit the patient and perform a colonoscopy the next morning. There is active bleeding from the polypectomy site.

What will you use to stop the bleeding in this case following hot snare polypectomy?

I think clips are still my choice. Usually, with clips you can focus your treatment. You will likely see a big ulcer and it's going to look ugly, but the culprit vessel is going to be very obvious and so typically one or two clips on the culprit vessel are going to be enough for hemostasis to occur. I wouldn't see a need to close the entire defect 7 days later, just treat the bleeding site because it's unlikely that anything else in that ulcer is going to bleed at that point.

References

1. Pohl H, Grimm IS, Moyer MT, et al. Clip closure prevents bleeding after endoscopic resection of large colon polyps in a randomized trial. Gastroenterology. 2019;157:977–984.e3.
2. Klein A, Tate DJ, Jayasekeran V, et al. Thermal ablation of mucosal defect margins reduces adenoma recurrence after colonic endoscopic mucosal resection. Gastroenterology. 2019;156:604–613.e3.
3. Mehta D, Loutfy AH, Kushnir VM, et al. Cold versus hot endoscopic mucosal resection for large sessile colon polyps: a cost-effectiveness analysis. Endoscopy. 2022;54:367–75.
4. Mangira D, Cameron K, Simons K, et al. Cold snare piecemeal EMR of large sessile colonic polyps >/=20 mm (with video). Gastrointest Endosc. 2020;91:1343–52.
5. van Hattem WA, Shahidi N, Vosko S, et al. Piecemeal cold snare polypectomy versus conventional endoscopic mucosal resection for large sessile serrated lesions: a retrospective comparison across two successive periods. Gut. 2021;70:1691–7.
6. Tate DJ, Awadie H, Bahin FF, et al. Wide-field piecemeal cold snare polypectomy of large sessile serrated polyps without a submucosal injection is safe. Endoscopy. 2018;50:248–52.
7. Pohl H, Grimm IS, Moyer MT, et al. Effects of blended (yellow) vs. forced coagulation (blue) currents on adverse events, complete resection, or polyp recurrence after polypectomy in a large randomized trial. Gastroenterology. 2020;159:119–128.e2.

Chapter 18
Rectal Incontinence

Ling Mei and Krupa Patel

*Case 1 A 73-year-old woman comes to your office complaining of rectal inconti-
nence that has occurred on five occasions. With each episode, she is aware of the
urge to defecate but can't "hold it" long enough to get to the toilet. There were a
number of other episodes when she felt the urge to defecate, but was just barely able
to get to the toilet on time. This all started about 3 months previously, after a bout
of "food poisoning."*

**Is this passive, urge, or seepage incontinence? What is the distinction
between the three forms, and why is it important?**

This is urge incontinence. Urge incontinence is the discharge of rectal contents
despite active attempts to retain them. Passive incontinence is the involuntary discharge of feces or flatus without awareness. Fecal seepage is involuntary seepage
with otherwise normal evacuation.

*The patient has a history of a complicated pregnancy when she was 20 years old,
which required an episiotomy. She has had no other anorectal operations and no
abdominal surgery. Her bowel movements occur once or twice a day, which is
unchanged from her norm. She denies urinary incontinence. Her last screening
colonoscopy was 4 years ago, when she was 69, which was normal, and no biopsies
were taken. Her physical examination is unremarkable except for the rectal examination, where she has a slightly diminished rectal tone.*

L. Mei (✉)
Department of Medicine, GI/Hepatology Division, Medical College of Wisconsin,
Milwaukee, WI, USA
e-mail: lmei@mcw.edu

K. Patel
Methodist Medical Group, Dallas, Texas, USA
e-mail: KrupaRpatel@mhd.com

© The Author(s), under exclusive license to Springer Nature   121
Switzerland AG 2023
W. H. Sobin et al. (eds.), *Managing Complex Cases in Gastroenterology*,
https://doi.org/10.1007/978-3-031-48949-5_18

Can you describe how you do your rectal examination in someone with incontinence?

The digital rectal examination is a very important aspect of the physical examination in a patient with incontinence. Here is a description of the full rectal examination:

1. Ask the patient to lie in the left lateral position.
2. Inspect the perineum and external anus by spreading the buttocks after donning a pair of gloves, to look for any dermatitis, scarring, skin tags, hemorrhoids, rectal prolapse, fistulas, or fissures.
3. Stroke the skin around the anus using a Q-tip to assess the anocutaneous reflex. When the reflex is acting normally, sensory stimulation of the skin around the anus leads to anal sphincter contraction (anal wink). A normal anocutaneous reflex indicates an intact sacral reflex arc and pudendal nerve innervation of the external anal sphincter.
4. Ask the patient to strain to evaluate the presence of perineal descent, prolapsed hemorrhoids, and rectal prolapse.
5. Assess the resting tone by gently inserting your index finger into the anal canal. This is best measured *after waiting a few seconds to allow for accommodation*. The resting tone is predominantly attributable to the internal anal sphincter. A reduced tone may indicate weakness of the internal anal sphincter, while the presence of increased tone may contribute to difficulty with defecation.
6. Have the patient perform a voluntary anal squeeze to evaluate the external anal sphincter tone. Reduced anal squeeze pressure may suggest weakness of the external anal sphincter.
7. Palpate the posterior rectal wall to evaluate for any pain. If this is present, it suggests puborectalis muscle tenderness.
8. Have the patient strain and try to push your finger out. Normally, the anal sphincter should relax associated with *perineal descent while bearing down*. If the sphincter muscles seem to tighten and there is no perineal descent, this may suggest dyssynergic defecation.

What are the causes of anal incontinence we are most likely to encounter?

Fecal incontinence may be caused by altered bowel habits and a variety of conditions that affect the ability of the rectum and anus to hold stool. Causes of fecal incontinence may include diarrhea, fecal impaction, obstetric or surgical sphincter muscle injuries, pelvic floor injury, neuropathy resulting from diabetes or stroke, spinal cord injuries, and some inflammatory conditions [1].

What evaluations would you do? Would you do anorectal manometry? If so, is it high resolution? Would you do an MRI? An endoscopic ultrasound? A balloon expulsion test? A colonoscopy?

If incontinence occurs in the setting of constipation or diarrhea, we have to manage the bowel disturbance first. We usually begin with an abdominal X-ray to evaluate stool burden.

If diarrhea is a concern, the work-up often includes a colonoscopy, with random biopsies to assess for microscopic colitis.

If fecal incontinence persists despite managing bowel disturbance, the next step is to perform anorectal manometry with assessment of rectal sensation and a rectal balloon expulsion test. We prefer to do high-resolution manometry, which is a novel, solid-state manometric system, which provides more accurate resolution of intraluminal pressure and greater anatomical detail compared to water-perfused manometric systems. The balloon expulsion test is a simple test to screen for a defecation disorder.

If a weak anal sphincter is identified during anorectal manometry, further evaluation with endoanal ultrasound or MRI can be considered to evaluate for muscle damage, especially when surgery is being considered. EMG can also be considered, depending on center availability.

MRI is superior for visualizing external sphincter defects, atrophy, and patulous anal canal. This should only be ordered if there are concerns about defects.

How do you like to manage patients like this?

We would first treat underlying causes such as constipation or diarrhea. For patients with fecal impaction with an overflow component, I would start a bowel regimen with a fiber supplement (psyllium) and a daily laxative program. For patients with diarrhea, we would initially start with dietary modifications, such as eliminating foods with artificial sweeteners (e.g., lactose, fructose, and sorbitol), spicy food, and caffeine-containing beverages. We will observe for any improvement in bowel habits and stool leakage. Anti-diarrheal agents, such as loperamide (non-prescription) or Lomotil (prescription), can be used to reduce loose stool. Loperamide is usually taken 30 min before meals or after each loose stool. The maximal dosage is 16 mg/day. Studies have shown that loperamide can also improve incontinence by increasing resting anal tone [2]. Other medications such as bile acid binders can be used in patients with IBS-D or post-cholecystectomy diarrhea.

Are there any surgical options you might recommend?

If the above measures have failed, then surgical options can be considered. I would initially recommend a sacral nerve stimulator, in which the nerves that supply the rectum and anal sphincters can be activated by a stimulator [3]. In selected patients, injection of bulking agents into the anal sphincter is another approach that may improve the anal seal [3]. A surgical sphincteroplasty can be considered in women with a sphincter defect resulting from vaginal delivery [3]. However, long-term outcomes with this procedure are mixed, with about 50% of patients having recurrence of symptoms [4]. In severe cases of incontinence that are debilitating and significantly affecting quality of life, a colostomy can be considered.

Can you describe the process of sending patients for sacral nerve stimulation?

Sacral nerve stimulation can be considered in all patients who fail conservative management. This is a two-stage procedure. First, a temporary nerve stimulator is attached and used for 2 weeks. Patients whose symptoms respond to the temporary nerve stimulator are then sent for permanent subcutaneous implantation of the device. There is about 80% therapeutic success and 40% complete continence at 3-year follow-up [5, 6].

Do you have any experience with biofeedback therapy?

This is the mainstay of treatment for patients who fail medical treatment. Pelvic biofeedback training by combining pelvic floor exercises and visual feedback from anal manometry or surface EMG can strengthen anal sphincters and improve rectal sensation. For patients having fecal incontinence due to dyssynergic defecation, biofeedback therapy, using a different technique, can improve the coordination between abdominal muscles and the pelvic floor and subsequently improve rectal emptying. Satisfaction has been reported in up to 70% of patients in prior studies [7].

Are there any particular areas you are personally researching in anal incontinence?

We have been researching the ability to exercise the external sphincter and puborectalis muscles beyond simple Kegel exercises with added resistance training via an exerciser balloon in the anal canal. We first evaluated the ability of the muscles to fatigue more with added resistance [8]. Muscle overload and subsequent neuromuscular fatigue are necessary requirements for any successful strength training as shown in rehabilitative exercises [9, 10]. We then assessed the ability to strengthen the muscles using pre- and post-anorectal manometry after 6 weeks of resistance training in patients suffering from fecal incontinence. Our preliminary results have shown improvement of symptoms and sphincter muscle contractility demonstrated as an increased anal resting and squeeze pressure after 6 weeks of resistance training [11].

Case 2 *A 75-year-old woman has occasional "accidents" where she is unaware that she is having a bowel movement until she smells stool in her panties, or feels wetness.*

What are some possible etiologies for this?

This patient has passive fecal incontinence. Passive incontinence can occur in the setting of neuropathy resulting in loss of rectal sensation and weakness of the internal anal sphincter. This may be seen in systemic illnesses such as diabetes. It can also be seen in patients with spinal cord injury, stretch injury, or obstetric trauma.

What might the rectal examination show?

Rectal examination might show poor resting sphincter tone.

What would you be looking for on a neurologic examination, and what other systems might be involved?

Neurologic examination may reveal decreased perianal pin-prick sensation, lower extremity weakness if related to an underlying spinal cord injury, or reduced sensation in the setting of neuropathy. The urinary system may also be involved with incontinence.

What findings would you expect on anorectal manometry?

Anorectal manometry may reveal reduced rectal sensation and/or resting sphincter tone. Squeeze pressure could be normal or reduced.

How would you manage this patient's problems?

Management would be different based on the cause of symptoms. In most cases, we recommend increasing stool consistency by adding fiber supplements and having scheduled bowel movements. Enemas or suppositories may be helpful in scheduling bowel movements.

We would also recommend biofeedback for rectal hyposensitivity if some degree of rectal sensation is still preserved. Biofeedback is usually not effective for isolated internal anal sphincter weakness; in which case, we might consider a bulking agent (such as dextranomer injection) and/or sacral nerve stimulation.

In some patients, the Eclipse system (in which a vaginal balloon compresses the rectum) or Renew insert (in which an anal plug is worn) can be considered on a PRN basis to reduce fecal leakage.

Case 3 *A 64-year-old woman has problems moving her bowels and will go several days without a bowel movement. In spite of difficulties with constipation, she has occasional episodes where liquid stools pass of their own volition. She has minimal warning but then feels the stool in her panties or down the side of her legs. Prior screening colonoscopy, 5 years earlier, was negative. There is abdominal fullness on the examination, presumably due to increased stool. On the rectal examination, there is adequate sphincter tone and some stool in the vault, although not a large rectal impaction.*

How would you recommend managing this situation?

It appears the patient has constipation with overflow diarrhea. We would first recommend an abdominal X-ray to assess the stool burden. After confirming increased stool, we would recommend a bowel regimen to regulate the bowel movements. We often recommend starting with a colon purge followed by a daily bowel regimen.

How do you respond when patients complain that the laxatives are only worsening their incontinence?

You are less likely to have this problem if you start out with a colon purge, attempting to get the colon cleaned out initially. In these patients, the incontinence is likely related to fecal retention/impaction, and once you correct this, you've corrected their incontinence. We would follow this with a daily laxative regimen. We also encourage patients to consume adequate daily fiber (25–30 g/day for adults). We encourage them to include psyllium in their daily bowel regimen. We might also do anorectal manometry to evaluate the defecatory disorder.

Will you ever use a full colon lavage, like 2 or 4 liters of Golytely?

We do usually recommend a colon purge before starting a daily bowel regimen. If choosing Golytely for the colon purge, we will start with 2 liters first. If the patient does not feel adequately emptied after the half dose of Golytely, we will then advise the patient to complete the second half. Alternatively, a colon purge using a bottle of MiraLAX or magnesium citrate is also an option if the patient is unable to obtain or tolerate the Golytely.

Case 4 *A 67-year-old man has had a stroke with left-sided weakness. He tries to schedule his bowel movements once a day in the morning and is successful about half the time. Recently, he has had episodes of rectal incontinence.*

What are some possible explanations for this?

There are multiple possible reasons for his altered bowel habits and incontinence. His immobility can be associated with reduced GI motility and incomplete evacuation/stool retention, which may subsequently result in overflow incontinence. Since he is post-stroke, his neurologic deficit may be associated with reduced rectal sensation and decreased sphincter strength, which may also contribute to his incontinence.

What might you find on the rectal examination?

We may feel the retained stool in the rectum. He may have reduced perianal sensation and reduced anal sphincter tone.

How would you manage his problems?

We will recommend a colon purge if the patient is able to cooperate. We will recommend a routine bowel regimen including adequate daily fiber intake and adding a laxative if his stool is hard (Bristol 1 or 2). We will recommend a scheduled bowel movement using a suppository or enema in the morning if the patient does not have a spontaneous bowel movement. If his symptoms do not show significant improvement with the bowel regimen, we will obtain anorectal manometry to further evaluate anorectal function.

Case 5 *A 54-year-old female psychotherapist is embarrassed because of occasional episodes where she has stool involuntarily soiling her pants. Her bowel movements seem normal, and she feels like she is totally emptying her rectum with each bowel movement. Afterward, she tries to clean herself very well. In spite of that, as the day goes on, she notices stool soiling her underpants almost every day.*

What are some possible explanations for this?

This patient has anal seepage, which is defined as staining or streaking of underwear. Anal seepage can occur if the rectum is not fully emptied after a bowel movement, something which is seen in dyssynergic defecation, rectocele, radiation therapy, and with prolapsed hemorrhoids. It responds to different treatments as compared to fecal incontinence.

Are there dietary or behavioral precautions she could take?

She should maintain a high-fiber diet to help bulk up her stool. We recommend avoiding excessive wiping after defecation and using alcohol-free wipes. We will advise the patient to place a cotton ball at the anus to act as an occasional wick. Some women may benefit from a splinting technique during defecation, particularly if a rectocele is present. The splinting technique involves placing a finger in the vagina to push against the rectum to help stool to empty.

Are there medications that might be helpful?

Anal suppositories can be tried to help with emptying the rectum. Patients with hemorrhoids can try topical steroids to shrink the hemorrhoids and reduce the irritation.

Are there any other sorts of intervention?

Patients with dyssynergic defecation may benefit from pelvic biofeedback retraining. Patients with a rectocele may need surgical consultation.

References

1. Menees SB, Almario CV, Spiegel BMR, Chey WD. Prevalence of and factors associated with fecal incontinence: results from a population-based survey. Gastroenterology. 2018;154(6):1672–81 e3.
2. Read M, Read NW, Barber DC, Duthie HL. Effects of loperamide on anal sphincter function in patients complaining of chronic diarrhea with fecal incontinence and urgency. Dig Dis Sci. 1982;27(9):807–14.
3. Whitehead WE, Rao SS, Lowry A, Nagle D, Varma M, Bitar KN, Bharucha AE, Hamilton FA. Treatment of fecal incontinence: state of the science summary for the National Institute of Diabetes and Digestive and Kidney Diseases workshop. Am J Gastroenterol. 2015;110(1):138–46.
4. Glasgow SC, Lowry AC. Long-term outcomes of anal sphincter repair for fecal incontinence: a systematic review. Dis Colon Rectum. 2012;55(4):482–90.
5. Meurette G, Siproudhis L, Leroi AM, Damon H, Urs Josef Keller D, Faucheron JL, French Faecal Registry Study Group. Sacral neuromodulation with the InterStim™ system for faecal incontinence: results from a prospective French multicentre observational study. Color Dis. 2021;23(6):1463–73.
6. Rao SS. Current and emerging treatment options for fecal incontinence. J Clin Gastroenterol. 2014;48(9):752–64.
7. Norton C, Cody JD. Biofeedback and/or sphincter exercises for the treatment of faecal incontinence in adults. Cochrane Database Syst Rev. 2012;7:CD002111.
8. Mei L, Patel K, Lehal N, Kern MK, Benjamin A, Sanvanson P, Shaker R. Fatigability of the external anal sphincter muscles using a novel strength training resistance exercise device. Am J Physiol Gastrointest Liver Physiol. 2021;320(4):G609–16.
9. Marques A, Stothers L, Macnab A. The status of pelvic floor muscle training for women. Can Urol Assoc J. 2010;4(6):419–24.
10. Johnson VY. How the principles of exercise physiology influence pelvic floor muscle training. J Wound Ostomy Continence Nurs. 2001;28(3):150–5.
11. Patel KML, Lehal N, Benjamin A, Sanvanson P, Kern M, Shaker R. External anal sphincter strength training exercise using a novel continence muscles resistance exerciser device results in improved anal sphincter contractility in patients with fecal incontinence. Gastroenterology. 2020;158(6):S-388.

Chapter 19
Diverticulitis

William Berger, Keely Browning, and W. Harley Sobin

Case 1 *A 54-year-old man presents to the ER with LLQ pain of 6-h duration. He has a temp. of 99, WBC is 14,000, and CRP is 30. A CT scan is performed that reveals mild uncomplicated diverticulitis.*

How would you manage this patient? Would you consider treating without antibiotics?

Browning: Treatment considerations for uncomplicated diverticulitis include antibiotics and patient disposition. Hospitalization should be considered for patients who cannot tolerate oral intake, have a fever, or have excessive vomiting. Outpatient management includes bowel rest, liquid diet, and oral antibiotics [1].

The AGA recommends consideration of liquid diet for patient comfort, but evidence suggests it is not necessary, and if patients would like to advance their diet, they should be allowed to. However, if they are unable to tolerate advancing the diet in 3–5 days, they should be re-evaluated [2]. The two most common antibiotic regimens are quinolone with metronidazole or amoxicillin-clavulanate for 4–10 days [1].

However, several studies have shown that antibiotics do not always accelerate recovery, nor prevent complications or recurrence. Due to this, the AGA recommends antibiotics be used selectively for patients with uncomplicated diverticulitis, including those who have comorbidities, frailty, immunocompromised state, refractory vomiting, CRP >140 mg/L, WBC >15 × 10^9 cells/L, or who have CT findings of a fluid collection or longer segment of inflammation on CT [2]. Patients

W. Berger · W. H. Sobin (✉)
Division of Gastroenterology and Hepatology, Medical College of Wisconsin,
Milwaukee, WI, USA
e-mail: wberger@mcw.edu; hsobin@mcw.edu

K. Browning
Madison Medical Affiliates, Milwaukee, WI, USA
e-mail: Keely.browning@ascension-external.org

© The Author(s), under exclusive license to Springer Nature
Switzerland AG 2023
W. H. Sobin et al. (eds.), *Managing Complex Cases in Gastroenterology*,
https://doi.org/10.1007/978-3-031-48949-5_19

with uncomplicated diverticulitis without comorbidities do not necessarily require antibiotics [1, 2].

Berger: I would only briefly consider treating without antibiotics. I know that the new literature is supposed to show that there's no difference, but when I have something that looks like a bacterial infection, I usually do start antibiotics and patients seem to respond. When antibiotics aren't started, the process seems to go off and on for a longer period of time before it resolves itself. I have a preference for using metronidazole, partly to avoid pseudomembranous colitis. Along with metronidazole, I use cipro. I am not a fan of Augmentin because of cases of pseudomembranous colitis that I've encountered using that.

I give the patient a follow-up call after 5 days, and if they're not better, I will give them a longer course of antibiotics or occasionally switch to a different antibiotic. If they're still not improving, I usually choose to do some more imaging.

What if you're dealing with a patient who has had repeated episodes of diverticulitis treated with antibiotics as an outpatient, but hates taking the antibiotics because of adverse symptoms, and comes in now with one more typical recurrence (mild, uncomplicated). Would you consider managing without antibiotics?

Sobin: I have had a few cases like this where a patient had repeated mild episodes that we reflexively treated with antibiotics. After a couple of times, the patient started pleading to skip antibiotics after another bout of diverticulitis, because of severe intolerance. These were mild cases, and because the literature supports withholding antibiotics in cases like this, I managed the cases without antibiotics and the patients did fine.

Berger: No. Actually, if this is a patient who is in his 40 s, 50 s, or 60 s, I would give antibiotics and suggest elective surgery after resolution of the acute episode. There is something focally wrong with that colon, and this person will be fighting this problem for the rest of his life. They just need that sigmoid in a bucket. Now if they're 85, the risk of surgery will far exceed any potential benefit, but no, I would rarely pass on giving antibiotics for recurrent/chronic diverticulitis to cool it down so we can get on with the appropriate therapy.

Case 2 *A 48-year-old man presents with an episode of sigmoid diverticulitis and is started on outpatient metronidazole and ciprofloxacin. However, after a week of antibiotics he still complains of pain and so a second 7-day course is administered. After 2 weeks, he returns to his doctor's office with ongoing LLQ pain and low-grade fevers to 100.5. Because his WBC is 18,000 and CRP is 75, a CT is ordered. The CT shows ongoing inflammation in the sigmoid. How would you manage this?*

Browning: Diverticulitis is the most common complication of diverticulosis. Prior estimates suggested that diverticulitis occurred in 10–25% of patients, but more recent studies suggest that the incidence is much lower, about 4% based on population studies [1].

Smoldering diverticulitis is a complication of acute diverticulitis where patients have continued abdominal pain with the presence of inflammation on imaging in spite of treatment with antibiotics [1, 2]. Based on systemic signs of inflammation like fever and elevated inflammatory markers, I would start IV antibiotics.

Berger: I would start IV antibiotics to cool things down. Now, we do IV antibiotics at home, and I think that's a very reasonable thing to try in an appropriate patient. I would also call a surgeon because this patient is going to have trouble again.

As I get older and more experienced, my threshold for operating on these patients becomes lower, but it is a balanced calculation, having to do with how old they are and how many comorbid health conditions they have. This is weighed against how severe, recurrent, and symptomatic the diverticulitis is.

However, on balance, I'm tipping a little bit more toward surgery. For one thing, the complications using laparoscopic or robotic surgery are so much less, and the recovery so much better than the old open surgical techniques.

Sobin: I agree. I would also bring the patient in for IV antibiotics and consult a surgeon.

Case 3 *A 45-year-old patient presents with his third episode of sigmoid diverticulitis in 12 months. He has been on a high-fiber diet and remains in good general condition.*

Would you recommend elective surgery at this point? If not, when?

Berger: After three episodes, you can be pretty sure they're going to have more, particularly at this young age. If you know you're going to end up having surgery, the earlier you have it done the better. You're healthier, and your nutrition's going to be better. You don't have to wait for complications of the disease. Everything just works better with earlier surgery if you know you're going to need it eventually. If you wait until you're older, you get less benefit out of it and are much more likely to have complications.

Three is generally my magic number for recommending diverticulitis in the younger patient, not the 84 years old.

There was a recent report in JAMA surgery [3], where they followed a group of patients who had a sigmoid resection vs conservative therapy for recurrent complicated, persistent, or painful diverticulitis. Mortality and complications of surgery were virtually nil. The quality-of-life assessment after 2 years was much better in those who had a sigmoid resection. It is interesting, though, that those with elective sigmoid resection still had a 10–18% risk of recurrent diverticulitis.

Now, in the conservative management group, about 20% ended up needing surgery anyway, but they had a much higher complication rate than the group that had elective surgery.

Browning: Due to recent data showing that there were fewer deaths and colostomies and better cost-effectiveness if surgical resection was delayed until the fourth episode rather than the second, both the American Society of Colon and Rectal Surgeons (ASCRS) and the AGA recommend a case-by-case basis for elective surgical resection. These factors include immune status, severity of diverticulitis, patient preference, patient age, and operative risk [2]. For example, young patients with diverticulitis tend to have more severe disease and fewer complications following surgical resection and therefore may be considered for earlier surgical resection [1]. In this case, I would refer to a surgeon given multiple episodes in a relatively short time and relatively good health of the patient.

If you had a 30 years old who had their first episode of sigmoid diverticulitis, would you recommend surgery?

Berger: Oh, no, because the first incident is a one-off, and the second is a coincidence, but three is a pattern. By the time you hit three, you'll know what you're in for.

Sobin: I agree. I would hold off on surgery after the first episode. I might recommend surgery after the second, if it is a severe attack, otherwise, probably after the third.

How do you advise your patients on a way to avoid recurrent diverticulitis? Any dietary or physical activity suggestions?

Browning: Diverticulosis is very common, and it is estimated that 2/3 of adults will have diverticula by the ninth decade of life [1]. Most people are asymptomatic, and thus, the prevalence of diverticulosis may be underestimated. The etiology of diverticula is debated. Traditionally, diverticula were thought to form from low-fiber diets leading to smaller caliber stools and constipation. This causes higher intraluminal pressures leading to herniation of colonic mucosa and submucosa [4].

Diverticula typically form between the taenia coli, which are the three bands of longitudinal fibers of the colon. Diverticula form along the sites of penetration of the vasa recta. Circular muscle layers thicken and taeniae shorten, causing the colon to appear thickened with luminal narrowing [1]. Evidence for this can be seen when people immigrate to regions with a Western diet, they develop a higher incidence of diverticula [4]. Most diverticula in the western hemisphere are actually pseudodiverticula, as the herniation only reaches the submucosa. In Asian countries, diverticula tend to be in the right colon and can be true diverticula involving all layers of the colonic wall [1].

Other known risk factors include smoking, alcohol, vitamin D deficiency, high red meat diet, physical inactivity, obesity, and genetic factors. Non-steroidal anti-inflammatory drugs (NSAIDs), steroids, hormone replacement therapy, and opiates increase risk of diverticula and diverticulitis, while calcium channel blockers and statins were found to be protective [1, 5].

Traditionally, it was recommended that patients with a history of diverticulitis should avoid nuts and seeds. However, studies have shown that there is no increased risk of diverticulitis and nuts and seeds may actually lower the risk. The AGA does not recommend a particular diet [2]. Unfortunately, there is no strong evidence to suggest medications to prevent recurrence of diverticulitis, and risk of diverticulitis is largely due to genetic factors. Although dietary changes are debated, due to absence of side effects, I would propose that this patient stick to a high-fiber diet or consider daily Metamucil. I would counsel him to avoid NSAIDs if possible, encourage regular exercise, and continue cessation from smoking.

Berger: I encourage everybody, whether they've had diverticulitis or not, over the age of 30 to 35 to be taking two scoops of Metamucil every morning for the rest of their lives.

That will reduce their chance of getting diverticulosis. It will also help reduce their cholesterol and their chance of developing colon cancer or colitis. Yes, I'm a big fan of fiber. Is it going to turn things back after you have somebody who already has a significant diverticular disease? Not really, but it may minimize symptoms and complications.

I think everybody ought to be on fiber anyway because of our diet. Do you remember the story about Denis Burkitt of Burkitt's lymphoma? He went to Uganda and not only discovered Burkitt's lymphoma, but he also noted that colon cancer, diverticular disease, and colitis were rarely seen in Uganda, and he attributed all of that to fiber. In Uganda, they eat huge amounts of very fibrous food, and he found that they would have four to five soft bowel movements every day. In contrast, the average Irish stool was round and hard and was produced once a day or even once every other day, and he concluded that it was the fiber that made the difference in their colonic health.

What do you think about NSAIDs increasing the risk of diverticulitis?

Berger: When I see NSAIDs causing an issue, it's usually something in the terminal ileum or proximal colon. I don't usually see them causing a problem downstream, in the sigmoid. So, from my experience I'm not big on that one.

Sobin: In my experience, it has not been a significant contributing factor. In spite of that, I recommend NSAID avoidance in patients with a history of diverticulitis.

Case 4 *A 47-year-old man has had one episode of sigmoid diverticulitis. He is treated, and all inflammatory markers resolve. However, months later, he has ongoing pain in the same region. His WBC and CRP are normal. A repeat CT scan shows no active inflammation.*

Is this SUDD (symptomatic uncomplicated diverticular disease)? Is this a real, distinct entity? If so, how would you treat it?

Browning: If abdominal pain is present in patients with diverticulosis, in the absence of diverticulitis or clinical bleeding, they may have SUDD. Some think of this as a continuum of irritable bowel syndrome (IBS), with benign physical examination and colonoscopy (other than diverticula), normal inflammatory laboratories, presence of abdominal fullness symptoms, and symptoms that improve with defecation [1].

Several medications have been used for prevention of recurrent diverticulitis or management of SUDD. Proposed regimens include mesalamine 800 mg twice daily for 3 months to help prevent SUDD relapse, rifaximin 400 mg twice daily for 7 days, or combination therapy with mesalamine and rifaximin. Most studies resulted in symptomatic improvement, but these studies were open-label. A Cochrane meta-analysis in 2017 reviewed the use of mesalamine for prevention of diverticulitis. They did not find evidence that mesalamine prevented recurrent diverticulitis, although the trials were heterogeneous [6].

Sobin: My bias is to manage these patients as if they have IBS, with visceral hypersensitivity. In fact, some have suggested that diverticulitis may predispose to IBS. There may be an entity of post-diverticulitis IBS, along the lines of post-infectious IBS. I would not be inclined to try mesalamine unless they were not responding to IBS therapy (which could include rifaximin).

Case 5 *A 47-year-old woman presents to the ER with severe LLQ pain, a fever of 101, and marked tenderness on examination. Her WBC is 21,000, and a CT scan shows phlegmonous sigmoid diverticulitis with an adjacent abscess, 4 cm in size. She has no past history of diverticulitis.*

Are patients with diverticulitis more likely to have perforations, and other complications, after their first episode or subsequent ones?

Browning: Complicated diverticulitis is defined by abscess, fistula, obstruction, or free perforation. Complicated diverticulitis should be suspected when there is persistent pain, fever, and leukocytosis despite IV antibiotics. Complications are more likely to occur with the first episode than subsequent episodes [2]. The Hinchey classification was developed to stratify patient management [1]. Stage I is confined pericolic abscess, stage II is distant abscess, stage III is generalized peritonitis due to rupture of pericolic/pelvic abscess, and stage IV is fecal peritonitis due to free perforation of diverticulum.

Complicated diverticulitis is treated with hospitalization, IV antibiotics, surgical consultation, and co-management. When patients develop worsening sepsis or have recurrent abscess, it means that they have failed antibiotic treatment and should be considered for drainage [7]. In general, if an abscess is greater than 3 cm in size, percutaneous drainage is recommended in addition to IV antibiotics [7].

Berger: My bias is that I tend to see complicated diverticulitis in elderly patients who have had problems before. In my experience, the first episode may not be the worst.

On a per-episode basis, first may be most likely to be complicated, but on a per-patient basis, I worry most about the elderly patients with multiple prior episodes. Tick, tick, tick.

Sobin: I believe the literature that says perforation is most likely with the first episode. I tell patients who have had multiple admissions for diverticulitis that I am less worried about them needing emergency surgery for perforated diverticulitis.

Case 6 *A 46-year-old man with a history of prior diverticulitis comes in for screening colonoscopy. He is found to have moderate inflammatory change limited to an 8-cm length of sigmoid with moderate diverticulosis, where the inflammation seemed to spare the diverticula themselves. Biopsies did not suggest chronic colitis.*

Do you think this may be SCAD—segmental colitis associated with diverticulosis?

Browning: Segmental colitis associated with diverticulosis (SCAD) is an inflammatory process affecting regions of colon that have diverticula [8]; SCAD can mimic the presentation of inflammatory bowel disease (IBD), with clinical features including rectal bleeding, chronic diarrhea, cramping abdominal pain, and fever.

Systemic symptoms like fever, weight loss, or leukocytosis are rare. It is present in 1.5% of colonoscopies, with the majority of patients being male, with a mean age of 63 [1].

Pathogenesis of this condition is thought to be the effect of excessive mucosa from bowel shortening in the setting of diverticulosis, leading to mucosal prolapse and inflammation associated with this [6]. However, when examined microscopically, there can be chronic crypt changes such as crypt distortion, that mimic changes seen in ulcerative colitis. It has also been suggested that there may be bacterial stasis in diverticula leading to increased bacterial mucinase activity and mucosal injury.

Lastly, given the overall older age of presentation in SCAD, there is also a hypothesis of relative colon ischemia, leading to segmental mucosal inflammation. Interestingly, despite chronic inflammation, there is not a higher risk of diverticulitis or colon cancer [1].

There are four subtypes of SCAD: crescentic fold (A), mild-moderate UC-like (B), Crohn's disease-like (C), and severe UC-like (D). These are delineated at time of endoscopy, but importantly all have sparing of the diverticula and regions of colon without diverticula, which separates this disease from other conditions such as IBD [6]. Type A is most likely to present with chronic diarrhea, has no crypt distortion on histologic appearance, and appears as red round lesions 0.5–1.5 cm at top of mucosal folds. Types B and D have loss of vascular pattern with severe ulceration in type D and have crypt distortion on biopsy with goblet cell depletion. Type C mucosa has isolated aphthous ulcers and evidence of transmucosal inflammation on biopsy. Types C and D are more likely to have rectal bleeding. Types B and D tend to have a high risk of relapse [6].

Berger: Segmental colitis associated with diverticulosis? I have seen cases where a patient has a single diverticulum exuding pus, and even though some of these folks were asymptomatic, but others were mildly symptomatic, in these cases, there's that one tic and it's red and there's pus coming out of it, and I usually treat them with antibiotics if they have symptoms to see if they get better.

Then, on occasion, it's 5 years later and we're scoping them again. They have the same darn thing with the same pus coming out of the same tic, and they've never had any symptoms, and in cases like that it's hard to justify treating that, unless of course you had somebody who was about to undergo chemotherapy.

And sometimes, I'll be working with the fellows, and we'll be coming through a really tight sigmoid with a lot of tics and very thick muscular haustra, and there will be these red splotches. Then, the fellow will say "Oh, that's colitis," and sometimes, I even say, "Okay, go ahead and take a biopsy of it," and it comes back with nothing, and that's because it's prolapsed, and you usually see the prolapse in the setting of a sigmoid that's also full of tics, and presumably there's a high-pressure zone that's causing the tics and the hypertrophy and the prolapse. Just because it's red doesn't mean it's inflamed. Mucosa isn't skin.

Sobin: I've primarily seen these mucosal changes on routine surveillance colonoscopy, and I believe that it's a residual change from prior diverticulitis. In a few cases, I have seen this pattern that looks like IBD, but there's sparing of the diverticula themselves, and the inflammation is limited to a short segment of sigmoid diverticula. Generally, these patients were asymptomatic, and before the designation of SCAD came about, I thought this was mild ischemia or mild Crohn's with just an unusual sparing of the diverticula themselves.

Browning: For patients who have more severe SCAD, with significant symptoms, treatment regimens have been based on case series and extrapolation of experience from IBD.

One first-line regimen starts with ciprofloxacin 500 mg BID and metronidazole 400 mg TID for 7 days, followed by mesalamine 2.4–3.2 g/day for 4 weeks and then long-term maintenance dosing of 1.6 g/day of mesalamine. For patients not responding, second-line therapy that uses beclomethasone dipropionate (BDP) with VSL for 4 weeks with tapering dose for another 4 weeks has been tried, followed by maintenance mesalamine. Third-line therapy with high-dose prednisolone has been offered, with surgery for refractory cases [4].

However, in those cases where second- or third-line therapies have been necessary, one must consider a misdiagnosis, and the patient has IBD instead. In fact, some patients later develop IBD at the site of anastomosis when resection was needed for SCAD [4].

Case 7 *A 70-year-old man presents with his fifth episode of sigmoid diverticulitis. He has tried everything and has failed all conservative measures and is ready to have elective surgery. On colonoscopy and CT scan, it is clear that he has diffuse diverticulosis involving all portions of the colon (except the rectum). However, the documented episodes of diverticulitis have only involved the sigmoid.*

With this history do you think it is sufficient to recommend a sigmoid colectomy, or do you think the patient should have a subtotal colectomy?

Berger: I would recommend just removing the sigmoid colon. I look at the colon as two different organs, three if you include the rectum. The proximal and distal colons have different motility, different pressures, different blood supply, and nerve supply. The proximal colon is supplied by the superior mesenteric artery and is innervated by the vagus. It is more-thin walled, and its contractions are segmental contractions designed to mix and churn, to increase exposure of the bolus to the wall to help extract salt and water. The distal colon is designed to store and expel, and its motility is propulsive with much higher pressure, and it's innervated by the sacral outflow and the vascular system is the inferior mesenteric artery, and so, they're actually two different organs and I don't really see diverticulitis in the proximal colon. I will see more bleeding from proximal colon diverticula, probably because the superior mesenteric artery has more perfusion pressure than the inferior mesenteric artery.

Really, they are two distinct organs and if you have pandiverticulosis, the more likely to bleed is the proximal, but the more likely to get diverticulitis is far and away the distal, either the descending or the sigmoid, but the lower down you go, the more likely it is to occur. So, I'm comfortable having him remove the sigmoid, or the sigmoid and descending colon, leaving the rest intact.

References

1. Feldman M, et al. Sleisenger and Fordtran's gastrointestinal and liver disease. 11th ed. Elsevier - OHCE; 2020.
2. Peery AF, Strate SA, LL. AGA clinical practice update on medical Management of Colonic Diverticulitis: expert review. Gastroenterology. 2021;160:906–11.
3. Santos A, Mentula P, Pinta T, Ismail S, Rautio T, Juusela R, Lähdesmäki A, Scheinin T, Sallinen V. Quality-of-life and recurrence outcomes following laparoscopic elective sigmoid resection vs conservative treatment following diverticulitis: Prespecified 2-year analysis of the LASER randomized clinical trial. JAMA Surg. 2023;158(6):593–601.
4. Sheth AA, Longo A, Floch MH. Diverticular disease and diverticulitis. Am J Gastroenterol. 2008;103:1550–6.
5. Strate LL, Modi R, Cohen E, Spiegel BMR. Diverticular disease as a chronic illness: evolving epidemiologic and clinical insights. Am J Gastroenterol. 2012;107:1486–93.
6. Carter F, Alsayb M, Marshall JK, Yuan Y. Mesalamine (5-ASA) for the prevention of recurrent diverticulitis. Cochrane Database Syst Rev. 2017;10:CD009839.
7. Hall J, Hardiman K, Lee S, Lightner A, Stocchi L, Paquette IM, Steele SR, Feingold DL. The American Society of Colon and Rectal Surgeons clinical practice guidelines for the treatment of left-sided colonic diverticulitis. Dis Colon Rectum. 2020;63:728–47.
8. Schembri J, Bonello J, Chrisodoulou DK, Katsanos KH, Ellul P. Segmental colitis associated with diverticulosis: is it the coexistence of colon diverticulosis and inflammatory bowel disease? Ann Gastroenterol. 2017;30:257–61.

Chapter 20
Pancreatic Cysts and Recurrent Pancreatitis

Phillip Chisholm

Case 1 *A 49-year-old man has a CT scan for LLQ pain. The CT reveals mild sigmoid diverticulitis and an incidental 3-cm cyst in the tail of the pancreas. The pancreas otherwise appears normal. He has no history of pancreatic disease, does not smoke, and reports only occasional alcohol use. Once he completes antibiotic treatment for his diverticulitis, he sees you about the pancreatic cyst. His CBC, LFTs, and lipase were all normal..*

Is a 3-cm cyst large enough to warrant a workup, and if so, how would you proceed?

When a patient like this is referred to us, we always review the history trying to tease out any symptoms that may have been missed and any significant social or medication history. We want to know, was there an episode of pain earlier that might signal unrecognized pancreatitis? In a young patient like this, we want to make sure there wasn't more significant alcohol intake. Is there a medication that might have caused pancreatitis, or a family history of pancreatic disease? We try to identify any old imaging of the pancreas to compare with the latest study. The differential for a cyst like this includes non-communicating pancreatic cysts that might be mucinous or serous, pancreatic pseudocysts, and branch-chain IPMNs.

After reviewing the history, physical and any laboratories previously performed we will generally order a dedicated pancreatic radiologic examination, either a dedicated pancreatic CT (which includes fine cuts, non-contrast, and timed contrast administration) or an MRCP. In our institution, we generally prefer the CT because a number of our patients have claustrophobia or can't hold still long enough to get a high-quality MRI. Another advantage of CT is that it can pick up fine pancreatic calcifications. Pancreatic calcifications won't be seen on MRI. On the other hand, an MRCP has the advantage of lack of radiation, which is important in patients who may have serial surveillance examinations. In addition, the MRCP is better at picking up IPMNs and is better at picking up subtle mural nodularity.

P. Chisholm (✉)
Department of Medicine, GI/Hep Division, Medical College of Wisconsin,
Milwaukee, WI, USA
e-mail: pchisholm@mcw.edu

© The Author(s), under exclusive license to Springer Nature
Switzerland AG 2023
W. H. Sobin et al. (eds.), *Managing Complex Cases in Gastroenterology*,
https://doi.org/10.1007/978-3-031-48949-5_20

139

Another laboratory we occasionally order is a serum CA 19–9. A high CA 19–9 may be found in high-grade dysplasia or cancer of the pancreas. However, we are selective with which patients we order the test, since an elevated CA 19–9 is not specific for pancreatic malignancy (elevated CA19–9 may be seen in cases of biliary obstruction, pancreatitis, liver cysts, and hepatitis). Also, some pancreatic cancers don't produce CA 19–9 so a normal result doesn't rule it out.

In most patients, we generally do an EUS and FNA on all cystic lesions larger than 2–3 cm in size. With the FNA, we want to see if the fluid is mucinous, and we order a CEA and glucose. A mucinous lesion is much more likely to be neoplastic, while a serous lesion or pseudocyst is very unlikely to be neoplastic. An elevated cyst fluid amylase suggests that the cyst is in communication with the pancreas—either a pseudocyst or a branch-chain IPMN. An elevated CEA suggests that the lesion is mucinous, either a dysplastic lesion or neoplasm. The cutoff for abnormal CEA is >192 although the specificity of elevated CEA is much higher when we use a cutoff of 1000. We also send off cytology, although the utility of cytology on these aspirates is low, there are many false-negative results.

When we aspirate these lesions, we draw off as much fluid as possible—until the cyst collapses. We make sure we have enough fluid for the CEA, glucose, amylase, and mucin stain and then send off whatever is left for the cytology. Hopefully, a larger volume of fluid may increase the sensitivity of the cytology examination. We hope to draw off at least 3–5 cc, and part of the reason we don't investigate smaller cysts is that it is difficult to draw off sufficient fluid.

With a mucinous cyst greater than 3 cm, we generally call in a multidisciplinary pancreatic team. Assuming the patient is a surgical candidate, most of these patients should have surgical resection since the risk of cancer in a mucinous cyst is relatively high. If the fluid is serous or suggestive of a pancreatitis related pseudocyst, we assume this is a benign cyst that does not require any follow-up, and repeat radiologic examinations are not indicated.

Case 2 *A 42-year-old woman presents to her primary care physician complaining of gradually increasing pain and fullness over the past 10 days. Her physician orders an ultrasound followed by a CT scan that shows cholelithiasis and a 7-cm cyst off the body of the pancreas. The pancreas otherwise appears normal. The common bile duct is not dilated. Her liver enzymes and lipase are normal. Five weeks earlier, she had an episode of severe pain that woke her in the middle of the night but resolved by morning.*

She has no history of alcohol use, prior pancreatitis, or family history of pancreatic disease. The distinct possibility of an episode of gallstone pancreatitis 5 weeks earlier is raised.

Is it necessary to do an EUS to evaluate this cyst?
In this case, we suspect the cyst could be a pancreatic pseudocyst. In considering other etiologies, we want to make sure there wasn't a prior history of weight loss, abdominal pain, or any new-onset diabetes, all of which could suggest neoplasm or chronic pancreatitis. If the symptoms continue to improve and the cyst gets smaller, we would simply observe the patient and repeat imaging studies in 1–2 months.

Assuming any pancreatitis has resolved, you would want to order a cholecystectomy to prevent any repeated gallstone pancreatitis.

If the cyst does not get smaller, and symptoms don't abate, it would be reasonable to do an EUS and FNA. A cyst aspirate fluid with an amylase greater than 1000 and CEA < 192 would be compatible with a pancreatic pseudocyst.

If the cyst did not decrease in size, draining the cyst, perhaps with an Axios stent, would be called for.

Case 3 *A 48-year-old man is seen for abdominal pain. He has a history of cigarette smoking of 28-year duration and has 2–3 drinks a day, 4–5 on weekends. A CT scan reveals a dilated pancreatic duct. MRCP is performed, showing cystic dilation of the pancreatic duct without proximal stricture, suggesting a main duct IPMN in the body of the pancreas.*

How do you manage a patient with pancreatic IPMNs?

IPMNs are mucous-producing tumors of the pancreatic duct that result in cystic dilation of either the main pancreatic duct, a side branch, or both. There is an important distinction between main duct IPMNs, which have a much higher malignant potential than branch-chain IPMNs. Diagnosis of IPMNs can be challenging, and radiologic examinations may confuse main duct IPMNs and chronic pancreatitis, both of which can cause cystic dilation of the pancreatic duct. MRCP is better than CT at picking up IPMNs but can miss the calcifications seen in chronic pancreatitis, which are well seen on CT. An EUS is best at identifying any solid component to the cysts or mural nodules in the IPMNs, and you can often see mucous extruding from the ampulla, the so-called fish-eye appearance. However, calcifications can interfere with EUS evaluation. Therefore, we frequently employ multiple imaging modalities if thee is clinical uncertainty. If the diagnosis of main duct IPMN is confirmed, we generally refer the patient to a multidisciplinary pancreatic team for evaluation for surgery because of the high malignant potential.

Branch-chain IPMNs, on the other hand, have a much lower malignant potential. These lesions are being identified more frequently in our senior population. In studies of patients who had an MRI for non-pancreatic problems, the frequency of pancreatic cystic lesions in patients over age 70 is 40%. In general, we don't investigate these lesions unless they are at least 2 cm in size, in which case we do our standard EUS with FNA with mucous stain, CEA, glucose, and amylase. Surgery and amylase. Surgery would only be recommended if there were high-risk findings on EUS or FNA.

"Idiopathic" Recurrent Pancreatitis

Case 4 *A 53-year-old man is admitted for his second episode of pancreatitis. His first episode was 3 months earlier. Prior to the first episode, he was a social drinker on weekends only. Since that episode, he has had no alcohol. During each episode, his liver enzymes were normal. His lipase was 1100 on admission with the first epi-*

sode and 700 for the second. His triglycerides were 350 during the first episode with normal calcium. An US shows a normal gallbladder. There is no family h/o pancreatic disease, and he is on no meds that would cause pancreatitis.

How do you evaluate a patient with recurrent idiopathic pancreatitis?

Remember, the vast majority of cases of pancreatitis, 70%, are due to gallstones (40%) or alcohol (30%). So, it's important to investigate whether there actually is significant alcohol use in the history, and if not, gallstones are going to be the most common etiology. Of course, in a 53 years old presenting with idiopathic pancreatitis we always want to consider, and rule out, a pancreatic neoplasm, particularly if the patient has a history of weight loss or new-onset diabetes.

Ultrasound is our first test looking for cholelithiasis. After that, we do our dedicated pancreatic imaging. In this instance, MRCP might be more sensitive for evaluating occult cholelithiasis and pancreatic ductal abnormalities. If these studies are unrevealing, we would do an EUS to rule out an occult neoplasm and look for evidence of microlithiasis, and sludge in the gallbladder (with the proviso that if the patient has been NPO for a number of days' sludge might form as a result of fasting and be a red herring).

If, after these investigations, an etiology is not discovered, we would generally recommend a cholecystectomy anyway, because many of these cases of recurrent "idiopathic" pancreatitis are due to occult microlithiasis.

What about a genetic etiology for recurrent pancreatitis?

This is a 53-year-old patient, and genetic pancreatitis usually presents earlier in life. If the patient was a 25 years old with recurrent pancreatitis, we would order genetic tests early on. After discussing the risks and benefits of genetic testing, we would order a genetic panel that includes CFTR, SPINK1, PRSS1, and CTRC. Most patients with genetic pancreatitis don't have a family history. If there is a family history of pancreatitis, the more common genetic abnormality is PRSS, which is autosomal dominant, while the other genetic diseases are autosomal recessive.

This patient has a negative MRCP and EUS, and cholecystectomy is performed. He presents 2 months later with a third episode of pancreatitis.

How would you proceed now?

In the patient with negative imaging who has had a cholecystectomy, we would order a secretin-stimulated MRCP to look for subtle ductal abnormalities. Following that, we consider an ERCP for the possibility of sphincter of Oddi stenosis or pancreas divisum, which we discuss further in the next two cases.

Case 5 A 57-year-old woman has gone to the ER four times for acute pancreatitis over the past 8 months. There is no significant alcohol use. She had gallstones, and a cholecystectomy was performed after the first episode. In spite of that, she presents with two more episodes of pancreatitis.

After the third episode, she had an MRCP that suggested a pancreas divisum.

There are no medications that should produce pancreatitis, and there is no suggestion of autoimmune pancreatitis.

How would you manage this patient?

MRCP is fairly accurate at picking up pancreas divisum, but the finding of pancreas divisum does not necessarily make it the culprit, the cause of the recurrent pancreatitis. However, in this case, other etiologies appear unlikely—the patient had a cholecystectomy, and there is no suggestion of autoimmune pancreatitis nor medication-induced pancreatitis. Because of her age, we would first offer her an EUS to rule out any subtle suggestions of malignancy. Assuming that is negative, we would recommend proceeding to ERCP. The marked frequency of the episodes—four episodes in 8 months, dictates the more aggressive management. We would suggest an ERCP with minor ampulla sphincterotomy. This would likely end the cycle of recurrent pancreatitis.

Case 6 *A 38-year-old woman presents with recurrent pancreatitis. One year earlier, she had suspected biliary pancreatitis treated with cholecystectomy. She has occasional alcohol and does not smoke. She presents in the ER with acute abdominal pain. Examination revealed marked abdominal tenderness, decreased bowel sounds, and increased tympany. She had a lipase of 600, white cell count of 10,000, AST of 220, ALT of 350, alkaline phosphatase of 240, and bilirubin of 1.4. Ultrasound revealed a dilated CBD of 11 mm.*

How would you manage this patient?

If available, you'd like to know the post-cholecystectomy ductal diameter as a baseline. In this case, you're questioning a possible sphincter of Oddi dysfunction (SOD), most likely type 1, vs a retained stone. We would order a secretin-stimulated MRCP. Secretin increases pancreatic secretions and relaxes the pancreatic sphincter. If there is a problem with the pancreatic sphincter or sphincter of Oddi, the pancreatic duct dilates. Secretin-stimulated MRCP could help rule out choledocholithiasis and provide evidence for any sphincter dysfunction. We no longer do biliary manometry to evaluate for SOD because of the high risk of post-ERCP pancreatitis, without much benefit. While in the past we did more isolated pancreatic duct sphincterotomies, it has been found that a routine biliary sphincterotomy will benefit most patients whether the defect is in the pancreatic sphincter or biliary sphincter.

Case 7 *A 47-year-old man is referred with a history of intermittent abdominal pain accompanied by episodes of elevated lipase. There is no significant history of alcohol use, smoking, or family history of pancreatitis. A CT scan reveals enlargement of the head of the pancreas, a sausage-shaped pancreas, with atrophy of the pancreatic tail, and some surrounding lymph nodes that are mildly enlarged. The diagnosis of autoimmune pancreatitis is questioned. You send off an IgG4, and it comes back negative.*

Do you think this is autoimmune pancreatitis?

If the IgG4 had returned positive, the treatment would be clear-cut. This would almost certainly be type 1 autoimmune pancreatitis, and high-dose steroids would be indicated. In this case, the IgG4 returns negative and management is more complicated. We do look for other diseases that would suggest IgG4-associated disorder like cholangiopathy, parotid disease, or retroperitoneal fibrosis. If those are absent, we have two choices. One is an empiric high-dose steroid trial with repeat imaging in 1–2 months. Alternatively, we could do an EUS with FNA looking for histologic diagnosis of type 2 autoimmune pancreatitis and to rule out occult neoplasm.

With a large head of the pancreas and enlarged lymph nodes, neoplasm has to be considered in the differential. While pancreatic adenocarcinoma is uncommon in someone this young, these X-ray findings could be seen with pancreatic lymphoma. The fact that pancreatic lymphoma is somewhat steroid-responsive can also complicate diagnosis in this case.

If the decision was made to proceed with an FNA and the results were non-diagnostic, we would probably do the steroid trial. If there was no response to steroids, we would repeat EUS to confirm the absence of neoplasm, but in the patient with ongoing symptoms, elevated lipase, in whom we don't have a diagnosis, it is extremely tricky but we would probably have to refer the patient for surgery.

Chapter 21
Chronic Pancreatitis

Srivats Madhavan

Case 1 *A 45-year-old man who is a chronic alcoholic is referred to your office with a history of chronic abdominal pain and weight loss. He has a history of three admissions to the hospital for pancreatitis over the past 6 months. He was drinking heavily before the first admission, cut back drinking, and then after a second episode quit entirely. He had no alcohol at all for the 2 months leading up to his third admission for pancreatitis. On each admission, he has characteristic pain, an elevated lipase, and he has CT scans that show mild bile duct dilation and calcifications in the pancreas. Although his pain subsided after his first and second admission, it has become chronic since his third admission. He has cut back on meals because eating seems to worsen his pain. In addition, he is having increased frequency bowel movements that appear foamy, with oil droplets. His examination is remarkable for abdominal tenderness and some muscle wasting. His Hbg is 12, WBC 4.8, lipase 180 (normal—60), ALT 50, AST 75, Alk phos 110, Bili 1.8, and glu 108 (fasting).*

When you see a patient like this with a past history of significant alcohol consumption do you consider other etiologies for exacerbation of pancreatitis or just assume that it is alcohol?

I think it's a good idea to consider other etiologies for pancreatitis especially since he has had another episode in spite of quitting alcohol. At the very least, I would want to rule out gallstone pancreatitis and make sure the patient is not on medications that might cause pancreatitis. We want to review whether there is any familial pancreatitis and review the scans to see if the patient has developed a pancreatic duct problem that might be causing recurrent pancreatitis.

S. Madhavan (✉)
Department of Medicine, Division of Gastroenterology and Hepatology, Medical College of
Wisconsin, Milwaukee, WI, USA
e-mail: smadhavan@mcw.edu

© The Author(s), under exclusive license to Springer Nature
Switzerland AG 2023
W. H. Sobin et al. (eds.), *Managing Complex Cases in Gastroenterology*,
https://doi.org/10.1007/978-3-031-48949-5_21

145

Are there other diagnostic tests you might order?

Occasionally, I will check IgG4 levels, and if there's any family history of pancreatitis we do a genetic panel, although, in general, these are low yield. We may also do a secretin-stimulated MRCP.

How does the secretin-stimulated MRI help you?

The secretin stimulation causes an increase in pancreatic ductal secretion, which helps elucidate the morphology of the pancreatic duct and helps to demonstrate any strictures on MRI. There is another scan, the quantitative secretin-stimulated MRCP, which can be used to evaluate pancreatic function by measuring the amount of bicarbonate secreted after secretin stimulation. This is a noninvasive way of demonstrating pancreatic insufficiency.

Would you do an EUS in this patient?

The main reason for doing EUS would be to diagnose pancreatic cancer. At forty-five, he is young to have pancreatic cancer although the risk is higher because of his history of chronic pancreatitis, but in general we find the yield of EUS in acute recurrent and chronic pancreatitis to be fairly low, and it doesn't add much to what we get from CT and MRI.

How often do you see recurrent pancreatitis/chronic pancreatitis in someone who has quit drinking?

Yes, we do see this occasionally, just a few cases each year. Most patients do fairly well if they stop drinking.

How do you manage the pain in chronic pancreatitis?

The patients who have chronic pain are referred to pain management. In terms of a celiac axis block, I don't advocate for it in chronic pancreatitis because there is always recurrence of pain down the road. At best, pain relief may last for three to 6 months. However, I do advocate for celiac axis neurolysis for patients with chronic pain from pancreatic cancer.

In patients with chronic pain from chronic pancreatitis what do you think about managing pancreatic ductal strictures or stones with endoscopic therapy?

The overall data suggest that long-term pain relief is better with surgical drainage of the duct rather than endoscopic drainage. There are only a few, select patients, in whom we recommend endoscopic therapy.

If I'm going to consider a patient for endoscopic therapy for a pancreatic stricture, the stricture has to be unifocal, or else a couple of strictures close together. They have to be located in the proximal pancreatic duct, near the ampulla, and the duct needs to be large enough that drainage makes sense.

Treating pancreatic stones is more complicated than treating choledocholithiasis. The stones in CP mold to the pancreatic duct and its branches, so it's not something that will slide out of the duct easily. These stones have a lot of extensions growing into the side branches of the pancreatic duct and anchoring them in place like dendritic processes reaching into the side branches, which is why they are difficult to remove. If a stone is more than 5–6 mm in size, it will require extracorporeal shock wave lithotripsy (ESWL) to break it up before we can remove it. The idea of using a spyglass scope as used in cholangioscopy is not feasible for pancreatoscopy.

Directed lithotripsy using this approach is usually not possible because the spyglass is about ten French in diameter, making it difficult to introduce into the pancreatic duct without causing a lot of trauma, since the proximal duct is only 2–3 mm in diameter. If there is a stone located beyond the neck of the pancreas, it is not feasible to remove it unless you are doing ESWL. Note that with ESWL you also have to do a pancreatic duct sphincterotomy to get those fragments out.

Our preference, if the patient quits drinking and the surgical anatomy will allow, is to send the patient to surgery. These patients are generally younger, in their forties and fifties, and often are candidates to undergo surgery. So, I will refer them to a surgeon that I trust, but some patients may not be good surgical candidates because they have portal vein thrombosis, or have portal hypertension from alcoholic cirrhosis. In these patients, we may offer endoscopic treatment and this may involve ESWL, but for lithotripsy to be successful the pancreatic stone has to be large enough to be visualized on X-ray, usually at least 5 mm in size.

We have seen good results from the surgery. The choice of operation comes down to the individual surgeon's preference and the patient's anatomy. The two that are generally offered are the Frey and Puestow procedures. It really comes down to how much disease there is in the head of the pancreas, and the Puestow is not as beneficial if you are trying to drain areas in the head of the pancreas. Total pancreatectomy with islet cell transplant is available in a few centers across the nation, but not at our institution. We will occasionally refer patients with chronic pain for this procedure.

Here the patient has weight loss and it sounds like he may have steatorrhea. How do you evaluate patients for pancreatic insufficiency?

We use stool elastase and spot fecal fat. If the stool fat is positive and the elastase is <200 that is sufficient to diagnose pancreatic insufficiency. We do not ask patients to collect 48-h stool fats. If the spot stool fat is negative but the elastase is low and the patient has typical symptoms, I will give a trial of pancreatic enzyme replacement. We usually give Creon because most insurances will cover it. I usually don't put them on a low-fat diet, since they are already struggling with weight loss. I generally give 72,000 lipase units of Creon (two 36 K tablets) with each meal. If there is a high-fat snack, then I recommend one Creon tab with the snack.

Do you do surveillance for pancreatic cancer in these patients?

They are at some increased risk because of chronic pancreatitis. However, they tend to get scans quite frequently because of new symptoms or to monitor the course of the pancreatitis. I have a low threshold for ordering scans if they have new symptoms, but I don't put them in a specific pancreatic cancer screening program.

What are the biggest mistakes you see primary care doctors and some gastroenterologists in the community making?

I see doctors putting patients on Creon for unnecessary reasons. Say, they've had one episode of acute pancreatitis, or they've had an episode of gallstone pancreatitis, and, without any evidence of pancreatic insufficiency, they're sent home on Creon. For those who actually have pancreatic insufficiency, there is a tendency to send them home on too low a dose of Creon, so under-dosing is another problem.

We used to give patients with painful chronic pancreatitis Viokase, an uncoated pancreatic enzyme, to try to suppress CCK stimulation of the pancreas. Is that something you find efficacious to help relieve chronic pain?

When I've tried it, I have not found it to be helpful, and the latest studies bear that out, it is no longer recommended.

Case 2 A 43-year-old man presents with abdominal pain and weight loss. He has one or two beers a weekend but was never a heavy drinker. He has no history of acute pancreatitis. However, his abdominal CT scan shows pancreatic calcifications suggestive of chronic pancreatitis, and his stool elastase is decreased at 55.

When you encounter a patient with apparent chronic pancreatitis who is not a drinker what differential diagnosis comes to mind?

We occasionally see a patient who presents with pancreatic calcifications and signs of chronic pancreatitis without any past history of acute pancreatitis. First, we want to know if he is a never-drinker or if he used to drink heavily and then quit. Second, it's important to get a good family history and find out whether there is a family history of pancreatitis. You want to know the patient's ethnicity and where they grew up. In South Asia, where I went to med school, we saw a number of patients with tropical pancreatitis, and some of these patients have SPINK mutations. With tropical pancreatitis, there is a wide spectrum of disease severity but a number of patients develop chronic pancreatitis with pancreatic insufficiency and also insulin-dependent diabetes. They also have an increased risk of pancreatic cancer.

In evaluating the patient with chronic pancreatitis with no history of significant alcohol use, no family history, and born in the USA with no travel history, I get a right upper quadrant ultrasound to rule out stones, and I order an IgG4, a lipid panel, and a genetic panel. You want to know about medication and smoking history and alcohol. Of course, gallbladder disease does not tend to lead to chronic pancreatitis although it might cause acute recurrent pancreatitis.

Autoimmune pancreatitis can present as chronic pancreatitis. Note that you can have autoimmune pancreatitis with a negative IgG4 and you can be IgG4 positive and not have autoimmune pancreatitis (SLE, IBD, etc.).

Cystic fibrosis is often associated with chronic pancreatitis, and the CFTR gene mutation can contribute to pancreatitis in patients without cystic fibrosis.

While we used to do EUS in idiopathic and chronic idiopathic pancreatitis, we have shied away from it because it has a low yield. Of the past forty patients, I did an EUS on with idiopathic pancreatitis and the only positive was one patient with microlithiasis.

Does the finding of pancreatic calcifications make chronic pancreatitis almost a certainty?

Pancreatic calcifications can occasionally be seen in patients with a history of abdominal trauma and occasionally splenic artery calcification may be misinterpreted as chronic pancreatitis. So, no, the reading of calcifications over the region of the pancreas is not pathognomonic for chronic pancreatitis.

Do you see much recurring acute pancreatitis or chronic pancreatitis from medications?

We are seeing a number of patients with checkpoint inhibitor-induced pancreatitis that acts in a similar fashion to autoimmune pancreatitis. Most of these patients respond to steroids. After 2–3 months of steroid therapy, we try to taper the steroids and transition to azathioprine or mycophenolate.

We have also seen patients with recurrent pancreatitis from ACE inhibitors and ARBS, also from HIV drugs.

How do you address patients with chronic pancreatitis who are asymptomatic?

We have some patients referred to us because in the evaluation of alcoholic cirrhosis they are found to have X-ray findings of chronic pancreatitis. They are often asymptomatic and have no signs of pancreatic insufficiency. Of course, we encourage alcohol abstinence and want to know about any future symptoms, but in the patient who is asymptomatic we generally don't recommend any intervention.

Chapter 22
GI Oncology

Ben George

Case 1 *A 67-year-old woman presents with iron deficiency anemia and has a colonoscopy that reveals adenocarcinoma of the ascending colon. Following right hemicolectomy, it is determined that she has stage 3 colon cancer.*

Is it true that most stage 3 and some stage 2 colon cancers should receive adjuvant chemotherapy and that the adjuvant therapy of choice is usually oxaliplatin and a fluoropyrimidine?

All localized colon cancers at the time of surgery should be tested to see whether the tumors are mismatch repair-deficient, or mismatch repair-proficient.

In general, all stage three colon cancers require adjuvant chemotherapy. Adjuvant chemotherapy can be for a duration of 3 months or 6 months. The chemotherapy agents most commonly utilized are a combination of oxaliplatin and a fluoropyrimidine so that will be FOLFOX or CAPOX.

Looking first at stage 3, there are a number of decisions to be made. Should the duration of therapy be 3 months or 6 months? Should everyone get the fluoropyrimidine and oxaliplatin combination, or, for older people, are there ways in which we can de-escalate the chemotherapy? How do we deal with chemotherapy side effects in these patients? Are there patients in whom we should shorten the chemotherapy program?

In general, patients who have early stage 3 disease-like T3N1 can get away with 3 months of chemotherapy. In general, the treatment of choice is CAPOX, capecitabine, and oxaliplatin. Any patient with T3N2 or higher should receive 6 months of adjuvant chemotherapy, which can be either CAPOX or FOLFOX.

B. George (✉)
Division of Hematology and Oncology, Department of Medicine, Medical College of Wisconsin, Milwaukee, WI, USA
e-mail: bgeorge@mcw.edu

While we are still discussing stage 3 disease, how do we manage older people? Patients who are 70 and older may have problems handling doublet chemotherapy. In these patients, I think it is reasonable to administer leucovorin-modulated fluoropyrimidine alone for a total duration of 6 months.

In the younger patient who starts out with adjuvant chemotherapy including fluoropyrimidine and oxaliplatin, if rate limiting peripheral neuropathy develops in 3–4 months, it is reasonable to de-escalate to fluoropyrimidine alone (if the neuropathy is relatively severe, grade 3 or 4).

Adjuvant chemotherapy in stage 2 disease is generally restricted to those patients who are deemed to have high-risk disease. It is high risk if you have a perforated tumor, an obstructing tumor, inadequate lymph node dissection (less than 12 lymph nodes), or a poorly differentiated tumor. Lymphovascular invasion and margin positivity would be considered high-risk features as well. Ideally, anyone with high-risk stage 2 colon cancer should receive 6 months of adjuvant chemotherapy with either single-agent fluoropyrimidine, or, preferably, combination of fluoropyrimidine and oxaliplatin, FOLFOX. If you're using CAPOX, you can get away with 3 months of CAPOX in high-risk stage 2 colon cancers. If you're using FOLFOX, you need 6 months.

Now, there are a couple of exceptions to the rules. We started out saying that all tumors should be checked to see whether they are mismatch repair-deficient, or mismatch repair-proficient. If the tumor is stage 2 and it is mismatch repair-deficient, then you can get away without any adjuvant chemotherapy simply because the risk of metastasis is very low. In the stage 3 setting, even if the tumor is mismatch repair-deficient, we prefer to give the full prescribed course of chemotherapy.

There are other new ways in which you can risk stratify stage 2 colon cancers over and beyond the pathologic features. One tool we are using is oncotype DX, a genomic panel to help with risk stratification. If deemed high risk on oncotype DX, it is better to receive chemotherapy but if low risk, surveillance alone following surgery is appropriate. If you're high risk, you're better off with combination chemotherapy.

Another tool available for risk stratification in the adjuvant setting is minimal residual disease (MRD)assessment in the circulation. It is a blood test using DNA from the patient's tumor. If MRD assay is positive, the risk of relapse is high. For stage 2, colon cancers with positive MRD adjuvant chemotherapy is a reasonable option. How long should it be given to these patients? Should chemotherapy be administered until the MRD assay returns negative? Should we change the adjuvant chemotherapy agents if the MRD is not impacted? We still don't know. There are trials that are addressing this question, which summarizes the adjuvant chemotherapy landscape for stage 3 and stage 2 colon cancer.

Can you discuss the differences between 5FU, leucovorin, and capecitabine?

5FU and leucovorin are administered together as an IV infusion. Capecitabine is a pill formulation of 5-FU. 5FU, when it is infused, is a continuous infusion over a duration of two days. Capecitabine is cycled as a 2-week on, 1-week off, regimen, where you take the pills morning and night. There are some subtle differences between their side effect profiles in that capecitabine tends to cause more hand-foot skin reaction than 5FU and leucovorin, but, otherwise, the side effect profile is fairly similar. Secondly, with capecitabine, you need to do dose modifications for kidney and liver dysfunction. With 5FU and leucovorin, you don't need to make any dose adjustments for liver or kidney dysfunction, though cautious use is recommended in the setting of kidney/liver dysfunction. Capecitabine is more convenient, since it is a pill, while 5FU needs to be administered IV through a port.

Is leucovorin always given as an adjunct to 5FU?

Yes, you don't need leucovorin along with capecitabine, but leucovorin is given as an adjunct to 5FU, more as a catalyst to stabilize the interaction of 5FU with thymidylate synthetase, thereby facilitating the function of 5FU. It helps form a ternary complex that enhances drug action.

Is there something about adenocarcinoma of the GI tract where it responds better to fluoropyrimidines and platinum drugs? I know these are used in esophageal and pancreatic adenocarcinoma and colon cancer.

Yes, but we don't necessarily have a great explanation for why tumors in the GI tract respond better to these agents. In fact, there are some subtle differences in that among the platinums, the only platinum that is active in colon cancer is oxaliplatin. The other platinum drugs used in oncology, cisplatin and carboplatin, are active in both pancreas and gastroesophageal cancer, but not so much in colon cancer. We don't have a good explanation for why these agents, in general, are active in GI cancers.

Is it true that patients with KRAS mutations respond poorly to EGFR inhibitors?

First of all, KRAS mutations in general are thought to be negative prognostic indicators in patients with colon cancer, but the predictive value of KRAS has been rigorously validated in the metastatic setting, not so much in the adjuvant setting. We don't use anti-EGFR-directed therapy for stage 2 or stage 3 colon cancer, but we use it in the metastatic setting. In the metastatic setting, patients with KRAS mutations do not respond to anti-EGFR-directed therapy simply because the KRAS mutation is downstream of EGFR and therefore that pathway is already constituently activated with KRAS mutation. So, blocking EGFR does not necessarily help in that scenario.

Is it true that right-sided colon cancers respond better to VEGF inhibitors and left-sided respond better to EGFR inhibitors?

Yes, and in addition, the sidedness of colon cancer is both prognostic and predictive. Right-sided colon cancers in general tend to behave worse than left-sided colon cancer. Several reasons have been postulated to explain this, but we don't know the exact reasons completely.

We think left-sided colon cancers may get diagnosed a little sooner because of symptoms than right-sided tumors. The right-sided cancers may get diagnosed later in the disease course because you don't get into obstructive-type symptoms. Secondly, patients with right-sided colon cancer are more likely to harbor BRAF mutations, which have a negative prognostic effect as well.

Third, the embryonic origin of the right side of the colon is different compared to the left side of the colon and that could predispose to the different behavior.

If you're looking at a biologic therapy to be used in combination with chemotherapy, right-sided colon cancers respond better to VEGF inhibitors than anti-EGFR-directed therapy. So, for tumors in the right side of the colon, when you're combining a biologic agent with chemotherapy, anti-VEGF agents work much better than anti-EGFR-directed therapy. That may partly be because there is a substantial proportion of patients with right-sided colon cancers that harbor BRAF mutations, but even in tumors that are wild type for KRAS or BRAF we see that the anti-EGFR-directed therapies just don't work as well for the right-sided tumors (compared to left-sided colon tumors) for reasons that are not very clear.

Conversely, for left-sided tumors, anti-VEGF therapies work well in combination with chemotherapy, but for KRAS wild-type tumors, the anti-EGFR therapies may work a little better than anti-VEGF therapies. Anti-EGFR therapies for left-sided colon tumors are effective only in the KRAS and BRAF wild-type tumors.

In a patient with newly diagnosed metastatic disease would you use bevacizumab?

If a patient develops metastatic disease and it starts in the right colon, bevacizumab should be added to chemotherapy backbone (in the absence of contraindications to bevacizumab). For right-sided colon cancers that present with metastatic disease, the chemotherapy backbone would be either FOLFOX (5FU and oxaliplatin), FOLFIRI (5 FU and irinotecan), or FOLFOXIRI (5FU, oxaliplatin, and irinotecan), which is a triplet of the 3.

Case 2 A 48-year-old man is found to have a right-sided colon cancer and is suspected of having Lynch syndrome. Testing is ordered on tissue obtained during colonoscopy, and results show it is microsatellite unstable (MSI-H) and there is an MLH1 mutation consistent with Lynch syndrome.

Having these results would you suggest the patient have a more extensive operation (subtotal colectomy)?

Yes, first of all, when you see an MLH1 mutation in the tumor in a young man you certainly worry about Lynch syndrome, but you need to coordinate germline testing to make sure that this is truly a Lynch and not a sporadic MLH1 mutation. If the patient harbors a germline MLH1 mutation (Lynch syndrome), I think it is very reasonable to do a subtotal colectomy or even a proctocolectomy, after an informed discussion between the patient and the surgeon.

Assuming the patient is found to have stage 3 disease would you avoid using a fluoropyrimidine because they are less effective in Lynch syndrome?

That's a great question. There was a time when we thought that single-agent fluoropyrimidine was not effective in patients with mismatch repair deficiency. Therefore, we always advocated for combination therapy—fluoropyrimidine and oxaliplatin. As we see more data, it seems that fluoropyrimidines may actually be effective in patients with Lynch syndrome.

Would you choose to use a checkpoint inhibitor here because they are more effective in Lynch syndrome?

There are no mature data currently that suggest using checkpoint blockade in the adjuvant setting in a patient with Lynch syndrome, and there are ongoing trials trying to answer this question. However, it has certainly been found to be effective in the metastatic setting. In Lynch syndrome, the use of checkpoint blockade alone as a single agent results in high response rates.

Do you agree that for the same stage of colon cancer, patients with microsatellite unstable colon cancers have a better prognosis than patients with sporadic colon cancer?

It is very important to emphasize that mismatch repair deficiency/microsatellite instability can be germline (Lynch syndrome) or acquired. The percentage of patients with microsatellite instability incidence is about 15% in patients with localized colon cancer, but in the metastatic setting, that percentage is much lower, about 5%. This is because microsatellite unstable tumors do not metastasize as much. In addition, these patients are very often part of a screening program, and things get picked up sooner, but, regardless, they tend to have better disease biology, and better prognosis, stage for stage than sporadic colon cancer.

Case 3 *A 68-year-old woman with alcoholic cirrhosis (abstinent for 5 years) was having routine surveillance USA and AFP every 6 months but then missed follow-up for 18 months. She is found to have two hepatomas, one 4 cm in size and another one is 5 cm. AFP is 600. TACE is performed, and both lesions decrease in size to 3 cm. However, the AFP rose to 700. The patient's functional status is good.*

Can you discuss the use of systemic chemotherapy in this setting?

An important question here is whether this woman could potentially be a transplant candidate. With tumor downsizing after TACE, the patient meets Milan criteria—a set of criteria that determines transplant eligibility.

So, let's think about it in two different ways. First, let's say the patient is deemed not to be a transplant candidate after medical evaluation by the transplant team. If she is not a transplant candidate, the best systemic therapy options for this patient are either a combination of bevacizumab + atezolizumab or tremelimumab (anti-cytotoxic T lymphocyte-associated antigen 4) plus durvalumab (anti-programmed cell death ligand-1).

Prior to receiving bevacizumab + atezolizumab, patients need to undergo an EGD to assess for varices and undergo variceal banding.

The other frontline systemic therapy options include lenvatinib and sorafenib, but certainly the preference would be either bevacizumab + atezolizumab or tremelimumab plus durvalumab on account of their efficacy and toxicity profile.

If the patient is a transplant candidate, immunotherapy should be avoided in the pre-transplant setting. The optimal systemic therapy options would be lenvatinib or sorafenib but preferably lenvatinib due to the higher objective response rates.

Has lenvatinib largely supplanted sorafenib in patients who have contraindications to immunotherapy and get tyrosine kinase inhibitor therapy?

Yes, lenvatinib has for the most part supplanted sorafenib, because of improved efficacy. That said, the side effect profile is not necessarily more favorable than sorafenib, it's just different.

Are checkpoint inhibitors felt to be less effective in HCC associated with alcohol? associated with NASH?

We don't have prospective data addressing that specific question. However, the available data certainly seem to indicate that checkpoint inhibitors are more effective in viral-induced (hepatitis B and hepatitis C) HCC compared to sorafenib. The magnitude of benefit with checkpoint inhibitors appears to be less compared to sorafenib in patients with hepatocellular carcinoma due to non-viral etiologies.

Right now, we are not prioritizing treatment based on etiology of HCC, but this may become part of routine clinical practice in the future as more data emerge.

Case 4 *A 67-year-old man presenting with dysphagia is found to have adenocarcinoma of the esophagogastric junction (EGJ). EUS shows positive lymph nodes. Tumor markers are sent off and the tumor has HER-2 overexpression.*

Do you manage adenocarcinoma of the esophagus the same as adenocarcinoma of the stomach?

Yes and no. For all intents and purposes, the chemotherapy agents that are active in adenocarcinomas of the stomach and the esophagus/EG junction are very similar. However, there are some key differences between tumors of the distal esophagus/EG junction, and tumors in the stomach, particularly as it pertains to treatment for localized disease. From a staging perspective, a diagnostic laparoscopy to look for peritoneal carcinomatosis is mandated for T2 or higher tumors in the stomach while that is not done routinely for tumors of the distal esophagus/GE junction (dictated by patterns of spread). In terms of neoadjuvant/peri-operative treatment, radiotherapy is more commonly utilized in tumors of the distal esophagus/EG junction than tumors of the stomach. Surgical approaches are different for these entities as well.

There are some biological differences between these entities as well. We know that tumors in the EG junction are more likely to overexpress HER2/neu than tumors in the stomach. Similarly, tumors that originate in the EG junction are more likely to respond to immunotherapy than tumors that originate in the stomach based on available data (this has not been prospectively validated).

At a molecular level, tumors in the distal esophagus/EG junction and stomach are classified into four distinct subgroups: (a) chromosomally unstable (CIN), (b) genomically stable, (c) microsatellite unstable, and (d) the EBV-positive.

The EG junction tumors tend to belong to the chromosomally unstable subtype (characterized by alterations in the signal transduction pathway) and the EBV-positive subtype (characterized by alterations in thePI3 kinase pathway and greater likelihood of response to immunotherapy).

Microsatellite unstable tumors tend to be present throughout the stomach, with a preponderance in the distal stomach while the genomically stable subtype correlates very closely with linitis plastica or diffuse gastric cancer.

Why might trastuzumab be useful in the above patient, with HER-2 overexpression?

Trastuzumab is a monoclonal antibody that binds to ERBB2 (Her-2) preventing the dimerization with ERBB3 and inhibiting downstream signaling that contributes to cancer progression. So essentially, it's a targeted agent that improves treatment response and prolongs survival in patients with metastatic EG junction/gastric cancers with a very favorable toxicity profile.

Can you discuss the general approach to treatment of localized adenocarcinoma of the esophagus (and stomach)?

For localized tumors of the esophagus and EG junction, we typically use neoadjuvant chemotherapy and radiation, followed by surgery for curative intent treatment. For tumors of the stomach, we use neoadjuvant or perioperative chemotherapy and surgery for curative intent therapy. The role of radiation in tumors of the stomach is controversial and it's not routinely used.

Is there a role for checkpoint inhibitors?

Yes, there is a role for utilizing a checkpoint inhibitor in the treatment of metastatic disease regardless of the PD-L1 expression. Typically, the frontline systemic therapy program for tumors of the stomach and distal esophagus/EG junction includes a fluoropyrimidine, a platinum, and a checkpoint inhibitor, if the tumor does not over express HER2/neu. If HER2/neu overexpression is present, we utilize a combination of fluoropyrimidine, platinum, trastuzumab, and a checkpoint inhibitor.

Case 5 *A 71-year-old woman presents with abdominal pain, weight loss, and new-onset diabetes. A CAT scan reveals probable cancer of the body of the pancreas. EUS shows malignant appearing lymph nodes and FNA is positive for adenocarcinoma. Genetic testing is performed that includes MSI testing and homologous recombination deficiency (HRD) testing.*

Is it true that when we talk about HRD testing we are checking for mutations in all of these genes: *BRCA1/2*, *PALB2*, *ATM*, *BAP1*, *BARD1*, *BLM*, *BRIP1*, *CHEK2*, *FAM175A*, *FANCA*, *FANCC*, *NBN*, *RAD50*, *RAD51*, *RAD51C*, and *RTEL1*?

We are interested in assessing the HRD status of pancreas cancers to help make treatment decisions. Assays that determine the HRD status of tumors use different methods, and the parameters tested vary based on the assay that is utilized. It is true that many of the above genes play a key role in DNA damage repair.

Is it true that if a pancreas cancer is found to have HRD you will turn to a platinum-based therapy like FOLFOX or FOLFIRINOX?

Yes, we will utilize platinum-based chemotherapy if a pancreatic adenocarcinoma harbors HRD.

Are all patients with pancreatic cancer getting this genetic testing done?

We offer germline testing to all patients with pancreatic cancer, and it has been incorporated in national guidelines.

Is gemcitabine commonly used anymore-alone or with nabpaclitaxil?

Yes, gemcitabine is used quite a bit both in the treatment of metastatic and localized pancreatic adenocarcinomas. Gemcitabine can be used as a single agent or in combination (with Nab-paclitaxel or Nab-paclitaxel and cisplatin). Gemcitabine is also utilized as a single agent for purposes of radio-sensitization in patients who undergo concurrent chemoradiotherapy.

When do you use a PARP inhibitor and how does it work?

PARP inhibitors are used currently in patients with pancreatic adenocarcinoma who have germline pathogenic alterations in BRCA1 and BRCA2. It is utilized for maintenance therapy in patients with metastatic pancreas cancer who are platinum-responsive. Olaparib is the PARP inhibitor approved for use in pancreatic adenocarcinoma., The idea behind treatment with the PARP inhibitors is that they cause synthetic lethality in the cancer cells of patients who have BRCA1 or BRCA2 germline alterations. Normally, PARP helps in the repair of single-stranded DNA breaks and PARP inhibitors prevent that. So, DNA in cancer cells that are exposed to DNA-damaging drugs undergo single- and double-stranded DNA breaks, and PARP inhibitors prevent the cancer cells from repairing them, causing increased cancer cell death.

Are you using checkpoint inhibitors in pancreatic cancer?

There are a lot of clinical trials in this space. Currently, there is no proven role for checkpoint inhibitors in pancreas cancer other than in the 1% of tumors that have a deficient mismatch repair gene status. There is also a very small percentage of pancreatic adenocarcinomas with an elevated tumor mutational burden that may respond to checkpoint inhibitors as well.

Are there any other points about pancreatic cancer management that you would like to emphasize for the community gastroenterologist?

One point I'd like to stress is the importance of a metallic common bile duct stent (as opposed to a plastic stent)—once tissue diagnosis is established—in patients with pancreatic head adenocarcinomas that cause biliary compromise. This helps decrease the incidence of stent occlusion and cholangitis in patients with pancreatic adenocarcinoma while on treatment.

Chapter 23
Issues in Therapeutic Endoscopy

Kulwinder Dua

Management of Refractory Benign Esophageal Stricture (RBES) Including Placement of Esophageal Stents

Case 1 *A 70-year-old man has prolonged NG tube insertion after a complicated colon resection for diverticulitis. Following that, he develops dysphagia. An EGD shows a tight stricture in the mid-to-distal esophagus from 27 to 37 cm, and biopsies are benign. He has received several endoscopic dilations but continues to re-stricture and is referred to you.*

How do you manage a patient with a refractory benign esophageal stricture?
The definition of RBES is that one cannot achieve an esophageal luminal diameter of ≥14 mm despite one dilation done every 2 weeks × 5 or if the patient requires one dilation every 4 weeks to maintain a diameter of ≥14 mm. In this patient, the stricture is due to prolonged trauma from the NG tube and damage from acid refluxing alongside the tube (like capillary action) for prolonged periods. Some of the other causes of RBES include corrosive ingestion, pill injury, radiation-related, post-endoscopic mucosal resections and ablations, and surgery.

In patients with RBES, besides etiology, it is important to know the diameter to which the patient was dilated previously, the frequency of dilations, and how soon the patient developed recurrent dysphagia. Based on this, one can decide on a treatment plan. Let's say you are dilating every 4 weeks and you can only achieve a diameter of 12 mm, then you need to dilate every 2 weeks. If you are going two steps forward and then two steps backward every 2 weeks, then you need to dilate

K. Dua (✉)
GI and Hepatology Division, Dept. of Medicine, Medical College of Wisconsin,
Milwaukee, WI, USA
e-mail: kdua@mcw.edu

© The Author(s), under exclusive license to Springer Nature
Switzerland AG 2023
W. H. Sobin et al. (eds.), *Managing Complex Cases in Gastroenterology*,
https://doi.org/10.1007/978-3-031-48949-5_23

every week. One can also consider injecting steroids (triamcinolone) into the stricture to delay fibrosis and recurrence. There is no limit to how many times you inject triamcinolone. If the stricture keeps closing up after each dilation, I would inject at every dilation.

At each dilation session, assess how much the stricture has regressed and then decide whether you need to increase or decrease the frequency of dilations (two steps forward and one step backward), but even though you are making progress you never want to leave the patient for more than 2 weeks without repeat dilation until you have achieved your goal. Once a diameter of 14–18 mm is achieved and maintained at weekly or every 2-week dilations, lengthen the interval between dilations. If the stricture continues to regress, one can consider other interventions, such as stent insertion, electrocautery incision, or both.

What sort of stents do you place?

The self-expanding stent has to be a fully covered stent so that it can be removed at a later date. If the stent is uncovered or partly covered, it will get embedded in the esophageal wall and may not be easy to remove. The only fully covered stent that is FDA approved and available in the USA for benign esophageal stricture is a plastic expandable stent (Polyflex® stent). This stent is difficult to load, has a high migration rate, and tends to cause chest pain. As a result, most gastroenterologists are using fully covered metal expandable stents, off-label.

For precise placement such as when the strictures are near (<2 cm) the UES, as we sometimes see in head and neck cancers after radiation therapy, non-foreshortening stents (laser-cut) are preferred. More often, we tend to use electrocautery and avoid placing stents in this location if the stricture is short and like a shelf.

When the stricture is in the lower esophagus and failed dilations, we will use stents, even if they need to bridge the LES. However, patients are predisposed to having significant gastroesophageal reflux that can create a considerable aspiration risk. Therefore, we have to use strict anti-reflux measures in these cases.

Stents for RBES are usually left in for 2–4 weeks. After removing the stent, reinstitute regular esophageal dilations. For those who fail the above approach, we offer them surgery (in many cases, this may not be possible) or train them to do self-dilation.

How do you teach self-dilation?

All patients get apprehensive when told about self-dilation. Good discussion with the patient and showing them videos of those who have successfully adopted this approach help. Patient is initially dilated to a diameter of 16–18 mm endoscopically. A week or so later, the patient is taught to self-dilate holding a non-wire-guided weighted dilator (such as the Maloney® dilator) of around 15 mm diameter, sitting on a chair, and watching the dilator go down under fluoroscopy (biofeedback), and immediately repeat without fluoroscopy. After that, the patient takes the dilator home and dilates himself once or twice a day. Initially, patients like to use some viscous lidocaine, but after a week or two it's no longer necessary. If, after a while, the patient finds it is once again becoming more difficult to pass the dilator because the stricture is tightening, we bring the patient back and dilate them endoscopically to 16–18 mm and after that they find the 15-mm self-dilation go easily again.

How do you decide what type of dilator to use in treating a benign esophageal stricture?

In talking about the type of dilator used, there are balloon dilators that have good radial force and there are bougies that have both radial and longitudinal force. In expert hands, the safety profile is equivalent. It is a good idea to use a bougie in cases where the stricture is long, or multifocal as bougies cause pan-esophageal dilation. These kinds of strictures are usually encountered with corrosives, radiation, and prolonged NG tube use. Balloon dilators are certainly acceptable for short strictures, such as anastomotic strictures, or short peptic strictures.

Case 2 *A 72-year-old smoker presents with dysphagia and is found to have a tight stricture of the mid-esophagus caused by esophageal squamous cell cancer. Chemoradiation is planned.*

Is there a role for a stent in this malignant esophageal stricture?

Generally, no; the initial enthusiasm for stents as a bridge to surgery for those receiving neoadjuvant therapy or even for those receiving palliative chemotherapy has been dampened by the high rate of adverse events and side effects from stents that may interrupt chemo-/chemoradiation treatments. With the tumor regressing and becoming "softer" with chemo-/chemoradiation treatments, stents can migrate, cause ulcers and bleeding, and perforate the esophagus.

Stents, however, are very effective in immediately relieving dysphagia. Therefore, if we have a patient with severe dysphagia (barely able to swallow liquids or total dysphagia), we will communicate with the oncologist and find out how long a delay they anticipate before chemoradiation will be started and how long a lag period between initiation of therapy and when tumor response is anticipated. If therapy is being delayed for a month and response will probably take 2 weeks, we may decide to place a temporary stent if the patient is suffering from severe dysphagia. In this instance, we will consider placement of a fully covered metal stent as a temporary bridge so that the patient can swallow and plan on removing it around the time chemo-/chemoradiation therapy is being initiated to avoid delayed stent-related adverse events. If the dysphagia is just for solids, I would not place a stent because I am fine with the patient simply swallowing a soft diet or liquids, such as Ensure and milkshakes.

Covered stents are the treatment of choice for those who have esophageal-airway fistulae or perforations. In these patients, available options, including stenting, should be discussed in a tumor-board or multidisciplinary meeting.

What about using an esophageal stent for a malignant stricture where the patient refuses chemoradiation?

It is important to discuss the expectations the patient may have about stents. The best one can eat with a stent is a soft-liquid diet, not a normal diet. So, do not place stents in those who are eating a soft diet at baseline.

In patients receiving a stent for palliation, it is important to counterbalance the benefits of the stent vs the side effects/adverse events. If the patient does not want any palliative chemoradiation, then optimally one can place a partially covered stent where the upper and lower ends of the stent are uncovered. This will allow tissue ingrowth and embed the stent, which will prevent migration, but if the patient changes his/her mind and decides to go for chemoradiation, removing the stent will be difficult (if not impossible). Therefore, one should have a frank discussion about this with the patient before placing the stent. Alternatively, fully covered stents with fixing devices to prevent migration can also be used in these patients for potential removal in the future if needed.

The other problem with the partly covered stent, along with the fact that it is not easily removed, is that you tend to get tumor ingrowth, which may eventually lead to secondary dysphagia.

In most cases of malignant stricture, we are reserving stents for patients who can barely handle liquids. We are placing stents in patients with severe, grade 3 or 4 dysphagia, but will not consider them with mild (grade 1 or 2) dysphagia.

Case 3 *A 67-year-old man receiving radiation therapy for metastatic lung cancer with enlarged mediastinal lymph nodes has a tight extrinsic compression of his mid-esophagus. The esophageal mucosa itself appears normal.*

What is the role of an esophageal stent in a case of extrinsic, malignant obstruction?

The best approach for extrinsic compression will be to treat the underlying cause, which may not always be easy or possible. However, if there is hope that planned chemoradiation or surgery will resolve the extrinsic pressure, one can consider placing a removable stent for the patient with grade 3 or 4 dysphagia.

A concern about stenting an extrinsic compression is that the mass may be pressing on the left or right main stem bronchus or trachea, and the moment the stent expands, it may cause occlusion of the airways. With upper esophageal cancers or obstruction from a mediastinal mass, it is very important to get and review a good quality CT scan of the chest to ensure that there is no impending airway compression.

If you have a patient who will be getting treatment and is not at risk of airway obstruction, one can place a fully covered stent and fix it in place, or place a partially uncovered stent based on long-term outcomes as discussed above.

Nutrition Needs

Although stents relieve dysphagia and allow feeding, often patients don't eat enough secondary to either chest discomfort or anorexia from chemotherapy. In these patients, one can consider alternatives such as placing a G- or a J-tube to supplement nutrition, while the stent improves quality of life, allowing the patient to take oral feeding.

Pancreatic Cancer

Case 4 *A 68-year-old man comes in with painless jaundice. He has no history of alcohol use, diabetes, or gallbladder disease. On examination, he is jaundiced; examination is otherwise unremarkable. His laboratory findings include: Bili 5.6, Alk phos 320, ALT 70, AST 55, and lipase 300.*

An ultrasound shows a dilated common bile duct, a normal gallbladder and liver, and a questionable mass in the head of the pancreas.

In a case of painless jaundice, what imaging studies do you like to start with?

If the patient has no contraindication (renal insufficiency or dye allergy), the preferred study will be a pancreas protocol CT scan with IV contrast. This provides accurate staging of the disease and must be done before other procedures such as EUS-FNA/B or ERCP, as these other procedures can result in pancreatitis, and then, CT staging can get clouded. If CT with contrast cannot be done, then MRI can be considered. One would also like to order a CA 19-9 on the patient.

The community gastroenterologist plans on doing an ERCP on this patient to decompress the bile duct with a plastic stent and do diagnostic brushing of the bile duct for tissue diagnosis. What do you think of this approach?

No, this is the wrong approach. This decision is based on two faulty premises. The first is the fear that if a patient is jaundiced from presumed pancreatic cancer, the patient is at a high risk of getting cholangitis. Patients with malignant obstruction of the bile duct rarely develop cholangitis. The second is that doing an ERCP and cytology brushing is an efficient way of making a tissue diagnosis, but it is not. An EUS-FNA is far superior. Moreover, EUS-FNA-ERCP-metal stent ("one-stop shop") all can be done in one setting with rapid on-site rapid cytology (ROSE) evaluation by a cytopathologist. Hence, if one does not have EUS-FNA and ROSE available, one should not do ERCP and, instead, refer the patient to a tertiary care center. Moreover, placing plastic biliary stents (because metal stents for durable biliary drainage should not be placed without tissue diagnosis) carries an increased risk of recurrent cholangitis. In addition, the patient will have to have another ERCP to exchange for a metal stent if the brushing came back positive for cancer, hence, all the more reason to refer these patients to centers with expertise.

Even in those with resectable pancreatic cancer, this approach of "one-stop shop" is being widely used, as more and more patients with resectable pancreatic cancer are getting neoadjuvant therapy rather than early surgery. Tissue diagnosis and durable biliary drainage are essential prerequisites for neoadjuvant therapy, and if, indeed, the patient is being considered for early surgery, biliary drainage before surgery is not required and can be detrimental. Hence, in this patient, ERCP should not be done.

Case 5 *A 65-year-old man presents with an episode of acute pancreatitis. There is no history of diabetes. He does not drink much alcohol. An ultrasound shows a normal gallbladder. A pancreas protocol CT shows pancreatitis but no mass or no stone. A CA 19-9 is sent off and returns 50 (normal is up to 35).*

What do you do when you suspect a patient may have pancreatic cancer but there is no mass on US or CT?

Not every case of obscure pancreatitis is pancreatic cancer. Some patients may have microlithiasis, etc., but when we see a patient who comes in out of the blue with pancreatitis we worry about pancreatic cancer, while keeping the rest of the differential in mind. Also, there can be a nonspecific rise in CA 19-9 with pancreatitis.

In the face of active pancreatitis, an EUS is less helpful as pancreatitis will show up as diffuse or focal hypoechogenicity of the pancreas, and a cancer can be missed. So, in a number of these cases, where one is concerned about possible pancreatic cancer, it is best to wait and let the inflammation settle down in 4–6 weeks and then repeat the pancreas protocol CT scan and CA 19-9. Then, one could consider EUS.

We recently saw a patient referred by one of our pancreatic surgeons because the patient had a dilated upstream pancreatic duct that stopped abruptly at the neck of the pancreas. This patient did not have pancreatitis and had undergone two MRIs and three CT scans in the last 5 months, and no mass was identified. On EUS, there was a half-cm hypoechogenic mass at the site of pancreatic duct obstruction that on FNA turned out to be a mucinous adenocarcinoma.

Here's another scenario. A patient with elevated liver enzymes is seen who doesn't have pancreatitis, but does have a bile duct that is mildly dilated. A CA 19-9 can be elevated in patients with bile duct obstruction. There is no mass in the pancreas in this patient. Could the dilation be due to stones? Could this be a cholangiocarcinoma along the wall of the bile duct? In these situations, we do an EUS, even if there is no mass identified on imaging studies.

Are there any red flags that make you worry that someone with some subtle findings could have pancreatic cancer when others aren't suspecting it?

I worry about this in an elderly person with unexplained weight loss or an unexplained attack of pancreatitis. I also worry if I see someone with an elevated CA 19-9. If normal is around 35 but I see a patient who is smoldering around 110, but nothing is showing up on the pancreas protocol CT scan, I still worry. Then, there are cases where someone has a family history with two members who had pancreatic cancer or a family member who had breast or ovarian cancer and was BRCA positive. In all these cases if pancreatic protocol CT is negative, we still do an EUS. In families with a worrisome history, we may do EUS and MRI in alternate years as part of our screening process.

Similarly, patients with pancreatic cysts/dilated main pancreatic duct with worrisome or high-risk features do merit an EUS (at times, these patients get operated upon based on these worrisome features).

Sometimes, we have the opposite problem, where the CT scan and EUS definitely show a lesion that looks like cancer but repeated FNA is negative for cancer. A recent patient presented with jaundice and a mass on CT scan; CA 19-9 was 900, and EUS with FNA/B was repeatedly negative. Everyone thought this was pancreatic cancer, but the oncologist would not give neoadjuvant therapy without a positive tissue diagnosis. Whipple surgery was being considered. However, prior to surgery a therapeutic trial of oral steroids was given, and sure enough, the "tumor" melted away and the CA 19-9 dropped precipitously. The jaundice resolved without a stent. Apparently, this patient has autoimmune pancreatitis, but had there been no response to steroids early Whipple would have been appropriate.

.

Chapter 24
GI Pharmacology:

Elizabeth Pieper

Eosinophilic Esophagitis

Case 1 *A 26-year-old man is diagnosed with presumed eosinophilic esophagitis (EOE) after an EGD is performed to remove a food impaction. Biopsies are done which confirm the physician's impression of EOE. The patient is started on PPIs empirically. A repeat EGD is performed 2 months later because of ongoing dysphagia, and repeat biopsies show a decrease in the eosinophil count from 90/hpf to 50/hpf, but because of the continued eosinophilia the request is made to start steroids.*

What steroid preparations do you have available for your patients, and what are the problems with insurance access?

The drug we've used the longest is fluticasone with patients swallowing the inhaled form. With fluticasone, the standard dose is 440 mcg twice a day. The hardest part though is to ensure the patient understands how to administer it, because the natural response is that everyone wants to inhale the contents. It's difficult to conceptualize that you are actually spraying it into your mouth and putting up your tongue to block it from going into your lungs so that you can swallow the liquid.

Regrettably, most pharmacists in the community who are filling these prescriptions are not necessarily familiar with EOE because this condition is not regularly taught in pharmacy school. Therefore, staff may inappropriately educate the patient thinking this is being used for asthma. I advise that the provider includes the indication for EOE and that the patient is supposed to swallow contents and not inhale it to prevent administration errors.

E. Pieper (✉)
Department of Gastroenterology and Hepatology, Froedtert Hospital, Milwaukee, WI, USA
e-mail: Elizabeth.pieper@froedtert.com

© The Author(s), under exclusive license to Springer Nature Switzerland AG 2023
W. H. Sobin et al. (eds.), *Managing Complex Cases in Gastroenterology*,
https://doi.org/10.1007/978-3-031-48949-5_24

Additionally, the fluticasone inhaler is a branded medication; therefore, insurance coverage can sometimes be a problem. When this is an issue, we may use budesonide slurry, which is available as a generic (as a respule) and works well. Once again, we are taking a product that is normally inhaled and putting it in a form that can be swallowed. We do this by opening up budesonide respules and then mixing the liquid with a vehicle that allows it to adhere to the esophagus. We ask the patient to mix 1mg of budesonide suspension with ten Splenda packets so that it creates a slurry that is very thick and syrupy and have the patient swallow that. Otherwise, you can mix the budesonide in one or two teaspoons of agave nectar, or chocolate syrup, or applesauce. Basically, you are looking for things that are thicker and will just stick to the esophagus. I have also used honey in a few cases. The team ultimately needs to work with the patient to determine what they can best tolerate.

So, due to insurance or out-of-pocket cost, many of our patients have easier access to generic budesonide respules than branded fluticasone inhalers. Some patients may opt to use a compounded form of budesonide suspension if they do not like to mix the slurry themselves and it is not cost-prohibitive. Unfortunately, most compounded medications are not covered by insurance, or each individual ingredient has to be billed separately through the insurance, which can cause financial strain for the patient so we use compounded medications infrequently.

How long are patients able to continue taking PPIs and steroids in EOE?

In EOE, patients are generally refilling prescriptions for PPIs and steroids indefinitely. It is our experience that when the patient stops the steroids or the PPI, patients typically have a recurrence of symptoms if they were previously responsive to the medication(s). By maintaining them on PPIs and steroids long term, we are trying to prevent prolonged inflammation and damage to the esophagus. Ultimately, continuing medication(s) will improve the quality of life for those who are able to tolerate these medications. However, we may discontinue PPIs if a patient develops a contraindication, say recurrent C. difficile infections, or atypical fractures. Topical steroids may be discontinued if the patient is transitioned to a biologic for EOE or if the patient is unable to tolerate steroids (such as having systemic side effects). Otherwise, patients will be maintained on these drugs indefinitely.

Helicobacter Pylori

Case 2 *A 35-year-old woman was found to have a gastric ulcer on endoscopy that was helicobacter pylori-positive. She is sent to you to help manage her antibiotic regimen.*

Historically triple-drug regimens have been prescribed most commonly in the USA. However, the latest ACG guidelines suggest quadruple therapy. What do you prefer?

The major argument for using quadruple therapy is HP resistance to clarithromycin. We would like to study H. pylori resistance in our area, but currently antibiograms are not available.

I still prefer to use triple therapy as the first line because patient compliance is much better than with quadruple therapy. Triple therapy treatment is so much easier for patients to take since it is only twice daily versus quadruple therapy, which may need to be taken up to four times a day. Triple therapy also seems to be better tolerated in terms of GI side effects. Therefore, it is commonly prescribed first line as long as there are no contraindications to any of the treatment components. However, if a patient has a true penicillin allergy, is on medications that interact with clarithromycin, has cardiac issues, or if a patient failed an earlier case of triple therapy with clarithromycin, I commonly switch to quadruple therapy. So far, most patients who have taken triple therapy (from our clinic) and were adherent seem to have a good response and are able to clear the bacteria.

Will you use triple therapy in a patient who has received clarithromycin, or other macrolides for some other indication in the past?

If a patient has received clarithromycin, or other macrolides, for an URI or some other short-term indication, I will still try clarithromycin again, because I don't know how long the HP infection has been present, and whether this bacterium has, or has not been previously exposed to macrolides.

If there is previous exposure but I think that triple therapy will suit the patient best, I typically have a discussion with the patient regarding the pros and cons of the treatment including the potential of drug resistance and the possibility that the patient might require retreatment with a different regimen should the infection persist.

If a patient has a real penicillin allergy (not just GI discomfort with amoxicillin), I may use quadruple therapy instead. I do not switch out metronidazole for amoxicillin in the triple regimen, because the combined resistance to both metronidazole and clarithromycin is too high in the community and the estimated success rate is less than 70%.

What is your preferred method for providing quadruple therapy?

First, although prescribing Pylera may be easier, this combination is a branded product and is generally not covered by insurance, or it requires prior authorization and causes marked delays. For example, Medicare recipients who have to pay a percentage of the drug cost may have higher out-of-pocket copay compared to if the individual medications were ordered.

The second thing is that I prefer to avoid prescribing tetracycline. I live in a dairy state, and people love their milk, cheese, and yogurt. You are supposed to space out the use of dairy products (and other calcium-containing products) at least 2 h from tetracyclines, and since tetracycline has to be taken four times a day, it becomes a logistical nightmare. Therefore, I commonly use doxycycline instead of tetracycline. It only needs to be taken twice a day, and we see much better compliance than taking tetracycline. In addition, it is much cheaper than tetracycline. Two weeks of doxycycline might cost $20, in comparison with $100 for tetracycline.

In terms of bismuth, I order bismuth subsalicylate. Generally, patients have to buy this over-the-counter since insurances normally exclude coverage of OTC items. There are multiple OTC products that contain bismuth including Pepto-Bismol and Kaopectate. You have to check the label and verify that it is truly bismuth subsalicylate and to verify the dose of the product. Different Pepto-Bismol products might have different ingredients, but I educate patients that they will need to take 524 mg per dose. This may be two 262 mg tabs or generally 30cc of the 262 mg/15 ml liquid. Of note, there is a new formulation of Pepto-Bismol available that is branded, called Pepto-Bismol Extra, which has 524 mg in one tablet. So, when I provide education, I always stress that they have to check the labeling so that they take the right amount, and not too much, of the medication.

Have you used any regimens containing levofloxacin or rifabutin?

I typically use levofloxacin (with amoxicillin and PPI) as second-line therapy if the patient fails triple therapy (with clarithromycin) or quadruple therapy. The data suggest that levofloxacin-based regimens work better when it is used as second-line therapy. I have not had too many problems with patients tolerating the medicine, but we typically check an EKG prior to initiation to ensure that there is no evidence of QT prolongation if there are any risk factors (older age, h/o cardiac issues, females, on other QTc prolonging medications).

I also have prescribed rifabutin-containing regimens, these are usually the third line when patients have failed other regimens or if there are contraindications for the other therapy options. I usually prescribe rifabutin with amoxicillin, but may also combine rifabutin with moxifloxacin depending on the patient's situation.

Do you test for post-treatment clearance?

Yes, and we also call and check in with the patient about halfway through treatment to make sure he/she/they is taking the medicine appropriately. Nonadherence is a huge problem with HP treatment so we try to prevent it and, if needed, correct issues before therapy is finished. Once I verify that they have been taking the medicine correctly, we will arrange to get a Helicobacter pylori stool antigen (HPSA) 6–8 weeks after finishing treatment. Our nurses order the test and call to remind the patient to get the testing done when it is due.

Besides HPSA, we occasionally order the breath test for patients who have difficulty dropping off their stool expeditiously. In the case where patients need a follow-up endoscopy, then we will get biopsies to verify eradication.

The most important counseling point for these tests is to ensure that patients are off PPIs for at least 2 weeks prior to testing and antibiotics for at least 4 weeks prior to testing; otherwise, you may get a false negative. In terms of the breath test, there are more requirements to get a valid result, such as fasting and not smoking for more than 1 h prior to the appointment.

In using PPIs in treating HP, GERD, etc., do you think it matters which PPI is used?

I do not think all PPIs are created equal. While they may have the same mechanism of action, they differ in terms of enzymatic metabolism, excretion, and potency. I think that most people get prescribed omeprazole first, because in terms of potency it's smack dab in the middle, and it is widely used and accepted. In addition, it is available over-the-counter and it's not terribly expensive.

However, if a person has intolerance to omeprazole you can switch to another PPI. If omeprazole starts to lose effect, you might want to switch to a higher potency PPI such as esomeprazole or rabeprazole. However, these may involve some insurance hurdles.

Prescribers need to consider CYP interactions and drug metabolism for PPIs. For example, there are many patients on clopidogrel, which is metabolized by CYP2C19. If omeprazole is used concomitantly, it can decrease the serum levels of clopidogrel, thereby increasing the risk of a cardiovascular event. In this specific case, pantoprazole is preferred due to less CYP interactions. However, because of pantoprazole's lower potency, a higher dose may be needed to get the same therapeutic effect as omeprazole. In addition, if you know that someone is a CYP2C19 rapid metabolizer you would want to switch to one of the PPIs where CYP2C19 is a minor substrate—including pantoprazole, lansoprazole, or rabeprazole. Rabeprazole is the strongest of these three. Normally, patients have to fail other PPIs before their insurance will authorize rabeprazole.

IBS-C, IBS-D, and Chronic Constipation

Case 3 A 32-year-old woman is diagnosed with IBS-C. She has been taking metamucil and miralax with only minor relief.

Which of the IBS-C and IBS-D medicines do your practitioners tend to order, and what are the issues with accessibility for these drugs?

Linaclotide, plecanatide, and lubiprostone are the most commonly prescribed medications for IBS-C. Linaclotide tends to be used first, it has very good evidence to support its use, patients respond very well to it, and there are also good patient assistance programs available, so financial issues tend to be pretty minimal. However, if patients don't tolerate linaclotide, or they do not get the desired effect, then we will try lubiprostone or plecanatide. While tegaserod is approved for IBS-C, I do not see it commonly prescribed due to its limitation for use in females only and those without multiple cardiac risk factors.

For IBS-D, eluxadoline is approved, but we only put in a few requests for it, in part because it's difficult for patients to get coverage for the drug. In addition, eluxadoline should not be prescribed to patients who have had a cholecystectomy or who drink more than three alcoholic drinks a day because of the risk of pancreatitis.

Another medication approved for IBS-D is rifaximin. It is an incredibly expensive medication and a number of doctors are reluctant to use it for IBS-D because of its expense and limited supporting data. Now, if the patient also has small intestinal bacterial overgrowth (SIBO) in addition to IBS-D, there is more evidence to support its use. Additionally, the use of rifaximin for IBS-D involves cyclic treatment. The patient takes the medicine for 2 weeks and then stops it, and then, even if it works, you usually get a recurrence of symptoms, and you need to restart it. Therefore, in my mind, it may be better to give a different medicine that a patient can take consistently, rather than having to endure cyclic treatment with recurrent symptoms.

Alosetron is another drug available for females with IBS-D who have tried and failed other drugs. I have not seen it used very often because of problems with insurance coverage of this medication and that the prescriber must follow REMS requirements.

Prucalopride is FDA approved for idiopathic chronic constipation and is a 5HT-4 agonist. I see prucalopride prescribed often since it not only helps with CIC, but there is evidence for its use in patients who have both upper and lower GI motility issues. While it is not yet approved in gastroparesis, a number of our practitioners have prescribed it for patients who have gastroparesis along with chronic constipation. I hope that it will be FDA approved for gastroparesis in the future given its tolerability and our currently limited treatment options in this population.

In the past, when I had patients with chronic constipation who responded incompletely to linaclotide I would occasionally add misoprostol (excluding women of reproductive age) off-label as an add-on. Do you see any misoprostol being used?

We do not see it used much for constipation. However, if a prescriber did want to use it, I think the indication for use should be included on the prescription. Due to rulings from the Supreme Court and state laws, pharmacists will need to pay special attention to how the drug is being prescribed. If the indication is not on the prescription, the pharmacist will likely need to call the prescriber before dispensing it since misoprostol may be illegal if being used for abortive purposes depending on the pharmacy's state.

The antispasmodics, dicyclomine and hyoscyamine, have been commonly used in IBS, particularly IBS-D. However, the 2021 ACG guidelines said they no longer recommend the use of these drugs, because evidence of their benefit is weak. The latest 2022 AGA guidelines, just published, gave a conditional recommendation for their use. Are these able to be prescribed?

We have no problems getting these antispasmodics for our patients. I'm aware of the literature but it's one thing to be looking at guidelines and another thing when you are talking to a patient with IBS who is in a lot of pain and you are trying to improve their quality of life. With IBS, you generally cannot identify a specific trigger that will make the symptoms disappear and prescribing these drugs can help allow a patient to live his or her life with less suffering.

What about use of PAMORAs the peripherally acting mu-opioid receptors, used in patients with chronic constipation related to chronic use of opioids?

I have seen mostly naloxegol and methylnaltrexone prescribed. Naloxegol is only available orally, while methylnaltrexone is available both orally and SQ, so for a patient having problems with oral intake it may be beneficial to have an injectable medicine.

You also have to think about drug interactions when prescribing. Naloxegol is a CYP3A4 substrate and so there are many potential drug interactions. On the other hand, methylnaltrexone does not have as many interactions. Therefore, if you are dealing with a patient on a number of medications for different health considerations, Relistor might be preferable. I have yet to see naldemedine prescribed. In part, it is because it is so new, but it is also a CYP3A4 substrate, so it will have similar drug interactions as naloxegol.

Hepatitis C

Case 4 A 26-year-old man with a history of IV drug abuse is found to have elevated liver enzymes. A hepatitis panel is positive for HCV antibody, and a PCR test is positive with a viral RNA of 1.5 million.

After years of struggling with trying to clear HCV using PEG interferon, ribavirin, and protease inhibitors, now it would appear to be very simple treating HCV with the oral agents. Are there any complexities involved?

We tend to give almost every patient pibrentasvir/glecaprevir or sofosbuvir/velpatasvir. Both are pan-genotypic agents, and insurance generally covers these well. Occasionally, we will have an insurer insist that we prescribe sofosbuvir/ledipasvir in a patient who is genotype 1A, but this is becoming less common.

The two major barriers to treating hepatitis C are adherence and drug interactions. Overall, it is expected that >75% adherence should allow for viral eradication. However, missing consecutive doses (vs. sporadic misses) may also have a greater chance for lack of response. I always stress the importance of adherence at my teaching appointments and the risk of resistance if noncompliance occurs.

My other major role to support patients being treated is to review medication lists and make sure there are no drug interactions. In my experience, patients often take over-the-counter medications or herbal supplements and do not necessarily consider these true "medications"; hence, they may not disclose them to their doctors to add them to the medication list. Therefore, if medication lists are not adequately reviewed, drug interactions may occur causing treatment failure or safety issues. In terms of drug interactions, one of the most common adjustments that I make is acid-reducing medications when sofosbuvir/velpatasvir is prescribed. SOF/VEL requires gastric acid for absorption. During my consultations, I specifically screen for famotidine, PPIs, and/or antacids, all of which may decrease the effectiveness of sofosbuvir/velpatasvir if not dosed or spaced appropriately. Additionally, strong CYP3A4 inducers, such as carbamazepine, primidone, and phenytoin, can decrease the drug levels of hepatitis C treatment, thereby preventing viral eradication. So, prior to starting HCV treatment, prescribers need to weigh the risk versus the benefit of their continued use.

Hepatitis C medications may also increase the risk for toxicity. For example, we have heard of patients on pibrentasvir/glecaprevir who have developed myopathy because pibrentasvir/glecaprevir can significantly raise the concentration of statins in the blood. Additionally, the use of oral ethinyl estradiol combined with a protease inhibitor (in pibrentasvir/glecaprevir) can increase the risk of potential liver injury. Therefore, it is important to screen whether women are taking oral contraceptives before starting pibrentasvir/glecaprevir.

There is some ongoing controversy about whether an HCV genotype is necessary since we are generally prescribing pan-genotypic medications. What do you think?

I still find that most insurance companies will not cover HCV meds without a genotype. In addition, a number of patients who we are treating for HCV are still struggling with IV or IN drug use, and if they show up with an HCV infection after receiving treatment, a genotype may help establish if it is a new infection versus a recurrence of the old infection.

Hepatitis B

Case 5 *A 38-year-old Asian American man was being followed for immune-tolerant HBV for a decade. However, his latest liver enzymes show an elevation, marking a transition to immune active disease. His ALT is 150, AST is 130, and he is HBeAg positive, with an HBV DNA of 100,000.*

How are you treating your patients with chronic HBV?

Our patients are prescribed either entecavir or tenofovir because of the higher barrier to resistance. If we are using tenofovir, I prefer tenofovir alafenamide (TAF) because the side effect profile is much more preferable than tenofovir disoproxil fumarate (TDF). Entecavir is generic while TAF is still brand only. TDF is also generic. A lot of times, however, insurance will dictate what therapy we are able to use.

However, if I have a young patient, I do not like to use TDF because of the long-term side effects. Many of these patients will eventually need to be changed because of renal problems or osteopenia. So, if we are having problems with insurance authorizing TAF we will generally use entecavir, although we acknowledge the fact that tenofovir appears to be associated with lower rates of HCC development.

We are not using much lamivudine or other older HBV antivirals because of the low barrier to resistance and their side effect profiles.

Pancreatic Insufficiency

Case 6 *A 54-year-old man with a past history of years of alcohol abuse carries the diagnosis of chronic pancreatitis. He presents with weight loss and a history of frequent fatty stools, and work-up reveals steatorrhea and pancreatic insufficiency.*

What agents are available for treating pancreatic insufficiency?

Typically, our first-line agent is Creon, it works well, and, in addition, the manufacturer has a robust financial assistance program for those patients who have problems paying. Pancreatic enzymes can be quite expensive. Our second line is Zenpep. Often, the insurance will dictate what option we use though. Occasionally, if a patient is having side effect to one, we can try a different pancrelipase option to see if the patient tolerates it better

In the past, we would use uncoated pancreatic enzymes like Viokase to treat the pain of chronic pancreatitis. Are you seeing much of that done currently?

No, we are not seeing much Viokase used, and when it is used, it is generally because patients have an intolerance to Creon or ZENPEP. I do see a group of patients who do not tolerate these enteric-coated preparations, and it seems like it more commonly occurs in patients who are also taking PPIs. Creon and ZENPEP have a pH-mediated release and perhaps the patients on PPIs have more problems tolerating them because of the more proximal release of the enzymes causing gastric upset.

Inflammatory Bowel Disease

Case 7 A 28-year-old man, who recently quit smoking, presents with severe diarrhea and rectal bleeding and is found to have severe ulcerative colitis. Your doctor wants to start an anti-TNF.

Are you generally pressured to start with biosimilars?

There are an increasing number of insurance companies that do request that we start with a biosimilar. Additionally, there is potential for cost savings for the patient and the infusion center when biosimilars are administered because of the lower acquisition costs compared to originator formulations.

What is your regimen for premedicating patients before they're given an infusion?

We have a premedication protocol before administering specific biologics that includes IV steroids, famotidine, and acetaminophen for patients who had a drug holiday (for IFX) or who had a history of infusion reaction. Patients on infliximab receive acetaminophen prior to each infusion. For those with other reactions on other infusions, it is a case-by-case basis what we may use for premedication going forward (if the patient continues therapy)

Are there issues, from a coverage standpoint between choosing a drug given via infusion vs. injection?

Insurance coverage always needs to be considered when choosing a high-cost medication. Depending on whether the medication is billed through medical versus pharmacy insurance, it could mean a thousand-dollar difference in out-of-pocket expenses. For example, patients with Medicare commonly find that infusions (billed through part B ± supplement) may be less expensive compared to medications billed through part D (pharmacy benefits). Medicare supplements usually cover the remaining cost after Medicare part B pays for 80%. However, for SQ drugs such as adalimumab, the patient needs to pay for their deductible and then must pay up to 25% of the drug cost, which can be thousands of dollars. Additionally, patients with government-provided insurance do not qualify for copay cards. Depending on the patient's income, the patient may not qualify for patient assistance and thus be unable to get access to a medication.

What about the use of some of the other IBD medications?

We are seeing vedolizumab used in our institution, particularly in patients without extra-intestinal manifestations. Because vedolizumab is gut-specific, I think it is a worthy drug to use in cases where patients have isolated GI tract Crohn's or ulcerative colitis. Our doctors have generally turned to vedolizumab after trying anti-TNFs first, but it may be used first line depending on specific patient factors. We very rarely use natalizumab due to the risk of progressive multifocal leukoencephalopathy, especially in those who are JC (John Cunningham) virus-positive.

We are also using more small molecules for IBD, especially in those who may want to avoid injectable therapies. Tofacitinib also has been used first line as rescue therapy to avoid colectomy in patients who are hospitalized for severe ulcerative colitis. There is evidence that high-dose tofacitinib, being given in the hospital over three days followed by maintenance dosing, may be useful to prevent colectomy.

In terms of one of the newer drugs, ozanimod, we educate and monitor for cardiac complications since bradycardia is a potential side effect. However, prescribers also have to be on the lookout for signs of a hypertensive crisis, particularly when patients eat high amounts of tyramine-containing foods. Patients on ozanimod should avoid eating things like aged cheeses or consuming dark beers. So, with ozanimod, a lot of educating and monitoring has to be done, particularly if the patient has a history of heart issues. You also need to check for macular edema in those who have diabetes. Ultimately, prescribing ozanimod may require more effort on behalf of the provider to ensure safety of the patient.

The new Jak-Stat inhibitors (tofacitinib and upadacitinib) are good oral options for those patients with ulcerative colitis (and Crohn's disease for upadacitinib) and want to avoid injectable medications. However, it is important to screen for any history of thrombosis or cardiovascular issues prior to starting these medications since there is a warning for thrombosis and myocardial infarctions with this class of therapy.

Autoimmune Hepatitis

Case 8 *A 33-year-old woman presents with weakness, and anorexia and is found to have an ALT of 340, AST 280, ANA + 1:640, and ASMA + 1:160. A liver biopsy is consistent with autoimmune hepatitis.*

Are most of your providers using prednisone or budesonide to treat AIH? Are they using azathioprine as well? In what doses? For patients who don't tolerate azathioprine, what are they using second-line?

Most of our providers are using prednisone as their first-line agent. Our doctors are using budesonide more in patients who are having problems being weaned off prednisone or having intolerable side effects from it.

Most are also adding azathioprine to prednisone for its steroid-sparing effects. We are seeing most patients receiving azathioprine 50 mg a day. However, if liver enzymes are elevated or trending up, the dose of azathioprine may be increased. We may also check 6 TGN and 6 MMP to make sure that the rising LFTs are unrelated to the medication via the presence of 6 MMP metabolite.

For patients who do not tolerate azathioprine, or do not get the appropriate therapeutic response, our second-line agent tends to be mycophenolate mofetil. In terms of problems with mycophenolate, the most important one is that it's absolutely contraindicated in pregnancy. The other is that some patients receiving the mycophenolate mofetil may be more prone to side effects (i.e., diarrhea). In these patients, switching to the other formulation (mycophenolic acid) may eliminate the GI issues.

What are the questions the gastroenterologists in the clinic ask you most often?

The most common thing the gastroenterologists contact me about is drug interactions. A pharmacist is going to have a wealth of resources to help with navigating interactions. At the hospital that I work at, there are complex patients with multiple comorbidities and long lists of medications and supplements. Therefore, choosing the best treatment can be difficult to ensure efficacy but also minimizing safety issues. Pharmacists can screen for drug interactions, dose adjustments, and safety concerns that may affect other health conditions for the patient. Doctors also want to know which drugs are most likely to be covered or will be most affordable for patients. I also get questions about supportive care guidelines such as immunization recommendations since we commonly work with immunosuppressed patients.

Part II
IBD Compendium

Chapter 25
Introduction to the Inflammatory Bowel Disease Compendium

W. Harley Sobin

There are multiple management decisions we deal with in caring for our IBD patients. The cases in the chapters that follow cover many complicated issues. Topics that are discussed include the following: How best to evaluate the remainder of the small bowel when ileitis is found on colonoscopy? How long should you continue budesonide? The use of agents such as ozanimod, ustekinumab, risankizumab, and vedolizumab in patients who do not want to be on anti-TNFs; the use of anti-TNFs in a patient with a history of MI; the use of JAK inhibitors when patients fail anti-TNFs; whether to anticoagulate a hospitalized patient with IBD and rectal bleeding; the management of C. difficile in a patient with IBD; how to manage severe IBD in a patient not responding to anti-TNFs; managing post-op Crohn's; managing multiple pseudopolyps and the finding of dysplasia on a random biopsy during surveillance colonoscopy; options in the management of acute severe ulcerative colitis; treating refractory proctitis; how best to administer vedolizumab? Managing functional diarrhea in IBD; when is it best to postpone infusions? How to interpret and manage musculoskeletal complaints in a patient on anti-TNFs for IBD? How to treat pyoderma gangrenosum? How to manage patients who are squeamish about self-injection or taking rectal medications? How to treat a patient with UC who has a colon stricture? How to approach nonspecific ileal ulcers? Whether to prophylax against Pneumocystis jirovecii in patients on several immunosuppressants; management of microscopic colitis; and help with many other long-term decisions that need to be made.

W. H. Sobin (✉)
Internal Medicine, Division of Gastroenterology and Hepatology, Medical College of Wisconsin, Milwaukee, WI, USA
e-mail: hsobin@mcw.edu

© The Author(s), under exclusive license to Springer Nature Switzerland AG 2023
W. H. Sobin et al. (eds.), *Managing Complex Cases in Gastroenterology*,
https://doi.org/10.1007/978-3-031-48949-5_25

181

Chapter 26
Crohn's Ileitis

Preetika Sinh

A 25-year-old married woman whose family came to the US from Vietnam when she was 5 years old presented to her community gastroenterologist with a history of diarrhea of 2-month duration. Stool cultures were negative for C+S and C diff. She does smoke cigarettes. She is on no meds and takes no NSAIDS. Fecal calprotectin was elevated at 600, and CRP was elevated at 30. Colonoscopy was performed and revealed mild inflammation of the terminal ileum over 5–6 cm. Findings were felt to be consistent with Crohn's ileitis.

If you find Crohn's ileitis, how do you like to evaluate the remainder of the small bowel?

The options for imaging are CT enterography, MR enterography, and a capsule study. There are data comparing CT enterography to a capsule exam, and overall, they are pretty equivalent in making a diagnosis. However, with milder disease, the CT enterography will occasionally miss smaller ulcerations that will be detected on capsule study. But, with more severe penetrating, or fistulizing, disease CT is diagnostic while the capsule may miss these changes. It is always helpful so see whether the patient has ever had any cross-sectional imaging previously to serve as a baseline.

If you decide to do a capsule study in your Crohn's patients, will you always do a patency capsule first?

We have to consider whether there are risk factors for capsule retention, which include any prior history of abdominal surgery, or any obstructive symptoms. If the answer is no and there has been prior cross-sectional imaging done, then I don't think a patency capsule is necessary. Another factor is whether the terminal ileum (T.I.) was looked at during colonoscopy. If the T.I. has never been looked at, then I

P. Sinh (✉)
Division of Gastroenterology and Hepatology, Medical College of Wisconsin, Milwaukee, WI, USA
e-mail: psinh@mcw.edu

© The Author(s), under exclusive license to Springer Nature Switzerland AG 2023
W. H. Sobin et al. (eds.), *Managing Complex Cases in Gastroenterology*, https://doi.org/10.1007/978-3-031-48949-5_26

would be a little wary of doing a capsule because you are unsure whether there is a longstanding disease, causing narrowing that might be missed on a CT scan. In this particular case, the T.I. did not appear strictured, and there was acute onset of symptoms, all things that make me believe a capsule should pass without difficulty.

The patient has CT enterography that reveals ileitis but is otherwise negative. Her community gastroenterologist starts her on entocort (budesonide) 9 mg a day.

Do you agree with the use of budesonide here?

In this setting, I think that is very appropriate because, first, the inflammation was mild as seen on the colonoscopy. Second, the entocort will help us define how much response we will get with steroid induction. And third, the entocort, while working as an induction regimen, sets us up to discuss with the patient what the next step, maintenance therapy, will be.

The patient does well on 9 mg a day of entocort but every time you try to taper it the symptoms get worse.

How would you manage this scenario?

I generally plan on using entocort for only 8 weeks. I get the patient back in the clinic before then to start the discussion about what maintenance drug to use, either a biologic or immunomodulator, as our long-term treatment for Crohn's. We are only using entocort as the induction agent to get the patient into remission. If the patient remains in remission on the maintenance drug, then entocort can be simply stopped, it does not have to be tapered.

You would never think about keeping a patient chronically on budesonide alone, 3 mg, 6 mg, or 9 mg alone if it controls symptoms?

In a Crohn's patient, I would not maintain them on entocort alone. I have some patients who are on 3 mg or 6 mg of budesonide in addition to a biologic, who I can't wean off of steroids. No, whenever I start entocort, I have an exit strategy that includes switching to a different drug for maintenance.

Entocort is a steroid, but only 10% gets into the system after absorption and liver metabolism. Its side effect profile is much better than prednisone. But we still need to keep in mind that it's a steroid, and Crohn's disease is a long-term disease and assuming that we confirm Crohn's in this 25 year old, we need to use a steroid-sparing medication.

You suggest to the patient that she quit smoking. Have you had much success getting your Crohn's patients to quit smoking?

It depends on the patient population and it requires counseling, plus support with medication like Chantix or nicotine gum. Overall, I've had about 50% success. When I'm doing all the work myself, I've had very little success. Part of the time I work in the VA, and I've had less success with that population.

Is it almost invariably true that your smoking patients who present with IBD have Crohn's rather than UC?

I'd like to frame the question a little bit differently. I think there is something of a referral bias. We get referrals for Crohn's patients who are doing poorly, and frequently, it is those people who continue smoking. And then, there are patients who have UC who quit smoking, flare up, do poorly, and then get referred to us. So, partly it's because we're a referral center that we tend to see a lot of Crohn's patients who continue to smoke and so their Crohn's doesn't get better.

The patient is unable to quit smoking. She recounts that her mother smoked her entire life, including through her pregnancy. In addition, she relates that she wishes to get pregnant within the next 2 years.

Would you consider surgery as a preferred option in this patient?

If you asked me 7–10 years ago, the answer would have been no, we should treat it medically. If we went back 30 or 40 years ago, the answer would definitely have been yes, there were not great medical options. But now there are new data that suggest that if a patient has short-segment T.I. disease, confirmed on CT enterography (like the 5–6 cm this patient has), with no evidence for other disease involvement, patients may do better with surgery. It has been shown that a surgical resection in this setting decreases the likelihood of requiring an anti-TNF or other biologic agent in a patient at a 1-year mark.

However, in this case, surgery would not be my first option. With an acute onset, no past history of symptoms, and a colonoscopy that shows more inflammatory than fibrotic disease, I'm going to discuss medical therapy primarily and keep surgical options much lower on my list.

Every case is unique. This patient's symptoms seem to be of a short duration. Another patient may present with mild symptoms, but have a history of GI problems that have been present for their entire lives. That patient may have had subclinical Crohn's for years, and colonoscopy may show more fibrotic change in the T.I. In that case, the fibrotic component is not going to improve much with a biologic agent. So, in those situations, I consider short segment T.I. resection and refer them to a surgeon for their input.

What medical option would you prefer?

Since this is a young patient, given the long-term risks of other biologics, I think vedolizumab would be a reasonable first choice. There is just one dose for vedolizumab, 300 mg, and we start induction dosing at weeks zero, two, and six and then continue maintenance dosing every 8 weeks.

After I start vedolizumab, I aim to continue budesonide for another 8 weeks. At that point, I try to stop budesonide. We either stop it without tapering or decrease to 6 mg for a week then 3 mg for a week, then stop it completely.

Are you checking vedolizumab levels on these patients?

I tend to check vedolizumab levels in patients at the 14-week mark, which is the first maintenance dose. The reason I check them is because in Crohn's disease the induction response to vedolizumab can be slow, and I want to make sure there is adequate drug available. In Crohn's, there's only a 13% response at the end of induction, it's much higher in ulcerative colitis. But, after 1 year, the Crohn's patients became as responsive to vedolizumab as the ulcerative colitis patients. The explanation for this is that it takes longer for vedolizumab to act in Crohn's disease because it is a transmural inflammation and the mechanism of action of vedolizumab is as an anti-integrin molecule that starts working at the mucosal level. Previously, I used to evaluate the response at 3 and 6 months with fecal calprotectin or colonoscopy. If the response was inadequate, I would check vedolizumab levels and, if levels were low, increase the frequency of the infusions. Now, I tend to check proactively, rather than have to wait 6 months. In this case, I would repeat fecal calprotectin, and get vedolizumab levels and a CRP at 14 weeks.

Then, if the vedolizumab level is adequate, and the patient is doing well, all is good. But if the vedolizumab level is low, the fecal calprotectin is elevated, and the patient is symptomatic I increase the vedolizumab frequency to every 6 weeks or 4 weeks, depending on the levels and inflammatory markers.

The patient has adequate vedolizumab levels at 14 weeks but as budesonide was stopped her diarrhea started worsening, and she developed drainage by her rectum, with a perianal fistula. Colonoscopy is repeated and now she has proctitis along with inflammation of the cecum and the terminal ileum as well.

How would you manage her now?

It's important to know that the vedolizumab levels were adequate. On the one hand, the disease has progressed on vedolizumab; however, it doesn't necessarily indicate vedolizumab failure, since it may take longer to see a clinical response to vedolizumab.

There are several different management options. A shared decision making is the best way forward. One option is to give vedolizumab a while longer to act. The patient has an adequate vedolizumab level at 3 months, so you might just continue the same therapy a while longer. However, the disease has progressed to a point where the disease is not just mucosal, there is actually a perianal fistula. So, I would like to switch to a biologic, like an anti-TNF drug. There are much more robust data for treatment of Crohn's perianal fistulae with anti-TNFs.

How do you evaluate and manage these perianal fistulae?

I like to get an MRI of the pelvis to assess if there is any abscess. If there is an abscess, I always start antibiotics-usually ciprofloxacin and metronidazole. I also ask a surgeon to place a seton in patients with Crohn's and perianal fistulae. The management combines medical management of Crohn's disease, antibiotics, plus surgical intervention with seton placement or abscess drainage, if needed.

When you see a perianal fistula in a patient with Crohn's, is it usually an association with proctitis?

The inflammation associated with a perianal fistula tends to extend into the distal rectum, right above the dentate line, very close to the anal canal. This really isn't Crohn's proctitis. But you can certainly see perianal fistulae in association with isolated Crohn's ileitis or proximal colitis.

The decision is made to place the patient on an anti-TNF for the more aggressive disease. If you're starting an anti-TNF, would you like to add an immunomodulator?

I would probably add an immunomodulator. I would prefer to avoid methotrexate because of the teratogenic risk, seeing how she wishes to become pregnant

However, she is not currently pregnant, so, we could start methotrexate and if we can get the patient into remission switch to another immunomodulator, like azathioprine, which we are comfortable using in pregnancy [1]. We could also consider a different biologic with evidence in treating Crohn's fistulizing disease that does not require an immunomodulator.

However, you don't always need to add a second drug when you're using an anti-TNF. Although the initial Sonic trial showed that combination drug therapy is better than anti-TNF alone, when they looked at drug levels of those patients who were on optimized anti-TNF dosage, they did as well as the combination therapy. Therefore, you can also argue for using an anti-TNF alone, with optimized dosing, closely following drug levels.

There is another new blood test that we can use to predict how patients will do on anti-TNF monotherapy. It is called RiskImmune (Prometheus lab), which uses the HLA phenotype of the patient. It's been shown to predict, at the 3-year mark, which patients with the genetic variant have a higher risk of progressing and requiring surgery on anti-TNF monotherapy.

So, I would consider sending this test, with the disclaimer that it is a very new test, and if the patient does have that risk profile, then we will definitely add a second agent. It has been shown that if you use combination therapy in those patients, they have a better outcome. They have a higher risk of immunogenicity on monotherapy.

Because the disease has progressed quickly, I would be more inclined to add an immunomodulator, particularly since the patient is young. If I do add an immune modulator, I generally keep that on for about 1–2 years. I have a plan of switching over to monotherapy at that point, because of the risk of lymphoma and skin cancer, with the immune modulator. Those are the main, big words that people get scared of, but they don't come into the picture until the patient has been on immunosuppressant medications like azathioprine for 2–3 years. So, I would consider checking the RiskImmune, start an anti-TNF, and add an immunomodulator like Imuran for now.

If you're going to add azathioprine, would you do genetic testing for NUD 15 because she is Asian?

If I was practicing in Asia, I would definitely check a NUD-15 because any abnormality can cause toxicity at the 6TG metabolite level. I'm not sure how commercially available the test is. If it is not available, I would certainly still check the TPMT phenotype, and closely monitor the CBC and liver panel.

The medical team suggests treatment with infliximab and azathioprine but the patient does not wish to come in for infusions.

Would you allow the patient to get adalimumab or would you push the patient to receive infliximab?

I think that shared decision making is very important. I tell the patient that I would rather she be on the medication which she will stay on, rather than me trying to tell her to take a different drug which she won't comply with, which will only make her disease worse. For some patients, there are other priorities that come before treating their disease, so, we always try to be flexible, to help the patient stay on track. So yes, I would be inclined to work with adalimumab if infusions are not going to work with her lifestyle. In addition, the original Humira studies do show that adalimumab is a good drug for perianal fistulizing disease.

However, another important point to make is that in perianal Crohn's disease we need to have higher anti-TNF trough levels. The usual desired level is 5 mg but with perianal disease we want to get levels of 10–15 or even 20 ug/ml. It can be more challenging to achieve these drug levels using adalimumab. With infliximab, we can go up to 10 mg/kg every 4 weeks. With adalimumab, all we can do is increase the frequency to q weekly.

Reference

1. Mahadevan U, Robinson C, Bernasko N, Boland B, Chambers C, Dubinsky M, Friedman S, Kane S, Manthey J, Sauberan J, Stone J. Inflammatory bowel disease in pregnancy clinical care pathway: a report from the American Gastroenterological Association IBD Parenthood Project Working Group. Inflamm Bowel Dis. 2019;25(4):627–41.

Chapter 27
Ulcerative Colitis Refractory to Mesalamine

Daniel Stein and Salina Faidhalla

A 35-year-old woman with mild ulcerative colitis is not responding to mesalamine. The patient is a non-smoker with no family history of IBD and no other medical problems.

How do you manage a patient with mild UC who is not responding to mesalamine?

When there is a concern for no response/loss of response, there must be objective evidence of disease activity since many IBD patients can have nonspecific symptoms due to IBS, rectal scarring, etc. Loss of response can be defined by a worsening of clinical status, and evidence of active disease based on colonoscopy or at least inflammatory markers. After confirming disease activity, we always confirm medication adherence and rule out other possible etiologies, like infection.

Other options for mild UC include maximizing mesalamine dose if not already done, adding topical mesalamine or topical steroids (in enema, rectal foam, or suppository form), to induce remission prior to escalating to a biologic. In patients with only mild UC, we can also consider adding curcumin or fish oil.

If the above fails, then we can proceed with evaluation for other treatment options like anti-TNFs, other biologics, or the new small molecules.

The dosage of mesalamine is maximized and mesalamine enemas are added. In spite of this, there is no response and alternative therapy is needed. She has heard about the anti-TNFs and wants to avoid starting those.

D. Stein (✉)
Internal Medicine, Division of Gastroenterology and Hepatology, Medical College of Wisconsin, Milwaukee, WI, USA
e-mail: dstein@mcw.edu

S. Faidhalla
Department of Medicine Division of Gastroenterology and Hepatology, Medical College of Wisconsin, Milwaukee, WI, USA
e-mail: sfaidhalla@mcw.edu

© The Author(s), under exclusive license to Springer Nature Switzerland AG 2023
W. H. Sobin et al. (eds.), *Managing Complex Cases in Gastroenterology*, https://doi.org/10.1007/978-3-031-48949-5_27

Since she wants to take anti-TNFs off the table, can you discuss the choice between ozanimod, Ustekinumab, and vedolizumab in UC?

Vedolizumab (VDZ) binds α4β7 integrin on blood monocytes, inhibiting their ability to enter the intestinal epithelium. It is more gut selective. VDZ is an infusion administered every 8 weeks and an effective choice in UC patients who are anti-TNF naïve.

Ustekinumab (UST) is an interleukin inhibitor, targeting IL-12 and IL-23. Induction is an infusion followed by self-administered injections every 8 weeks. It is an effective medication in UC patients who have failed anti-TNFs, some data suggest that it is more effective in inducing and maintaining remission than VDZ.

Ozanimod is a selective sphingosine-1-phosphate receptor modulator that has been used for relapsing MS and was recently approved in patients with moderate to severe UC. The medication is in pill form with once-daily dosing. This is a newer medication with some limited data. However, it seems effective in patients with mild to moderate UC who are anti-TNF naïve. Some of the known side effects of ozanimod include infection, malignancy, macular edema, bradycardia, and elevated LFTs.

For the three treatment options outlined, there is no head-to-head comparison study, but a meta-analysis suggests that ustekinumab could be more effective than vedolizumab in inducing and maintaining remission in UC patients [1]. Limited data are available about ozanimod especially when comparing it to other biologics.

When it comes to choosing a treatment, we recommend discussing with the patient in detail available treatment options, their efficacy, side effects, and route of administration to reach a mutual decision.

In this young patient with mild UC, no previous anti-TNF exposure, and no chronic medical problems, ozanimod would be a reasonable choice. The fact that it is an oral med is a benefit. Vedolizumab would also be a reasonable option to start with, given its efficacy and favorable side effect profile. Ustekinumab is also a valid option.

What is involved with starting a patient on ozanimod?

Ozanimod is a safe, effective pill that can be used in mild-moderate UC patients who are TNF naive. During the induction and maintenance period of the ozanimod trial, the incidence of clinical remission was significantly higher in the ozanimod group when compared to the placebo group [2]. Improvement in the incidence of histologic remission also occurred with ozanimod therapy.

When deciding to start ozanimod, you need to document vaccination or immunity to varicella zoster virus prior to starting the medication. In addition, you need to obtain an EKG, and ask about any history of uveitis or DM, as these patients might need to see an ophthalmologist.

In women of reproductive age, it's important to remember that there are no data about ozanimod and pregnancy, and there is possible risk of teratogenicity in animal studies. We must discuss if there are any plans for pregnancy and if this patient is planning to become pregnant, we recommend against using ozanimod.

Ozanimod dosing: starter pack (7 days), Days 1-4 (0.23 mg), Days 5-7 (0.46 mg). Day 8 patients start the maintenance dose of 0.92 mg daily.

Some of the reported side effects of ozanimod are infections, malignancy, macular edema, bradycardia, and elevated LFTs. When it comes to bradycardia, ozanimod has been shown to have a lower risk of bradycardia on long-term follow than some other drugs in this class. This may be due to the selective nature of the drug since it targets S1P1 and S1P5 (notice that S1P 1-3 is highly expressed in the heart).

References

1. Welty M, Mesana L, Padhiar A, Naessens D, Diels J, van Sanden S, Pacou M. Efficacy of Ustekinumab vs. advanced therapies for the treatment of moderately to severely active ulcerative colitis: a systematic review and network meta-analysis. Curr Med Res Opin. 2020;36(4):595–606.
2. Sandborn WJ, Feagan BG, D'Haens G, Wolf DC, Jovanovic I, Hanauer SB, Ghosh S, Petersen A, Hua SY, Lee JH, Charles L. Ozanimod as induction and maintenance therapy for ulcerative colitis. N Engl J Med. 2021;385(14):1280–91.

Chapter 28
Managing Crohn's in a Patient with Prior MI

Preetika Sinh

Patient is a 58-year-old male smoker with a history of myocardial infarction 2 years earlier, who presents with bloody diarrhea. There is a strong family history of coronary artery disease. Stool cultures are negative. Colonoscopy is performed and demonstrates moderately severe colitis with ulcers involving the entire colon. The terminal ileum is normal. It is interpreted to be an indeterminate colitis.

Is there any role for using ANCA or ASCA antibodies in the diagnosis of indeterminate colitis?

I do not use ASCA/ANCA for diagnosis. I think we get more information from the clinical picture alone. But there is a role for ASCA and ANCA, in those patients who will require colectomy. The risk of pouchitis and pouch failure is much higher in patients who are ANCA positive.

Although it was an indeterminate colitis, it was felt clinically to be favoring Crohn's colitis.

Is there any role for mesalamine or sulfasalazine in milder Crohn's colitis?

I have only one or two patients on these drugs, I rarely start Crohn's patients on mesalamine. However, if I had a patient with mild Crohn's colitis who was not yet ready to start a biologic, I might start them on mesalamine. If someone is already on mesalamine and in remission, I would not insist on making changes.

The patient starts developing increased diarrhea and bleeding and is hospitalized for LGI bleeding, presumably related to colitis alone. His hemoglobin drops from 12 to 10.

P. Sinh (✉)
Division of Gastroenterology and Hepatology, Medical College of Wisconsin,
Milwaukee, WI, USA
e-mail: psinh@mcw.edu

W. H. Sobin et al. (eds.), *Managing Complex Cases in Gastroenterology*,
https://doi.org/10.1007/978-3-031-48949-5_28

You have a patient with Crohn's disease, and a history of an MI who's in the hospital with GI bleeding. Would you be willing to use lovenox for DVT prophylaxis?

Yes, we face this problem frequently. I will place the patients on lovenox unless they develop a more significant bleed, which we define as a drop in hemoglobin of two grams. In the case outlined here, I would hold the lovenox because there was a 2-point hemoglobin drop. In any other situation, it's very important to stay on lovenox, even if they have some amount of bleeding, because there is a sixfold increased risk of venous thromboembolism in patients who have inflammatory bowel disease, and the risk is even higher in those who have an active flare

So, in those other cases I will start lovenox, while keeping a close eye on the hemoglobin. If there was a significant Hbg drop, I would hold the lovenox but otherwise emphasize very emphatically to the primary team that patients should remain on lovenox.

Would you be willing to start an anti-TNF in this patient with a history of an MI?

Yes. The contraindication to using an anti-TNF in heart disease is heart failure. There's a black box warning from the FDA saying that anti-TNFs should not be used in patients with NYHA classification three or four heart failure.

This is based upon the ATTACH study, which looked to see if anti-TNFs could be used to treat heart failure because TNF levels have been shown to be increased in heart failure. However, in patients taking 10 mg/kg of the anti-TNF there was a higher mortality in CHF, leading to this black box warning.

However, this patient has a history of MI, but no history of clinical heart failure. Studies have not shown any increased mortality in MI so; therefore, this would not be a contraindication. Overall, the data on anti-TNFs in other chronic inflammatory disorders show that they might be beneficial to reduce cardiovascular events over time, in those patients who don't have advanced CHF.

You are thinking this indeterminate colitis is favoring Crohn's disease. How would you like to manage that?

So, for Crohn's colitis I would go with steroid induction first to get the disease into remission. And then, I would probably use an anti-TNF for maintenance.

How would you feel about using ustekinumab instead of an anti-TNF in this patient?

The patient is 58. If he was 65, or a 70-year-old, I would be more concerned about a higher risk of infection with anti-TNFs compared to ustekinumab in this older age range. But this patient is younger and is admitted for acute care and there is a lot of experience using anti-TNFs as the first line in hospitalized patients.

Have I started patients on ustekinumab in the hospital with an induction? Yes, primarily in patients who have had a prior anti-TNF failure.

The patient is placed on an anti-TNF, has quit smoking, and does very well for about a year. But then the patient starts developing diarrhea and bleeding. You check stool cultures for C diff and his NAAT is positive, but his toxin is negative.

How would you manage this?

First, I would try to go back and check if the patient ever had a c. diff check before, and usually we do check c. diff at the time of diagnosis. So that means that this patient, at some point in time, was not colonized by c diff.

But, now the c diff NAAT is positive. This could either mean colonization or active disease. But c diff in IBD behaves differently than in non-IBD patients. I think you have to look at the clinical picture here. We have a situation where the patient flares and now the c diff NAAT is positive. So, even though the toxin is negative, I would treat this patient as if he has active c diff.

The next question is how would we categorize his c diff? Is it fulminant, severe, or not severe? In severe c diff, the white blood cell count is >15,000 and the creatinine is >1.5. Fulminant infections are associated with severe hypotension or shock or toxic megacolon. Non-severe infections can be treated with vancomycin 125 mg, four times a day for ten days or fidaxomicin 200 mg, twice a day for ten days. Fulminant infections are treated with vancomycin 500 mg qid PO and IV metronidazole. Severe infections fall between the two.

The patient is clinically deteriorating and is hospitalized. Vancomycin 500 mg po QID and IV metronidazole are started. Colonoscopy is performed and he has a moderately severe diffuse colitis, looking like ulcerative colitis.

The patient had an indeterminate colitis that was originally diagnosed as favoring Crohn's disease. Since then, he quit smoking and clinically worsened. Do you ever change your categorization, your diagnosis, from Crohn's to UC?

When I said that the colitis was indeterminate but favored Crohn's over UC, it was with the understanding that there were never any granulomas on biopsy, there were never skip lesions, and there was never any extra-colonic disease. Had these things been present, it wouldn't be labeled as indeterminate colitis. So, it was never definite Crohn's disease. And now, the patient has quit smoking, and the fact that the disease flared when he quit smoking is more consistent with an ulcerative colitis phenotype. What is the significance of changing the diagnosis? This largely relates to the drugs you would use and the prognosis if you were to perform a colectomy.

So, the patient has been relapsing in spite of being on an anti-TNF. Do you think he is a candidate for a JAK inhibitor, is this permissible in this setting? After all, the original diagnosis was Crohn's, where JAK inhibitors are not approved, and he has a coexisting c. diff infection. Do we have any idea how JAK inhibitors perform in this setting?

He is a complicated patient, and we do have to keep the whole concept of active c diff infection in mind. I would add to the management options possibly treating his c diff with an FMT. It is not at all unusual that when a patient with IBD develops c diff the c diff flares up the colitis. We are frequently faced with bumping up the treatment regimen for UC as well as trying to get the c diff under control. We have to be cautious with our management of the UC, however. There have been patients maintained on high doses of steroids who were not tapered off prednisone at the right time, and their c diff infections flared and they underwent colectomies with a poor outcome.

But if we are treating the c diff and doing steroid induction and the patient is not responding, we can say that anti-TNF treatment is a failure. Then, we can switch to a JAK inhibitor. The benefit of JAK inhibitors is that they are small molecules and their response is not dependent on the albumin. Acutely ill patients in the hospital are more likely to have a low albumin level. There are data showing that when there is a low albumin level those patients are less responsive to anti-TNFs. This does not hold true for JAK inhibitors. And in treating acute (fulminant) UC, the data are better for using a higher dose of tofacitinib, 10 mg, three times a day for induction and as a rescue therapy, when anti-TNFs don't work.

Chapter 29
Managing Post-Op Crohn's

Amir Patel

A 57-year-old male is admitted with a bowel obstruction. He has no past history of IBD and has not had a prior colonoscopy. He ends up requiring surgery for the obstruction and is found to have an ileal stricture, which is resected, and found on pathology to be Crohn's. The patient is a non-smoker. There is no family history of Crohn's.

Does small bowel obstruction in Crohn's usually occur at the terminal ileum?

Yes, it is usually at the terminal ileum. I've had one or two where they were more proximal, usually in a younger patient who had a duodenal or jejunal stricture. But that's exceedingly rare. About 33% of patients with Crohn's will have just isolated ileal disease.

He's never had a colonoscopy. When would you perform that?

I would do it a month post-op. You really want to assess what their phenotype is. You want to make sure they don't have colonic involvement. For someone who has had prior colonoscopies, we would not repeat it at 1-month post-op; instead, we typically repeat the colonoscopy about 6 months to a year after surgery, because that's when we would see some type of recurrence.

One-month post-op you do a colonoscopy and find a normal appearing colon and distal 20 cm of ileum.

Would you put this patient on any medication for Crohn's at this time?

I would say he's probably low risk. He is a non-smoker and he's older. This is his first operation and theoretically it's a short, stricture. I don't know how long he's had his Crohn's disease; he might have had smoldering Crohn's disease since his twenties and it's just progressed to this point.

A. Patel (✉)
Dept. of Medicine, Division of Gastroenterology and Hepatology, Medical College of Wisconsin, Milwaukee, WI, USA
e-mail: ampatel@mcw.edu

W. H. Sobin et al. (eds.), *Managing Complex Cases in Gastroenterology*, https://doi.org/10.1007/978-3-031-48949-5_29

The high-risk individuals who I think really need biologics and thiopurines to be started postoperatively are the smokers, the patients that are younger than 30, those with a history of fistulizing disease, and those with a history of two or more surgeries or who have a shorter duration of disease prior to surgery.

If I have a patient who says, "I started having diarrhea about a month ago, and all of a sudden, I have a bowel obstruction," then I would say that person's at very high risk. For our patient, I'm not that concerned. Some practitioners do order genetic testing to see if their patient has a higher risk for postoperative recurrence, checking the NOD-2 or CARD-15 genes. Some of us will do that to see if the patient is at a higher risk for a recurrence. But for this gentleman, I think that his risk of recurrence is pretty low. You could potentially get away with not starting him on therapy right away and wait to see what the postoperative colonoscopy shows at 6 months to a year.

Chapter 30
Managing Pseudopolyps

Poonam Beniwal-Patel

A 45-year-old male with a 12-year history of ulcerative colitis is referred to you. His personal gastroenterologist performed a recent colonoscopy which once again revealed dozens of pseudopolyps scattered through the colon (last colonoscopy was 3 years earlier—with similar finding). None of these polyps looked like a conventional adenoma. Random biopsies were done throughout the colon and a few pseudopolyps were removed. The patient is referred to you because biopsies done in the right colon and a pseudopolyp in the transverse colon both showed dysplasia. The referring doctor did not anticipate these biopsy results and is referring the patient asking you how to manage this.

What is your standard approach to surveillance in patients with chronic UC?

In general, I begin dysplasia surveillance after a patient has had pan-ulcerative colitis for 8 years or left-sided colitis for 10 years. In patients who have been in sustained deep remission, without a history of colon dysplasia or large post-inflammatory polyps (PIP), I generally survey the colon every 3–5 years. In contrast, if a patient has had extensive disease or large PIPs, I bring them back in 2–3 years. Finally, those patients with concurrent primary sclerosing cholangitis are brought back annually for dysplasia surveillance.

In patients with multiple pseudopolyps are there any tips you have to detect which are true adenomas? Do you bring them in more often for colonoscopic surveillance?

I use a combination of endoscopic appearance and narrow-band imaging (NBI) to decide whether I am encountering a PIP versus an adenoma. The endoscopic appearance of a fibrin cap along with distinct appearances such as a mucosal bridge formed by a long polyp are more consistent with a PIP and do not need to be biopsied.

P. Beniwal-Patel (✉)
Medicine, Gastroenterology/Hepatology Division, Medical College of Wisconsin, Milwaukee, WI, USA
e-mail: pbeniwal@mcw.edu

One of the first natural history of PIP studies was published in 2019 [1]. About 500 patients with PIPs were followed for a median of about 5 years. This group was compared with patients without PIPs to evaluate the rate of developing colorectal neoplasia. There was no difference between these 2 groups. A more recent study confirmed these findings [2]. I survey patients with large PIPs closer and generally bring them back in 2–3 years for repeat colonoscopy.

It is important to carefully survey for flat polyps because these adenomatous polyps represent a more aggressive type of polyp in the setting of IBD. I utilize NBI to evaluate the pit pattern of a polyp and to delineate the borders of flatter lesions. It is important to biopsy the mucosa around such a polyp and place it in a separate bottle to evaluate for active IBD.

If you're removing one of these larger pseudopolyps, will you use cold snare or hot snare?

I generally do not remove PIPs because of the increased bleeding risk. If I do need to biopsy one, I often need to apply a hemoclip to achieve hemostasis.

What do you do when a random biopsy in a patient with chronic UC shows dysplasia?

First, I look at the pathology report to determine the type of dysplasia: low vs high grade vs. indeterminate. Low-grade/indefinite dysplasia can be indistinguishable from active inflammation in ulcerative colitis. In this scenario, if there is concurrent active disease, I would adjust therapy and bring the patient back in 6 months for a repeat colonoscopy.

In the case of high-grade dysplasia, if these were truly random biopsies without a focal lesion, I would repeat a colonoscopy with chromoendoscopy.

So, you are generally using NBI to look at the pit pattern. When will you actually do chromoendoscopy where you are spraying the mucosa?

The pendulum on whether and when to use chromoendoscopy keeps changing, each year. It is certainly warranted when there is high-grade dysplasia on random biopsies to better delineate if there's a focal lesion that can be intervened upon. In patients with concurrent PSC, chromoendoscopy can also be used to especially survey the right colon.

References

1. Lewis AE, Kirchgesner J, Dray X, Svrcek M, Beaugerie L. 305 Clinical significance of pseudo-polyps for patients with inflammatory bowel disease. Am J Gastroenterol. 2019;114:S179–80. https://doi.org/10.14309/01.ajg.0000590752.06064.e8.
2. Wolf T, Lewis A, Beaugerie L, Svrcek M, Kirchgesner J, Network S-AIBD. Risk of colorectal neoplasia according to histologic disease activity in patients with inflammatory bowel disease and colonic post-inflammatory polyps. Aliment Pharmacol Ther. 2023;57(12):1445–52. https://doi.org/10.1111/apt.17495. Epub 2023 Mar 31.

Chapter 31
Ulcerative Colitis Refractory to Anti-TNF

Daniel Stein and Salina Faidhalla

A 38-year-old man with moderately severe ulcerative colitis is not responding to infliximab. You are considering switching to a JAK inhibitor. He is mildly obese, a non-smoker and has no other medical problems.

How effective have you found the JAK inhibitors to be in patients who have failed anti-TNFs?

Currently, the FDA has approved two different JAK inhibitors, tofacitinib, a JAK 1-3 inhibitor, and upadacitinib, a JAK 1 inhibitor for use in moderate to severe UC patients who failed anti-TNFs. Both medications have been found to be effective in induction and maintenance of remission in patients with moderate to severe UC who failed other biologics including anti-TNF agents,

With tofacitinib, there is a rapid decrease in stool frequency and rectal bleeding, generally within days. The recommended induction dose is 10 mg BID for 8 weeks, which can be continued for another 8 weeks if there is no initial response. This is then followed by a maintenance dose of 5 mg BID. A maintenance dose of 10 mg BID can be used in patients with severe disease and in patients having failed anti-TNF therapy.

Upadacitinib has been recently approved for moderate to severe UC. It also has a rapid clinical response. The recommended induction dose is 45 mg daily for 8

D. Stein (✉)
Department of Internal Medicine, Division of Gastroenterology and Hepatology, Medical College of Wisconsin, Milwaukee, WI, USA
e-mail: dstein@mcw.edu

S. Faidhalla
Department of Medicine Division of Gastroenterology and Hepatology, Medical College of Wisconsin, Milwaukee, WI, USA
e-mail: sfaidhalla@mcw.edu

© The Author(s), under exclusive license to Springer Nature
Switzerland AG 2023
W. H. Sobin et al. (eds.), *Managing Complex Cases in Gastroenterology*,
https://doi.org/10.1007/978-3-031-48949-5_31

weeks followed by 15 mg daily maintenance dose. A higher maintenance dose of 30 mg daily can be used in patients with a higher disease burden or in those that have failed other advanced therapies.

Both medications are very effective in patients with moderate to severe disease who have failed TNF inhibitors, making them valuable treatment options in UC patients. Overall, the efficacy of both medications has been shown to be dose dependent with higher doses associated with higher response rates.

In our practice, tofacitinib efficacy has been comparable to the efficacy in clinical trials reaching up to 20% remission rates. The response rates for upadacitinib have been even higher, presumably because the medication is more selective.

In the OCTAVE induction trials, remission rates with tofacitinib were up to 18.8% compared to 8.2% in the placebo group [1]. And in the OCTAVE sustain trial, maintenance of remission rates at 52 weeks was 34% in the 5 mg group and 40% in the 10 mg group compared to only 11.1% in the placebo group.

For upadacitinib, in the UC1 trial, remission at 8 weeks was 26%, and in the UC2 trial, 8-week remission rate was 33% (higher than rates of tofacitinib). In the UC 3 trial [2], clinical remission at week 52 was achieved in 42% of patients receiving upadacitinib 15 mg once daily and in 52% of patients receiving upadacitinib 30 mg once daily.

When it comes to positioning these new medications, it appears that upadacitinib is more effective than tofacitinib, but this has yet to be validated in a head-to-head trial.

With JAK inhibitors there is no immunogenicity. There is an FDA black box warning about MACE events and thrombosis risk, based on observations in an RA population. MACE and VTE events were not seen more commonly in the trials studying ulcerative colitis.

In clinical practice, lowering the dose sometimes results in flare-ups, which we can usually overcome by increasing the dose. Although the lower maintenance dose is preferred, patients have been comfortable with continuing higher doses when needed to achieve and maintain remission.

Tofacitinib has been found helpful in treating acute severe ulcerative colitis (ASUC) in inpatients. We know that the most studied and effective options for ASUC are infliximab and cyclosporine. When a patient with ASUC has failed infliximab therapy in the past, tofacitinib has worked as a rescue therapy, knowing that despite rescue therapy up to 30% of patients with ASUC end up requiring colectomy.

In a retrospective case control study by Berinstein et al. [3], 40 patients, 85% of whom failed IFX in the past, received tofacitinib in addition to IV steroids for ASUC. These patients had a significantly lower risk of colectomy at 90 days when compared to the controls, with no increased risk of infection, VTE, or cardiovascular events in the 90-day period.

This suggests that high-dose tofacitinib plus IV steroids may be considered for treatment of high-risk biologic exposed patients admitted with ASUC.

If insurance will allow either drug, would you prefer to go with tofacitinib or upadacitinib?

There have been no head-to-head trials yet, but upadacitinib has shown higher absolute clinical remission rates during induction and maintenance in cross trial comparisons. In terms of side effects, upadacitinib was found to cause nasopharyngitis, and we see an increase in lipid levels, although usually not significant enough to stop treatment. Cardiovascular risks and increased VTE/PE risks in patients over age fifty have been documented in RA patients but not yet in the IBD population. Other risks include malignancies, particularly non-melanoma skin cancers.

We suggest using caution with these medications in older patients who have underlying cardiovascular disease or a history of VTE. However, we would still consider using them in patients with severe ulcerative colitis who failed other biologics because the risk of complications from active disease usually outweighs the risk of medication side effects. Also, if patients do have a history of VTE/PE and they are already anticoagulated, then we feel that you can safely start JAK inhibitors.

References

1. Sandborn WJ, Su C, Sands BE, D'Haens GR, Vermeire S, Schreiber S, Danese S, Feagan BG, Reinisch W, Niezychowski W, Friedman G. Tofacitinib as induction and maintenance therapy for ulcerative colitis. New Engl J Med. 2017;376(18):1723–36.
2. Danese S, Vermeire S, Zhou W, Pangan AL, Siffledeen J, Greenbloom S, Hébuterne X, D'Haens G, Nakase H, Panés J, Higgins PD. Upadacitinib as induction and maintenance therapy for moderately to severely active ulcerative colitis: results from three phase 3, multicentre, double-blind, randomised trials. Lancet. 2022;399(10341):2113–28.
3. Berinstein JA, Sheehan JL, Dias M, Berinstein EM, Steiner CA, Johnson LA, Regal RE, Allen JI, Cushing KC, Stidham RW, Bishu S, Kinnucan JAR, Cohen-Mekelburg SA, Waljee AK, Higgins PDR. Tofacitinib for biologic-experienced hospitalized patients with acute severe ulcerative colitis: a retrospective case-control study. Clin Gastroenterol Hepatol. 2021;19(10):2112–2120.e1. https://doi.org/10.1016/j.cgh.2021.05.038. Epub 2021 May 25. PMID: 34048936; PMCID: PMC8760630.

Chapter 32
Acute Severe Ulcerative Colitis

Amir Patel

A 34-year-old man presents with severe exacerbation of his ulcerative colitis. He was diagnosed with ulcerative colitis at age 30 and responded well to infliximab. He moved out of state for a new job, which involved doing a lot of traveling. He did not want to travel home and miss work to have infusions, and so he let them lapse.

You see him for the first time after he gets admitted. He has been having bloody diarrhea about 15 times a day. The diarrhea started 2 weeks earlier but is getting progressively worse. He is acutely ill, with a temp of 101, a BP of 90/60, and his heart rate is 110. His WBC is 19,000; his CRP is 85. Stool cultures are negative. You place him on IV steroids. An unprepped flex sig confirms severe colitis. After 3 days of steroids, he is still doing poorly. You get a surgical consult but decide to try a rescue therapy.

How do you manage acute severe UC in this case?

For this patient, there are three options. If he's in the hospital setting you can retry the infliximab at a high dose and see if he responds after 72 h. You could try cyclosporine. However, many of us are not using cyclosporine as much because there is a lot of monitoring to do and you can't give it to patients who have high blood pressure, renal disease, seizures, electrolyte abnormalities, or low albumin.

Another problem with cyclosporine is that you can use it in the hospital setting, but then you have to have some type of end game. What are you going to put him on once he gets out of the hospital? For this particular patient, I would probably try the infliximab, and if it doesn't work, then I would consider another therapy or surgery.

A. Patel (✉)

Dept. of Medicine, Division of Gastroenterology and Hepatology, Medical College of Wisconsin, Milwaukee, WI, USA

e-mail: ampatel@mcw.edu

The other therapy that has good data and a lot of promise is high-dose tofacitinib. This is for in-patients with severe UC, you give them 10 mg of tofacitinib three times a day. The tricky part with that is that after they leave the hospital, you need to make sure that they can continue on the Xeljanz on an outpatient basis.

But there are some robust data on using tofacitinib 10 mg three times a day, which is a high dose, to treat acute severe ulcerative colitis. We've had a couple of patients in the hospital recently where we were able to use it, and my colleague recently had a case where she tried to give Remicade rescue therapy but the repeat flex sig failed to show improvement. She gave high-dose tofacitinib, and miraculously, after 2 days, there was significant mucosal healing.

If you're giving the infliximab rescue, what dose would you give, would you pretreat with steroids, and would you give azathioprine along with the infliximab?

You're concerned about antibodies, but this patient's already on steroids. So, you don't really need to pretreat them. In terms of the dose of infliximab, it depends on the patient's albumin. If the albumin is low, I would probably give the 10 mg per kilogram dose of Remicade in the hospital setting.

I would plan on adding an immune modulator in the future, but we all know that it takes some time for that to build up in the system. But if it works for them, I would keep them on combination therapy going forward.

I would not necessarily start the immune modulator in the hospital. We're not sure which way he's going to go with the treatment, with the infliximab. I would probably start it a few days later, if they do respond to the infliximab.

If they respond to infliximab, when are you giving the second dose and the third dose?

It depends how they do clinically. If they do fine, and you're able to get them off of IV steroids, then I would just restart the induction doses at 0, 2, and 6 weeks. If they're in the hospital and they're having a partial response, some reduction in stool frequency and bleeding, sometimes I will give the second dose earlier. I might give it a week later or even within the same week.

The tricky part always is insurance coverage once they leave the hospital. But a lot of times we have a good prior authorization team that helps us with that.

Chapter 33
Resistant/Refractory Proctitis

Poonam Beniwal-Patel

A 38-year-old man is sent to you for a second opinion regarding proctitis. The patient started having bloody diarrhea and tenesmus 1 year earlier. His gastroenterologist performed a colonoscopy that revealed moderate severity proctitis, with a normal appearing colon proximal to 15 cm. Biopsies were consistent with ulcerative colitis. He was started on oral mesalamine and rowasa enemas and had only minor clinical improvement and is disappointed and frustrated. He wants to talk to an academic expert regarding his case.

In treating proctitis how do you decide whether to use suppository, enema, foam?

I actually tend to use suppositories very little for two reasons. One is that I'm not convinced that they have great distribution in the rectum, certainly compared to enemas or foams. And, anecdotally, I think the patient sometimes has a harder time holding in a small suppository versus the enema with the tip, or the foam where you spray it in.

The one occasion where I do use a suppository is if someone has a pouch, and they have cuffitis. Otherwise, I tend to use either an enema or the foam. I particularly like the foam; I think it's very user friendly. Patients can just spray the foam into the rectum and hold it and that way they don't have to mix the solution, hold the catheter in there, and distribute the solution the way you do with your traditional enema.

Therefore, if I have a patient who is having a flare, I like to use the foam. However, it is a steroid product, so it's fine for short-term use, for a flare. But if someone is going to be taking a long-term maintenance rectal treatment, I will use mesalamine enemas. I would rather not use the steroid product long term.

P. Beniwal-Patel (✉)
GI and Hepatology Division, Medical College of Wisconsin, Milwaukee, WI, USA
e-mail: pbeniwal@mcw.edu

Since the patient's proctitis clinically is not responding remarkably well to rectal medications, what would you do next?

I would restage him with a flexible sigmoidoscopy because the last scope was done a year ago, in order to assess whether there has been a change in severity or extent. If the repeat endoscopy shows persistent limited Mayo 2 disease, I sometimes consider adding oral mesalamine-4.8 g, along with enema/foam therapy. In select cases, we also try an oral budesonide or prednisone taper. If the disease has progressed to Mayo 3, if there's more extensive distribution, or if the patient is clinically not doing well, I would start biologic therapy. In that case, we might start with vedolizumab versus an anti-TNF.

I think a common misconception with proctitis, when I see patients who are coming in for a second or third opinion, is that, oh, it's *"just proctitis"*, how bad can it be? But it can really progress rapidly, and I've had several patients who've had Mayo three of just the distal 30, 40 centimeters who ended up in the hospital and got quite sick and almost needed surgery.

I think the key thing with resistant proctitis is making sure that we pull the trigger early enough, but not too early. We will usually start something like vedolizumab or an anti-TNF and that usually does the trick.

Chapter 34
Vaccinations in Newly Diagnosed IBD

Preetika Sinh

A 57-year-old woman, non-smoker, is seen for bloody diarrhea and found to have moderately severe UC involving most of the colon. She has not had any vaccinations in recent memory, perhaps none since she finished school.

How would you go about vaccinating this lady and does her lack of recent vaccinations alter your choice of therapy?

We always discuss the necessity of having up-to-date vaccinations, and in most cases, we can get patients to go along with that. We are talking about yearly flu vaccine, pneumonia vaccine, and tetanus every 10 years. We need to check hepatitis serology and vaccinate if not immune. In this patient, HPV is not clinically indicated. Shingrix is very important, particularly when JAK inhibitors are used.

IBD itself does not interfere with the ability of patients to respond to vaccinations but immunosuppressive drugs may. Ideally, we should wait for at least 4 weeks after vaccination to start our immune-suppressing drugs. But we often don't have time to wait, we have to start the drugs right away, and so we just get the patient rolling on their vaccinations. We do try to give the first Shingrix dose prior to starting an anti-TNF and particularly a JAK inhibitor.

But, no, I would not veto the use of anti-TNFs because the patient has not been vaccinated. The major infections associated with anti-TNFs are TB and fungal infections, and we can't vaccinate against those anyway. We do take age into account, however. There is an increased risk, with anti-TNFs, of infection, including serious infections, in those patients over 65.

P. Sinh (✉)
Division of Gastroenterology and Hepatology, Medical College of Wisconsin, Milwaukee, WI, USA
e-mail: psinh@mcw.edu

W. H. Sobin et al. (eds.), *Managing Complex Cases in Gastroenterology*, https://doi.org/10.1007/978-3-031-48949-5_34

In talking about JAK inhibitors, how does the new upadacitinib compare with tofacitinib?

Upadacitinib is a selective JAK inhibitor while tofacitinib is non-selective. There does not appear to be a different safety, side effect profile with either one currently. It is possible, in the long run, that the selective JAK inhibitor may have a better safety profile.

Upadacitinib appears to have a more rapid induction, the number of patients responding in the first 2 weeks is compelling. And these excellent results were seen not only in those who are biologic naïve, but also those who had been exposed to anti-TNFs previously. Would I switch a patient from tofacitinib to upadacitinib? No, not unless a new mechanism of action was present. But, if a patient is first being started on a JAK inhibitor, I would probably opt for the use of upadacitinib.

Chapter 35
Ustekinumab vs Risankizumab in Crohn's

Daniel Stein and Salina Faidhalla

A 28-year-old female smoker is found to have mild moderately severe Crohn's colitis without obvious small bowel involvement. She does not want to go on an anti-TNF and is wondering about going on ustekinumab or the new drug risankizumab.

Can you discuss how you would choose between ustekinumab and risankizumab if insurance coverage was not an issue.

Ustekinumab is an IL-12 and IL-23 inhibitor while risankizumab is an IL-23 inhibitor alone. Risankizumab was recently approved for use in moderate-to-severe Crohn's disease. It has endoscopic and histologic data supporting its efficacy.

Both medications start with IV infusion for induction followed by SQ injections. They have good efficacy and comparable side effect profiles; however, there are not enough data comparing the two medications since risankizumab was only recently approved. The safety profile overall appears to be similar; there might be a small risk of DILI with risankizumab since one patient developed liver injury in the trial.

Risankizumab may have increased efficacy compared with ustekinumab and clinically may be comparable to infliximab. Our clinical experience with risankizumab in Crohn's patients who failed multiple biologics has been similar to what was seen in the clinical trials. If insurance is not an issue, then we would generally choose risankizumab.

D. Stein (✉)
Department of Internal Medicine, Division of Gastroenterology and Hepatology, Medical College of Wisconsin, Milwaukee, WI, USA
e-mail: dstein@mcw.edu

S. Faidhalla
Department of Medicine Division of Gastroenterology and Hepatology, Medical College of Wisconsin, Milwaukee, WI, USA
e-mail: sfaidhalla@mcw.edu

© The Author(s), under exclusive license to Springer Nature Switzerland AG 2023
W. H. Sobin et al. (eds.), *Managing Complex Cases in Gastroenterology*,
https://doi.org/10.1007/978-3-031-48949-5_35

In comparing vedolizumab, ustekinumab, and risankizumab in Crohn's disease, what is your first choice, or which drug do you prefer in which situation?

Many factors, including age, disease severity, disease behavior (inflammatory, stricturing or fistulizing), location, the presence of perianal disease, extraintestinal manifestations, prior biologic exposure, history of malignancy, serious infections, and patient preference, play a role in choosing a biologic and must all be considered carefully.

VDZ is usually used to treat moderate-to-severe Crohn's patients with no extraintestinal manifestations, and no perianal disease since it is more gut selective. This is also a good choice in patients with a history of malignancy or serious infections given its favorable side effect profile. However, it does have a slower onset of action and possible delayed clinical response when compared to anti-TNF or UST.

That being said, there are some data supporting VDZ use in perianal disease. The exploratory analysis from the GEMINI 2 trial showed a greater percentage of Crohn's disease patients with draining fistulae achieving fistula closure by week 52 with vedolizumab compared to placebo [1]. There were similar findings in the ENTERPRISE study where >50% of patients with fistulizing CD treated with vedolizumab (with concurrent seton until week 14 and antibiotics until week 6) had >50% decrease in the number of draining perianal fistulae [2].

UST has been effective in Crohn's patients including those patients who are refractory to infliximab. While the data for use of UST for treating EIMs didn't show statistical significance, UST is effective in treating psoriasis and psoriatic arthritis. There are some data that suggest that UST can be effective in patients with perianal disease in CD. Notably, infliximab is the most effective and most studied drug for treatment of perianal disease in CD, but UST may be useful in CD patients not responding to infliximab who have refractory perianal CD. Being a self-administered injection is more convenient for patients.

As mentioned above, there is no head-to-head trial comparing ustekinumab and risankizumab. However, the absolute remission rates in separate trials were higher with risankizumab [3]. If we have the freedom of choosing between the two, we would start with risankizumab since it appears to be more effective than UST. We also have some clinical experience in using it in patients with TNF-resistant perianal disease with very good response. The safety profile for UST and risankizumab is comparable. They are both effective for perianal disease but not the first choice.

However, if we have a patient with Crohn's disease and EIM, we usually start with an anti-TNF; if the patient fails the anti-TNF, then we would consider UST or risankizumab.

If the patient was amenable to an anti-TNF, would you choose that over the other 3 drugs previously mentioned? How do you decide?

Anti-TNFs are long established with good efficacy and known safety profile in treating CD. Treatment with anti-TNF agents appears to be more effective when given earlier in the course of disease; rates of response and remission are higher if given within 2 years of onset of disease.

Anti-TNFs also target extraintestinal manifestations (EIMs) of CD and should be considered in such patients. IFX is very effective in patients with perianal and fistulizing disease.

In this young patient with mild-moderate disease, no EIM or perianal CD, and no previous biologic exposure, all options are reasonable and should be discussed in detail.

We recognize that choosing therapy in patients with Crohn's disease can be complicated. To shed some light on positioning therapy, a recent meta-analysis by Singh et al. [4] assessed the comparable efficacy and safety of biologics in patients with Crohn's disease and this may be a guide.

This study highlighted that treatment with anti-TNFs: infliximab or adalimumab, consistently ranked high for induction and maintenance of clinical remission. And infliximab in combination with azathioprine was the highest ranked treatment for induction of clinical remission and maintenance of long-term remission in biologic-naive patients.

It is also important to remember that anti-TNFs still play a crucial role in the treatment of patients with high-risk phenotypes such as fistulizing, penetrating, and stricturing disease and also TNF-sensitive extraintestinal manifestations.

IL-23 blockade might be the preferred mechanism of action in patients who have been previously exposed to TNF antagonists. Overall data suggest that both ustekinumab and risankizumab are effective after either primary or secondary loss of response to other biologics. Risankizumab and ustekinumab also appear to be more effective than vedolizumab in patients who have lost response or have intolerance to anti-TNF therapy.

It is also crucial to keep in mind that when you are dealing with a primary non-responder, the best strategy is to switch the class of drugs. In cases of secondary non-response, you can still try another medication within the same class.

References

1. Sandborn WJ, Feagan BG, Rutgeerts P, Hanauer S, Colombel JF, Sands BE, Lukas M, Fedorak RN, Lee S, Bressler B, Fox I. Vedolizumab as induction and maintenance therapy for Crohn's disease. N Engl J Med. 2013;369(8):711–21.
2. Schwartz DA, Peyrin-Biroulet L, Lasch K, Adsul S, Danese S. Efficacy and safety of 2 vedolizumab intravenous regimens for perianal fistulizing Crohn's disease: ENTERPRISE study. Clin Gastroenterol Hepatol. 2022;20(5):1059–67.
3. Ferrante M, Panaccione R, Baert F, Bossuyt P, Colombel JF, Danese S, Dubinsky M, Feagan BG, Hisamatsu T, Lim A, Lindsay JO. Risankizumab as maintenance therapy for moderately to severely active Crohn's disease: results from the multicentre, randomised, double-blind, placebo-controlled, withdrawal phase 3 FORTIFY maintenance trial. Lancet. 2022;399(10340):2031–46.
4. Singh S, Murad MH, Fumery M, Sedano R, Jairath V, Panaccione R, Sandborn WJ, Ma C. Comparative efficacy and safety of biologic therapies for moderate-to-severe Crohn's disease: a systematic review and network meta-analysis. Lancet Gastroenterol Hepatol. 2021;6(12):1002–14. https://doi.org/10.1016/S2468-1253(21)00312-5. Epub 2021 Oct 22. PMID: 34688373; PMCID: PMC8933137.

Chapter 36
Use of Vedolizumab in UC

Daniel Stein and Salina Faidhalla

A 67-year-old man who quit smoking 6 months earlier is diagnosed with new-onset left-sided ulcerative colitis that is mild to moderate in severity. He is started on oral and rectal mesalamine but does not respond. He continues to move his bowels 4–5 times a day with a small amount of blood mixed in his stool. He would like to try vedolizumab as his next course of therapy.

Is vedolizumab a reasonable option? If so, would you start steroids as well?

In patients with mild-moderate left-sided UC with active disease despite being on an adequate dose of oral and rectal mesalamine, we usually add budesonide 9 mg daily for 12 weeks for induction of remission. We prefer budesonide to prednisone due to its lower systemic side effects. We would start budesonide prior to escalating to biologics and assess response.

If the decision was made to proceed with VDZ, then we would start budesonide that clinic visit while waiting for the first infusion of VDZ. We would then continue budesonide for 12 weeks and stop without tapering.

Do you check vedolizumab levels early on?

There is some evidence that higher VDZ levels are associated with higher clinical response and mucosal healing especially in UC. In a recent systematic review and meta-analysis by Singh et al. [1], they reported that in UC patients, median vedolizumab trough concentrations were consistently higher in patients achieving

D. Stein (✉)
Department of Internal Medicine, Division of Gastroenterology and Hepatology, Medical College of Wisconsin, Milwaukee, WI, USA
e-mail: dstein@mcw.edu

S. Faidhalla
Department of Medicine Division of Gastroenterology and Hepatology, Medical College of Wisconsin, Milwaukee, WI, USA
e-mail: sfaidhalla@mcw.edu

© The Author(s), under exclusive license to Springer Nature Switzerland AG 2023
W. H. Sobin et al. (eds.), *Managing Complex Cases in Gastroenterology*,
https://doi.org/10.1007/978-3-031-48949-5_36

clinical remission or endoscopic remission. Based on their meta-analysis, they suggested that vedolizumab trough concentration >20 µg/mL at week 6 and >12 µg/mL during maintenance may be associated with better outcomes.

Some providers do proactively check VDZ levels but we don't do this routinely. We only do reactive drug monitoring in the case of primary non-responders or secondary loss of response. We don't think that there is enough evidence supporting proactive monitoring of the VDZ levels. We know what to do with anti-TNF levels but with vedolizumab you have completely different mechanisms of action. How high a level do you need to saturate those receptors? We don't know. We don't think that we necessarily know the full significance of our vedolizumab levels.

The patient is responding to combination budesonide and vedolizumab but when you stop the budesonide after 8 weeks his disease starts to flare. His vedolizumab levels are adequate.

How would you manage this?

Usually, when drug levels are adequate, and the patient's clinical response has been steroid dependent, the best next step is to switch therapy. However, in the case of VDZ it has been recognized that it can take longer to achieve the desired clinical response (6–8 weeks in UC, 10–14 weeks in CD).

In this patient who has been on the medication for 8 weeks, we would discuss the options of giving the drug more time and continuing budesonide vs switching to another agent. If at 10–12 weeks the patient still has no response, then we should switch to another agent.

Do you ever suggest to your patients who develop UC after quitting smoking that they go back to smoking a cigarette or two a day?

We wouldn't recommend that the risks of smoking outweigh the benefits, especially since we have so many options for treatment.

Are patients who develop UC after quitting smoking more difficult to get under control?

There are no data to suggest that.

If you decide to give vedolizumab more time to "kick-in" how much longer would you continue budesonide?

Maybe 10–12 weeks if they are primary non-responders, if they have partial response then up to 6 months. If there is no clinical response and active inflammation is confirmed with fecal calprotectin and/or CRP, then switching therapy to another agent is reasonable. If the patient is doing poorly, we would switch medication earlier.

The patient continues to show a lack of response to VDZ

What is your next choice for patients who choose vedolizumab but fail to respond to it?

In this patient with mild-moderate left-sided UC who failed mesalamine and VDZ, available options include anti-TNFs and UST. Ozanimod is another option for UC patients who are anti-TNF naive.

In this case, since this patient is older and has mild-moderate UC with no EIM we would probably start UST. Obviously, a discussion with the patient regarding treatment options is essential in choosing the next drug.

Reference

1. Singh S, Dulai PS, Vande Casteele N, Battat R, Fumery M, Boland BS, Sandborn WJ. Systematic review with meta-analysis: association between vedolizumab trough concentration and clinical outcomes in patients with inflammatory bowel diseases. Aliment Pharmacol Ther. 2019;50(8):848–57. https://doi.org/10.1111/apt.15484. Epub 2019 Sep 4. PMID: 31483522; PMCID: PMC7083298

Chapter 37
Functional Diarrhea in IBD

Amir Patel

A 32-year-old woman with a history of Crohn's involving the terminal ileum and right colon has been well controlled on Humira. She now comes in complaining of frequent watery diarrhea and rectal urgency. Her exam, CRP, stool cultures, stool calprotectin, and colonoscopy are within normal limits. Are there other tests you would want to run?

It sounds like her Crohn's is well controlled and the symptoms are either functional or bile acid related. How do you manage those patients?

We see that a lot. Many of our patients with Crohn's disease will have overlapping irritable bowel syndrome, and if they have ileal disease, we also think about bile acid diarrhea. In this particular patient, you would also like to know their underlying medical history, do they have a history of depression, anxiety?

But I probably would start them on cholestyramine first, to treat bile acid diarrhea. And if that doesn't help, I would wonder whether this could be irritable bowel syndrome. That, to me, is a little bit more difficult to treat. But some studies in our inflammatory bowel disease literature show that patients may do well with a low FODMAP diet.

The other thing you think about, if this patient has ever had any stricturing disease, is the possibility of small intestinal bacterial overgrowth. So, it would be fair to try a course of antibiotics as well.

A. Patel (✉)
Dept. of Medicine, Division of Gastroenterology and Hepatology, Medical College of Wisconsin, Milwaukee, WI, USA
e-mail: ampatel@mcw.edu

© The Author(s), under exclusive license to Springer Nature Switzerland AG 2023
W. H. Sobin et al. (eds.), *Managing Complex Cases in Gastroenterology*,
https://doi.org/10.1007/978-3-031-48949-5_37

When you use cholestyramine, do you tend to use it once a day or several times a day?

I typically use it once a day, mostly in the morning. I think that's when they get the most benefit from it. So, I start it in the morning with a low dose, and if they notice some improvement, I'll increase the dose incrementally, but I just give it once in the morning.

Chapter 38
When to Postpone Infusions

Poonam Beniwal-Patel

A 32-year-old man has UC well controlled on infliximab. He has a history of sinus infections in the past and feels like he has one now. He is due for his infusion tomorrow.

Would you postpone the infusion? In which situations do you feel it is necessary to postpone an infusion and why?

In the setting of a mild infection where a patient has been afebrile for 48 h, the infusion is given. If a patient is hospitalized with an infection, we will delay therapy given that source control is needed.

But this raises an interesting question. It used to be that the only biologic agents available were the anti-TNFs, and we would have to struggle with this dilemma. But now, if I have a patient who keeps getting recurrent sinus infections, in the absence of any anatomic defects, and we are really thinking that it's the infliximab that is increasing their risk of infections, I actually have changed them over to vedolizumab if they're in deep remission. It's nice that now, we have other options, other medications that may not increase the risk of things like sinus infections or folliculitis.

What are some other examples of patients where you've told them it's not a good idea to go ahead with their infusions?

With COVID, if someone was diagnosed within the last couple of days, we'll have them wait a week and make sure they haven't spiked a fever for a few days before administering an infusion. But outside of having a fever or a prolonged infection where source control with antibiotics hasn't been achieved there really are very few scenarios where we will postpone an infusion.

P. Beniwal-Patel (✉)
Medicine, Gastroenterology/Hepatology Division, Medical College of Wisconsin,
Milwaukee, WI, USA
e-mail: pbeniwal@mcw.edu

W. H. Sobin et al. (eds.), *Managing Complex Cases in Gastroenterology*,
https://doi.org/10.1007/978-3-031-48949-5_38

221

Chapter 39
Musculoskeletal Complaints in a Patient on Anti-TNFs

Amir Patel

A 35-year-old woman has been receiving infliximab for 2 years for Crohn's disease. Her ileocolitis has been under good control, but she comes in complaining of joint pain in her knees and fingers which is something new for her. On exam, her joints seem tender but not acutely inflamed.

When do you consider the possibility that a patient with IBD who develops new musculoskeletal symptoms might be experiencing an adverse reaction from their anti-TNF?

Arthropathy is common in inflammatory bowel disease. There are two types. Type one is generally peripheral, acute, and involves less than six joints. That type of arthropathy typically occurs at the beginning of the disease. It's self-limiting, non-erosive, and correlates with flares. So, if someone has active colitis, they typically complain of joint pains, commonly affecting the knees and elbows in my experience. Type two is more polyarticular. The MCPs, the small joints, are commonly involved. These do have active synovitis but this type of joint pain does not correlate with IBD flares and can happen years after the disease commences. That's one thing I think about, but if someone's been on an anti-TNF for a couple of years and now, they start having arthralgias, I do start wondering if this could be a side effect of the Remicade.

Usually, I see arthralgias as an adverse reaction to Remicade occurring early after initiation of therapy. If it starts up years later, then I do get concerned about conditions like drug-induced lupus, where I consider referring the patient to the rheumatologist.

A. Patel (✉)
Dept. of Medicine, Division of Gastroenterology and Hepatology, Medical College of Wisconsin, Milwaukee, WI, USA
e-mail: ampatel@mcw.edu

Drug-induced lupus is pretty low risk with your anti-TNFs compared to other medications, but it can happen. This usually occurs months or years after they've been exposed to the drug. If I am thinking about drug-induced lupus, I do get some blood work before I send them to the rheumatologist, including a CBC, CMP, anti-double-stranded DNA, anti-histone antibodies and complement levels, C3 and C4. And if any of those antibodies are elevated, I have them see the rheumatologist to determine whether they have to come off anti-TNF and go on some other medication.

The rheumatologist reports that it is possible these symptoms are related to the infliximab and she would like you to stop infliximab and switch to a different class of drug,

Which drug would you choose?

In a patient with arthralgias like this, I'd probably go with an IL-12,23 or an IL-23 inhibitor, so that's ustekinumab (Stelara) or risankizumab (Skyrizi). Those are the types of therapies I'd probably go with in a patient with Crohn's disease. Obviously, it also depends on the phenotype of their disease. If it's more severe and stricturing, then obviously I prefer the IL-12,23, and IL-23 over something like anti-integrin therapy, vedolizumab (Entyvio). If a patient has a lot of extraintestinal manifestations, I'll also go with Stelara or Skyrizi over Entyvio. Data suggest that Entyvio might not be the best drug for extraintestinal manifestations, including arthralgias.

With arthralgia and other extraintestinal manifestations, particularly psoriasis, we have found that the IL-12,23s and IL-23s have really helped. However, the one exception is in ankylosing spondylitis. In ankylosing spondylitis, the anti-TNFs are clearly superior and the anti-IL 12,23s and anti-IL23s have not been that effective.

Now, if it were ulcerative colitis and not Crohn's disease you could also consider switching to a JAK inhibitor like tofacitinib or upadacitinib. So far, these drugs are just approved for UC not Crohn's (upadacitinib was recently approved for Crohn's). But they are very effective second-line therapies.

Chapter 40
Use of Immune Modulators in Patients Being Started on Anti-TNFs

Daniel Stein and Salina Faidhalla

You have a patient with moderately severe ulcerative colitis who you want to start on an anti-TNF. He is a 32-year-old man who is a social drinker, having about 2 drinks on Saturday night and Sunday during ball games. No other medical problems.

Do you think immune modulators should be used in all patients on anti-TNFs or are you doing more anti-TNF monotherapy with close dose monitoring?

Combination therapy with IFX and AZA is superior to monotherapy. The benefit of adding an IM to adalimumab or a different anti-TNF is not well established. We are less likely to add AZA to Humira unless we are treating a patient with Humira who has had secondary loss of response and antibody to IFX.

On the other hand, close dose monitoring with monotherapy can be very effective in patients on anti-TNFs. We are more likely to employ this when using IFX in a patient over 60, to decrease the risk of bone marrow suppression and lymphoma. We know that very high drug levels of the infliximab are as protective against antibody formation than immunomodulators, if not more. So that's a different approach.

If you decide to use azathioprine, how would you use it in this young male, and for how long, noting concerns that exist about hepatosplenic T-cell lymphoma (HSTCL)?

Men under 35 years of age receiving long-term thiopurines (>2 years) are at a significantly increased risk of HSTCL, although the true incidence remains low. The risk of HSTCL in IBD patients on combination therapy is about 1:3500. This

D. Stein (✉)
Department of Internal Medicine, Division of Gastroenterology and Hepatology, Medical College of Wisconsin, Milwaukee, WI, USA
e-mail: dstein@mcw.edu

S. Faidhalla
Department of Medicine Division of Gastroenterology and Hepatology, Medical College of Wisconsin, Milwaukee, WI, USA
e-mail: sfaidhalla@mcw.edu

© The Author(s), under exclusive license to Springer Nature Switzerland AG 2023
W. H. Sobin et al. (eds.), *Managing Complex Cases in Gastroenterology*, https://doi.org/10.1007/978-3-031-48949-5_40

usually doesn't affect our decision to start the medication. But we always discuss the risk with the patient beforehand.

While we feel this is a small risk, one strategy to reduce the risk even further is to use a lower dose of azathioprine. We can target lower 6TG levels, a 6TG level of 100–120 is enough to prevent antibody formation.

We can also stop the azathioprine earlier. We think that once you get two years out that the benefit with combination therapy, probably isn't there. If you look at when people are going to get antibodies, they usually get it, within the first year. The cases of HSTCL have occurred in patients taking azathioprine for >2 years.

You can also do monotherapy with anti-TNF alone with close dose monitoring.

Do you ever use methotrexate as your immune modulator in treating IBD? How do you administer it?

In UC, there are limited data on using methotrexate in combination with anti-TNFs. Currently, MTX is not commonly used in adult patients with UC. However, in CD there are data supporting use of methotrexate to reduce immunogenicity and improving drug concentrations when used in combination with an anti-TNF agent. This may be the preferred immunomodulator for combination therapy in those at higher risk of adverse effects of thiopurines such as young men or those with multiple skin cancers.

We do use methotrexate occasionally in our practice for select patients.

For combination therapy, we use an oral dose of 12.5 mg per week. This low dose works to prevent antibody formation. The only time we use MTX IM or SC is when we use it as monotherapy in CD at a dose of 25 mg weekly.

Alcohol use in this case would make using methotrexate risky.

Chapter 41
Pyoderma Gangrenosum

Poonam Beniwal-Patel

A 27-year-old female presents with acute ulcerative colitis and a skin rash on her legs, which is diagnosed as pyoderma gangrenosum. Colonoscopy revealed a mild-moderate severity pancolitis.

Does someone have to have severe ulcerative colitis to develop pyoderma gangrenosum? What therapy would you use to treat the UC and the pyoderma in this patient? Is a dermatologist always involved?

You can see pyoderma gangrenosum in someone with mild IBD. We had one patient who had very severe PG and never had any GI symptoms. He had several colonoscopies that looked normal and revealed only minimal histologic evidence of ulcerative colitis.

PG severity does not have to correlate with bowel disease activity. I would say that about half of the patients I've seen with PG have severe colitis and half do not. The best treatment for PG is anti-TNF drugs. I prefer infliximab. So, even if they have just mild UC, I would treat them with an anti-TNF if they have biopsy-proven PG.

There is a dermatologist involved in the beginning to do a skin biopsy and make the diagnosis. But after that, they generally leave the management up to us, since treating the patient with anti-TNFs usually heals the skin lesions as well as the IBD. Occasionally, the dermatologist will use topical steroids, but the mainstay is the anti-TNF.

P. Beniwal-Patel (✉)
Medicine, Gastroenterology/Hepatology Division, Medical College of Wisconsin, Milwaukee, WI, USA
e-mail: pbeniwal@mcw.edu

© The Author(s), under exclusive license to Springer Nature Switzerland AG 2023
W. H. Sobin et al. (eds.), *Managing Complex Cases in Gastroenterology*,
https://doi.org/10.1007/978-3-031-48949-5_41

227

Chapter 42
UC in a Patient Who Failed Mesalamine and Anti-TNF

Daniel Stein and Salina Faidhalla

A 33-year-old female has moderate left-sided UC. She has tried and failed mesala-mine and Humira (with azathioprine) and needs a change of therapy to treat her symptoms.

How would you feel about each of these options in a patient with moderate UC who has failed an anti-TNF? (a) Vedolizumab (b) Ustekinumab (c) Ozanimod (d) Tofacitinib

UST is one option. It has proven effective in patients who have failed an anti-TNF. It is an injectable medication, which is convenient in patients who have work or school.

UST has been found to be more effective than vedo in inducing and maintaining remission as a second-line therapy in Crohn's disease in a network meta-analysis. So, vedo is not our first choice in patients who have failed an anti-TNF.

We would not recommend ozanimod in a patient who failed anti-TNF, since the original study population had only a small percentage of patients who failed anti-TNF.

Tofacitinib is a Jak1/JAK3 inhibitor that is approved for moderate to severe UC patients who have failed anti-TNFs. Upadacitinib is a specific JAK1 inhibitor, which

D. Stein (✉)
Department of Internal Medicine, Division of Gastroenterology and Hepatology, Medical College of Wisconsin, Milwaukee, WI, USA

Department of Medicine Division of Gastroenterology and Hepatology, Medical College of Wisconsin, Milwaukee, WI, USA
e-mail: dstein@mcw.edu; sfaidhalla@mcw.edu

S. Faidhalla
Department of Medicine Division of Gastroenterology and Hepatology, Medical College of Wisconsin, Milwaukee, WI, USA

© The Author(s), under exclusive license to Springer Nature Switzerland AG 2023
W. H. Sobin et al. (eds.), *Managing Complex Cases in Gastroenterology*,
https://doi.org/10.1007/978-3-031-48949-5_42

229

is also effective. Our clinical experience suggests that it is possibly more effective than tofacitinib, and there is some consensus that it has a more favorable side-effect profile, given that it's more selective. However, since this is a young female who may have plans for pregnancy, we would want to avoid any JAK inhibitor and ozanimod at this time, and we would probably choose UST.

IFX can be considered if the patient failed adalimumab; however, most of us are turning to the JAK inhibitors in patients who have failed anti-TNFs.

Chapter 43
Patients with IBD Who Are Squeamish About Rectal Meds and Self-Injection

Amir Patel

A 20-year-old college sophomore presents with chronic UC that previously involved the left colon to the splenic flexure. She had been doing well, taking mesalamine for a year but over the past month started having increased bowel frequency, urgency, and rectal bleeding. Her community gastroenterologist repeated her colonoscopy and noted active inflammation in the rectum, with the rest of the colon looking fairly normal. The woman is going to school 1000 miles away on a fairly rural campus. Her doctor recommends that she try rectal meds – either suppository or enema – but she gets squeamish thinking about this and doesn't want to try. He also discusses possibly using Humira, but she is frightened about self-injection.

This gastroenterologist, who frequently sends you patients for a second opinion, calls and curbsides you with these questions:

Do you have any tips for convincing a patient to try taking a rectal med? If so, are you more successful in getting them to take suppositories, foams, or enemas?

Do you have any tricks for dealing with patients who are reluctant to do self-injection?

A lot of our patients with proctitis don't want to take rectal suppositories for several reasons: first, they're uncomfortable; second, there's a stigma of putting something in the rectum; and third, sometimes it's really hard to retain suppositories or enemas, if there's significant inflammation, and they have a lot of urgency and diarrhea already.

A. Patel (✉)
Dept. of Medicine, Division of Gastroenterology and Hepatology, Medical College of Wisconsin, Milwaukee, WI, USA
e-mail: ampatel@mcw.edu

© The Author(s), under exclusive license to Springer Nature Switzerland AG 2023
W. H. Sobin et al. (eds.), *Managing Complex Cases in Gastroenterology*,
https://doi.org/10.1007/978-3-031-48949-5_43

231

Injections are another problem. We have a lot of young individuals diagnosed with IBD who don't want to self-inject or they're afraid of needles. This is sometimes very difficult to manage. What we typically do in the clinic is discuss with them the risks if their disease goes uncontrolled and what the benefits of our medications are. So, we have that risk and benefit talk. Because the truth is that if they don't get their proctitis under control, there's always a chance the disease may progress. There's an increased risk of flares. And, obviously, there's concern for the increased risk for cancer.

So, we have that discussion and see if they're willing to try the rectal suppositories or the self-injections. But unfortunately, I don't have any other tricks to convince them otherwise.

In terms of choosing between suppositories, foam, and enemas, if it's just proctitis involving the last 5 cm of the rectum, I think that suppositories are the ideal route. Typically, they can be easier to retain than enemas. If you're talking about more left-sided colitis, where there's involvement to the splenic flexure, then I would use enemas. And here I'm talking about mesalamine. Now, we do have hydrocortisone foams as well. And some patients feel that they can retain those better.

There is also a small subset of patients who may have a paradoxical response to mesalamine. So, if they try Canasa suppositories or Rowasa enemas, which are both mesalamine products, and they get a paradoxical response, you're typically going to switch them to hydrocortisone enemas or foams as a substitute.

Do you have any experience with tacrolimus suppositories?

Yes, tacrolimus suppositories have been around, and they're usually dosed at 2 mg twice a day. We typically reserve those for patients who are refractory to mesalamine or steroid suppositories. I use them rarely. There have been several studies, one was a head-to-head study looking at tacrolimus versus steroids, and while that study didn't find tacrolimus superior in controlling symptoms, there was another study of about 40 patients that did show a benefit. So, I am using it for those who are willing to take suppositories but haven't had a robust response to mesalamine or steroid suppositories. And I typically give it for about a month to see if it helps. But obviously, a lot of times, this is just a bridge until you find them an appropriate maintenance therapy.

Chapter 44
Colon Stricture in UC

Poonam Beniwal-Patel

A 58-year-old female with chronic ulcerative colitis managed with infliximab comes to see you for a surveillance colonoscopy. Her last gastroenterologist just retired, and her last colonoscopy was 3 years ago. Colonoscopy and random biopsies were unremarkable, showing chronic UC in remission. Now on colonoscopy, you find mild inflammation in the rectum, descending colon and transverse colon. But when you get to the ascending colon, there is narrowing, and you cannot advance the colonoscope to the cecum. There is minor inflammation in the ascending colon but no suggestion of a tumor or dysplasia. Biopsies distal to the narrowing and blind biopsies within the narrowed segment are unrevealing; there is no dysplasia found.

Do you feel compelled to investigate this "stricture" in some other way? If so, how?

Anytime a stricture is encountered, the diagnosis needs to be reevaluated. If there truly is a stricture present, this suggests a diagnosis of possible Crohn's disease instead of ulcerative colitis. This finding would warrant a review of prior colonoscopies and cross-sectional imaging. The next step would be a CT or MR enterography.

Can you really delineate fibrosis on an MR enterography?

There have been research studies showing that MRE can distinguish between active inflammation versus fibrotic lesions; however, this is not done as standard clinical practice.

Assuming there is a true colon stricture in a patient with IBD, do you feel compelled to send the patient to surgery? And, if you do, do you think it is sufficient for the surgeon to do a right hemicolectomy or is a more extensive resection indicated?

P. Beniwal-Patel (✉)
Medicine, Gastroenterology/Hepatology Division, Medical College of Wisconsin, Milwaukee, WI, USA
e-mail: pbeniwal@mcw.edu

233

I have encountered a number of patients with ascending colon strictures, and this is in the setting of people feeling well. So, then the question becomes what do you do? And in those patients, I actually have sent them to surgery, because you don't know what's on the other side of the stricture. You can't survey it for disease activity or, more importantly, dysplasia. And so, if someone truly has an ascending colon stricture, I would send them to surgery.

To answer the question how extensive a resection is necessary, there are cases (e.g., limited colonic Crohn's involvement), where a right hemicolectomy can be considered over a total colectomy. It really is decided on a case-by-case basis and includes consideration of several factors, such as which medications a patient has tried, disease trajectory, and overall health status.

Chapter 45
Nonspecific Ileal Ulcers

Amir Patel

A 35-year-old nonsmoking male is referred with chronic diarrhea. All stool cultures are negative. Diarrhea is watery and non-bloody. Stool calprotectin is 250. You decide to do a colonoscopy. The colon appears normal, but you enter the terminal ileum and find three or four small ulcers that are fairly nondescript. Biopsies of the colon are negative, and biopsies of the ulcers are nondiagnostic, with no granulomas present. You think these findings are not convincing for IBD. The patient does not routinely take NSAIDS but did take some one weekend, a month earlier, after a basketball injury.

What is the level of calprotectin that you will pursue?

It depends on the range at the institution, but at our institution, anything greater than 50 can be considered elevated. Now that being said, I think the range between 50 and 80 is a gray area. So, if it's in that low range, right below a hundred, I might consider repeating the fecal calprotectin in a few weeks just to see if it's still elevated. Some of the literature suggests that we'll see higher fecal calprotectin when there's significant colitis versus ileitis.

The value generally does not correlate with disease severity; however, if I see numbers in the thousands, that's when I get really concerned, and that result is probably more sensitive for inflammatory bowel disease.

A. Patel (✉)
Dept. of Medicine, Division of Gastroenterology and Hepatology, Medical College of Wisconsin, Milwaukee, WI, USA
e-mail: ampatel@mcw.edu

© The Author(s), under exclusive license to Springer Nature Switzerland AG 2023
W. H. Sobin et al. (eds.), *Managing Complex Cases in Gastroenterology*,
https://doi.org/10.1007/978-3-031-48949-5_45

When you see a patient with ulcers in the terminal ileum that you think are probably not Crohn's, how do you approach them? Will you do further small bowel imaging (capsule, SBFT, or CTE)? Will you give a trial of budesonide? Just follow them?

Although we've always been taught to look for granulomas, the actual finding of granulomas is pretty low, they're only found in a minority, perhaps 30% of patients with Crohn's disease. When you think about the different causes of ileal ulcers, it could be NSAIDs, or it could be Crohn's disease, and you always think about your bacterial infections, like yersinia and tuberculosis, but we're not seeing those in developed countries.

But when I see ulcers in the small bowel, I do want to consider further testing, just to make sure that we're not missing anything. So, your options include capsule endoscopy, CT, MRE, or the old-school, small bowel follow-through. We do know that capsule endoscopy is the most sensitive test because it can actually get direct visualization.

In Crohn's disease, we use scoring systems, like the Lewis scoring system, where we look at the villous appearance on a capsule, look for ulcers, and look for strictures. Capsule endoscopy has a pretty high negative predictive value; when you're looking at Crohn's disease, it's almost a hundred percent; I think it's around 95%. So, in this case, if the patient has never had bowel obstructions or any abdominal surgeries, I'd probably go with a capsule endoscopy to evaluate the remainder of the small bowel.

Now, if capsule endoscopy is not available, CTE and MREs have become more popular. And there have been studies looking at our ability to diagnose or define Crohn's disease using enterography studies. What you're looking for, on CTE, is mucosal enhancement, fat stranding, and hyper-enhancement as well.

Dynamic MRIs have also been used in our institution. When they're looking at the contrast in the ileum, they can actually see how well the ileum is moving. So, not only can they determine if there's an inflammatory component of the Crohn's, but they can actually see if there's any fibrotic appearance. So that's some exciting, new technology we can apply to our patients with Crohn's disease. But typically, I would do a capsule endoscopy in this case, but I think a CT or MR would be acceptable as well.

The patient has a capsule endoscopy, which is otherwise negative.

Would you do any further testing, do any treatment, or simply follow the patient at this point?

If I'm not concerned about Crohn's disease, I would simply tell the patient to avoid NSAIDs. NSAID damage can happen pretty quickly, within 10 days, according to the Crohn's disease literature. If I'm not concerned about Crohn's disease, I will not treat them. Some practitioners will give a course of Entocort, 9 mg a day, and try it for a couple of months. But I would only do this if I think the patient might have mild Crohn's disease and has ongoing symptoms.

Chapter 46
Concern About *Pneumocystis jirovecii*

Poonam Beniwal-Patel

A 32-year-old female presents with acute ulcerative colitis, requiring admission and a course of IV steroids. She improves markedly within a couple of days, and she is able to be discharged on prednisone 40 mg a day. You begin therapy with infliximab after sending off hepatitis serology, a QuantiFERON assay, and TPMT. A few days after the TPMT returns normal, azathioprine is added. The patient's dose of prednisone has been dropped to 20 mg.

Would you agree with adding azathioprine in a patient still receiving prednisone along with infliximab? Would you wait until prednisone is tapered off? If you do start azathioprine, along with infliximab and prednisone, would you start prophylaxis for pneumocystis (in the face of triple immunosuppressive therapy?)

The SONIC trial showed that starting patients on azathioprine when beginning infliximab led to higher steroid-free remission. Additional data has shown that the use of an immunomodulator with antitumor necrosis factor therapy decreases the risk of drug antibody formation [1]. Therefore, in a patient with aggressive disease who is starting infliximab, I would start azathioprine as an outpatient without waiting for prednisone to be completely tapered off.

However, over the last year or two, there have been studies that show that if you treat someone with infliximab monotherapy and then they develop antibodies, it is possible to add azathioprine at that time and usually be able to recapture them by eliminating their antibodies [1, 2].

That's really interesting data, because the question arises whether you really have to start azathioprine at the outset. Certainly, I will say that for patients with severe ulcerative colitis who are at high risk for a colectomy, I will definitely start

P. Beniwal-Patel (✉)
Medicine, Gastroenterology/Hepatology Division, Medical College of Wisconsin, Milwaukee, WI, USA
e-mail: pbeniwal@mcw.edu

© The Author(s), under exclusive license to Springer Nature Switzerland AG 2023
W. H. Sobin et al. (eds.), *Managing Complex Cases in Gastroenterology*, https://doi.org/10.1007/978-3-031-48949-5_46

azathioprine at the same time as infliximab. These patients, especially if they've been hospitalized, have proven that they have aggressive disease. We don't have time for them to develop antibodies and then reverse them.

So, in this patient, I would start azathioprine, start it at the same time that she receives infliximab, and not wait until prednisone is tapered off. With the long half-life of azathioprine, it actually takes about 8 weeks for it to reach its steady state. So, even though we're starting the azathioprine at the same time as the other two, it really doesn't kick in full effect until the prednisone dose is leveling off.

As to whether you need prophylaxis for PJP, there have been some small cohort studies, looking at the rate of PJP in patients who have IBD but do not have HIV. There was one study, about 10 years ago, that found the absolute risk to be only about 0.07% of developing PJP in non-HIV IBD patients [3].

In general, it is high-dose, long-duration prednisone scenarios in older patients where you want to prophylax against PJP. But in our patients, we really start tapering them after the first week. So, if it's a patient in whom I'm tapering off steroids, I do not prophylax them. On the other hand, if I have a patient who's older than 55 who I'm meeting for the first time and they've been on steroids for 3–4 months, then that's someone who I may consider doing a PJP prophylaxis, especially if they have underlying lung disease. So, it's really on a case-by-case basis. But most of the time, I do not prophylax. them.

References

1. Villareal EM, Yarur AJ. Better late than never: adding thiopurines after loss of response to infliximab monotherapy. Dig Dis Sci. 2021;66(9):2851–2. https://doi.org/10.1007/s10620-020-06681-w. Epub 2020 Oct 31.
2. Zeze K, Hirano A, Torisu T, Esaki M, Moriyama T, Umeno J, Kawasaki K, Fujioka S, Fuyuno Y, Matsuno Y, Kitazono T. Adding thiopurine after loss of response to infliximab versus early combination in treating Crohn's disease: a retrospective study. Dig Dis Sci. 2021;66(9):3124–31. https://doi.org/10.1007/s10620-020-06600-z. Epub 2020 Sep 13.
3. Sierra CM, Daiya KC. Prophylaxis for Pneumocystis jirovecii pneumonia in patients with inflammatory bowel disease: a systematic review. Pharmacotherapy. 2022;42(11):858–67. https://doi.org/10.1002/phar.2733. Epub 2022 Oct 25. PMID: 36222368; PMCID: PMC9828113.

Chapter 47
Bloating in Crohn's

Poonam Beniwal-Patel

A 42-year-old female with a history of Crohn's disease well-controlled on infliximab and azathioprine comes in for complaints of diarrhea and bloating. She had a prior terminal ileal resection (20 cm) for her Crohn's. Her CRP and fecal calprotectin are normal. A colonoscopy to the neoileum is normal.

Is there any treatment you would consider?

First, if there's significant diarrhea or bloating, and this is relatively new, I would do cross-sectional imaging, like a CTE or MRE, to make sure there's no upstream disease activity that we're not capturing on a colonoscopy.

If that comes back negative, then I'd be interested in knowing what kind of anastomosis they have, because patients who have a side-to-side anastomosis do have a higher rate of SIBO compared to those with an end-to-end anastomosis.

If there's no active disease on cross-sectional imaging, you could try cholestyramine. But be judicious with it; I would just give it once a day. Also, you could try treating with rifaximin, just empirically for SIBO, given that they have had an abdominal intestinal surgery, which is a risk factor for SIBO.

The patient is started on cholestyramine, 4 g, once daily, and diarrhea improves but bloating gets worse. A CTE shows some areas of small bowel dilation without significant stricture.

Would you consider doing a capsule in someone like this?

I think it would be reasonable to do, but I certainly would do a patency capsule before that. The interesting thing is that to have dilation, there's one of three things that could cause that. There might be a mechanical stricture, there could be

P. Beniwal-Patel (✉)
Medicine, Gastroenterology/Hepatology Division, Medical College of Wisconsin, Milwaukee, WI, USA
e-mail: pbeniwal@mcw.edu

© The Author(s), under exclusive license to Springer Nature Switzerland AG 2023
W. H. Sobin et al. (eds.), *Managing Complex Cases in Gastroenterology*, https://doi.org/10.1007/978-3-031-48949-5_47

aperistalsis at that point, or it could be that we're viewing the x-ray in the middle of a peristaltic wave and it's not truly a dilation. I would also consider a small bowel follow-through in order to get a functional assessment of the area.

Would you bother doing a breath test looking for SIBO or would you just treat with rifaximin?

In this case, because rifaximin is relatively low risk, I'd treat it empirically. If this occurs again, then I'd perform testing for SIBO before retreating.

Chapter 48
Severe Diarrhea in a Patient on Chemotherapy

Amir Patel

A 57-year-old male is admitted to the oncology service with severe diarrhea. He has been having diarrhea for weeks. The patient is on chemotherapy for metastatic lung cancer but is not receiving a checkpoint inhibitor. You look up the drugs he is receiving and see that they may cause diarrhea but do not tend to cause colitis. His chemo has been on hold since his diarrhea started, but his oncologists are anxious to restart it. His stool cultures are negative. He had his last screening colonoscopy 4 years ago, just before his lung cancer was first diagnosed, and it was unremarkable.

Obviously if you're consulted on a patient receiving checkpoint inhibitors and having bad diarrhea, you're going to do a colonoscopy, looking for the inflammatory bowel disease-type phenotype. Do you ever do that with patients who are on other chemotherapy?

We've been seeing a lot of checkpoint inhibitor therapy causing colitis in the last decade, but we have also found that some other chemotherapy medications that are not checkpoint inhibitors can cause an immune-mediated colitis as well.

So, a lot of times the oncologists will send these patients to us, and we will do a colonoscopy just to make sure that there's no immune-mediated colitis occurring. If that does happen, we treat it like checkpoint inhibitor colitis. The oncologists are pretty vigilant about this, and a lot of times when we see these patients, they're already on steroids. If they have a response to prednisone, that tells you that this is likely some type of autoimmune-mediated colitis, even if the biopsies are not specific.

A. Patel (✉)
Dept. of Medicine, Division of Gastroenterology and Hepatology, Medical College of Wisconsin, Milwaukee, WI, USA
e-mail: ampatel@mcw.edu

© The Author(s), under exclusive license to Springer Nature Switzerland AG 2023
W. H. Sobin et al. (eds.), *Managing Complex Cases in Gastroenterology*,
https://doi.org/10.1007/978-3-031-48949-5_48

241

Together, the oncologists and gastroenterologists have generated some guidelines and have good data on the use of anti-TNFs as well as anti-integrins. We tend to see a robust response to anti-TNFs and Entyvio for treatment of these medication-induced autoimmune immune-mediated colitis cases.

To treat checkpoint inhibitor colitis, usually it takes one or two doses of an anti-TNF, at the standard 5 mg per kg dosing of infliximab, 2 weeks apart. Sometimes, one dose alone is enough to knock out the colitis; sometimes you need two. And for vedolizumab, 300 mg IV, one to two doses can be quite effective.

I think the oncologists are actually looking at what they can do preventatively. There are no good studies on this, but they're studying this particular question: if someone is going to be put on a checkpoint inhibitor, should they be started on an anti-TNF or anti-integrin therapy prophylactically?

You decide to do a colonoscopy to evaluate the diarrhea, and you find mild diffuse erythema and some minimal friability involving portions of the colon. The appearance is nonspecific. Although it might be a milder IBD, the appearance is consistent with infection or possibly a drug-induced colitis. Biopsies are not diagnostic for IBD and are rather nonspecific.

Would you treat for IBD?

With these findings, I would not give therapy for IBD if the patient was not on a checkpoint inhibitor. We'll give them antidiarrheals, but a lot of times, if the diarrhea is really debilitating, the oncologist will be changing the choice of chemotherapy.

Chapter 49
Microscopic Colitis

Poonam Beniwal-Patel

A 67-year-old female presents with diarrhea. She had a screening colonoscopy 2 years earlier that was negative. Her only medical problem is hyperlipidemia. Her meds include simvastatin and baby ASA. A repeat colonoscopy is performed, which is grossly normal, but biopsies are positive for lymphocytic colitis. She is started on budesonide 9 mg a day, and her diarrhea resolves. After a month, her gastroenterologist tapers her dose to 6 mg, and she does well. But every time she tries to drop the dose further, the diarrhea worsens. She is referred to you for a second opinion.

What would be your initial approach upon seeing her, and would you stop her statin, since statins have been associated with microscopic colitis?

The first thing I think about, even though it sounds like she responded to budesonide initially, is to check a celiac panel, because patients with microscopic colitis are at increased risk of developing celiac disease.

Her celiac panel returns negative. Her IgA level is normal.

I would not stop her statin, because even though there is an association between statins and microscopic colitis, the statin clearly has cardiovascular benefits that are more important.

Would you keep a patient on budesonide 3 mg or even 6 mg long term?

Yes, sometimes I do; if we need to, then we need to. With lymphocytic colitis, sometimes they're flaring, and I'll keep them on 6 mg for 6 months, bring them back, and then try to drop them to 3 mg. So, it's definitely not a rapid taper. And I've actually had pretty good success with that. I find that keeping them on the higher dose for longer periods, not just a month, makes it much more likely they will stay in remission and are not as likely to rebound.

P. Beniwal-Patel (✉)
Medicine, Gastroenterology/Hepatology Division, Medical College of Wisconsin,
Milwaukee, WI, USA
e-mail: pbeniwal@mcw.edu

© The Author(s), under exclusive license to Springer Nature
Switzerland AG 2023
W. H. Sobin et al. (eds.), *Managing Complex Cases in Gastroenterology*,
https://doi.org/10.1007/978-3-031-48949-5_49

The other thing I will sometimes do in these scenarios is drop the budesonide dose and use loperamide for breakthrough diarrhea. And then, if this works, I'll wait 6 months before trying to bring the dose down further. I've had pretty good success with this strategy. However, there are some patients who develop bad diarrhea and electrolyte abnormalities, because their diarrhea is so severe. Those patients I'll just leave on higher-dose budesonide.

The good news is that there have been studies looking at metabolic bone disease with budesonide, and thankfully, budesonide really does not impact bone health significantly [1]. In patients with concurrent osteoporosis, I'll loop in an endocrinologist, and generally I've never had pushback regarding budesonide use.

Have you ever had cases where you've had to go to stronger medications?

Not for purely lymphocytic colitis. I can only think of one patient who had a family history of ulcerative colitis and was initially diagnosed with lymphocytic colitis. But then years later, things evolved. We repeated the scope, and now, it looked like it was ulcerative colitis. So, we ended up putting that person on a biologic. Rarely, there are indications for placing patients on a biologic, such as vedolizumab.

Reference

1. Reilev M, Hallas J, Thomsen Ernst M, Nielsen GL, Bonderup OK. Long-term oral budesonide treatment and risk of osteoporotic fractures in patients with microscopic colitis. Aliment Pharmacol Ther. 2020;51(6):644–51. https://doi.org/10.1111/apt.15648. Epub 2020 Jan 30.

Chapter 50
Miscellaneous Questions About IBD

Daniel Stein, Salina Faidhalla, and Amir Patel

1. Do you ever try a second anti-TNF if the first one didn't work? What if the first one was adalimumab? What if it was infliximab?

In a primary nonresponder to adalimumab, we would try infliximab but not the reverse. The thought is that the IV infusion and high-peak drug levels that we can achieve with infliximab are beneficial. In general, Humira seems to be underdosed in comparison with infliximab. We have much bigger dosing flexibility; with infliximab, you can really ramp those levels up. So, in general, if they failed infliximab, we won't really consider Humira. That being said, we do have some patients that are on Humira after failing infliximab and are doing well, but it's not something I would do today.

Now, if a patient has had a response to one agent and then developed antibodies, (a secondary nonresponder), we would try another anti-TNF, because there is no overlap with the antibodies. However, we would suggest adding an IM with the second anti-TNF.

D. Stein (✉)
Division of Gastroenterology and Hepatology, Department of Internal Medicine, Medical College of Wisconsin, Milwaukee, WI, USA
e-mail: dstein@mcw.edu; ampatel@mcw.edu

S. Faidhalla
Department of Medicine Division of Gastroenterology and Hepatology, Medical College of Wisconsin, Milwaukee, WI, USA
e-mail: sfaidhalla@mcw.edu

A. Patel
Dept. of Medicine, Division of Gastroenterology and Hepatology, Medical College of Wisconsin, Milwaukee, WI, USA
e-mail: dstein@mcw.edu; ampatel@mcw.edu

2. If patients are responding well to biologics, do you ever try to get them off these drugs?

We would consider dose de-escalation, if possible, for a patient who has been in deep remission for a long time (clinical remission is not sufficient). However, stopping the medication completely will risk flaring up disease, and the medication may not be effective if restarted.

The recurrence rate after stopping biologics is about 85% in 5 years.

In a large meta-analysis by Torres et al. [1], to evaluate the effect of de-escalation/stopping immunomodulators or anti-TNFs in IBD patients, relapse rates after cessation appear high across all therapeutic classes. After stopping IM, only 15%–37% of patients maintained clinical remission after 5 years.

That meta-analysis also showed that approximately 40%–50% of patients who discontinue anti-TNFs will experience a relapse within 2 years, and studies with longer follow-up of 7 and 10 years after withdrawal show only 35% and 12%, respectively, remain in remission at those time intervals [2, 3].

You can consider stopping biologics in patients who are in remission and have low drug levels, because their remission might not be drug related. This can be considered if they are in deep remission. On the other hand, for dose de-escalation, we usually let drug level guide that.

If the patient is insisting on stopping medication: then we need deep remission, at least two normal colonoscopies, with normal histology 2 years apart before stopping medication. Once the drug is stopped, we closely follow fecal calprotectin every 6–12 months and follow up colonoscopies every 2 years.

In general, we do not proactively stop anti-TNFs. But if a patient has concerns and wants to stop it, or if there's some borderline reason to stop it, for example, if someone is getting recurrent minor infections or recurrent UTIs where you wouldn't otherwise stop it, it might be worth trying.

But the caveat is that anytime you stop medications, it has to be somebody who you trust will follow up and be willing to have surveillance colonoscopies. So, in short, we avoid stopping biologic agents proactively and generally attempt to get patients off immune modulators first.

Amir Patel

It is accepted dogma that adding azathioprine to infliximab enhances benefit. But has adding azathioprine to adalimumab been shown to be beneficial?

The original Sonic study looked at the combination of azathioprine and infliximab and showed efficacy. They did not study adalimumab and azathioprine. But, more recently there was a study looking at Humira with azathioprine, which did show superiority compared to Humira alone [4].

When I use combination therapy, I'm typically combining anti-TNFs and immunologics in someone who has severe disease. So, for someone with fistulizing disease or severe colitis, we use combination therapy to reduce the risk of developing antibodies, and we know that adding the immunologics to the anti-TNFs can also boost the drug levels.

If a patient fails an anti-TNF in ulcerative colitis, it is my impression that ustekinumab is a good second choice, JAK inhibitors are a good second choice, but vedolizumab doesn't work. Do you agree?

I would ask: what is the severity of disease and what is the context? Entyvio is a great drug. It just doesn't have a lot of good induction data. It works slower. So that's why, if speed is of the essence in treating someone's disease, a lot of us will probably go toward an IL-23 or a JAK inhibitor as our second line.

Is your opinion about Entyvio as second-line treatment for patients who fail anti-TNFs in Crohn's the same as for UC?

A lot of us have the opinion that Entyvio works better for colonic disease. So, if someone has a stricture in the ileum or fistulizing disease, then Entyvio would not be our preferred choice.

Is infliximab superior to adalimumab in UC and in Crohn's?

There's been no head-to-head study looking at that question, but I would say that for ulcerative colitis, Remicade is probably superior to Humira. A lot of that is because with Humira, you're just giving a flat dose, while with Remicade, you can adjust the dose by weight. And some of these patients will have a protein-losing enteropathy, where they're losing albumin and protein and potentially the drug itself. So, for ulcerative colitis, I would say that there's no question Remicade is superior.

For Crohn's disease, I guess it would depend on the context of the disease itself.

So, if someone came to me and they had fistulizing disease and had multiple surgeries, then I would say, yes, Remicade is probably going to be a superior drug for that same reason and that you can give them a dose based on their weight and adjust it easier. The problem with Humira has always been that the only adjustment you can make is giving it weekly or every 2 weeks.

And the data on therapeutic drug monitoring with Humira is not as well validated as it is with Infliximab. That's why Remicade, in our opinion, has always been superior to Humira, in which you can always adjust the dose. They can get 10 mg every 4 weeks, or every 8 weeks. Some of us have gone as high as 15 mg every 4 weeks just to get them at this nice therapeutic drug range. A lot of us would probably say that Remicade is superior to Humira.

Do you feel relatively safe using AZA in young males for periods under 2 years?

Yes, I think I feel safe doing that. And a lot of that relates to the context of the disease. So, if a young man comes to me and he's had multiple surgeries and a history of fistulas, there's no question; I'm going to give him combination therapy, because the risk of the untreated disease far outweighs the small risk of that rare hepatosplenic T cell lymphoma.

Another question, and it's along a similar narrative, is when can we de-escalate therapy. So, for someone on combination therapy, when can we stop the azathioprine? And a lot of us would do it after 2 years, but there have been some recent studies on de-escalating therapy within a year.

So, someone's on combination therapy, and they're doing great. The colonoscopy shows deep remission, where they don't have any activity endoscopically or under the microscope. Then, the question is, can we just stop the azathioprine? And some of us will do that and that'll be based on drug levels.

Where do you stand on the newer drugs? How much do ozanimod, risankizumab, and upadacitinib add to the mix? Do you think they are a good addition?

Yes, a lot of the experts are very optimistic, particularly about risankizumab and upadacitinib. As a result, we have been using them a lot. In one of your earlier cases—the young lady with proctitis who didn't want to take suppositories—I was going to say that if she's away at college, you can offer her some of these new oral therapies, like ozanimod (Zeposia), tofacitinib (Xeljanz), or upadacitinib (Rinvoq). She would've been a perfect candidate for ozanimod because she was just failing mesalamine. And the studies actually looked at a subset of patients with colitis who had failed mesalamine, and patients on Zeposia did very well.

The reason why we're enthusiastic about Skyrizi and Rinvoq is because a lot of the studies these days are not only looking at how these patients respond clinically but how they respond histologically and endoscopically. So, more of the studies over the last decade have looked at mucosal healing as an endpoint, because we do know that if you can achieve that deep remission, it reduces the risk of flares, hospitalizations, and colon cancer risk, and some of the data on Skyrizi and Rinvoq have shown early induction data and the ability to heal the mucosa.

A lot of IBD experts are considering the use of Skyrizi first line for Crohn's disease and Rinvoq first line for ulcerative colitis. But we have to remember, Rinvoq right now is being marketed only for patients with colitis who have failed anti-TNF

Is vedolizumab a godsend because of its lack of side effects and concerns? Is it strong enough?

Yes, vedolizumab is a great drug because of its safety profile, but I think that the induction therapy is what concerns a lot of us. It takes a certain type of patient to consider Entyvio, someone with moderate ulcerative colitis or moderate Crohn's disease who isn't on the verge of needing surgery. Also, older patients who typically don't present with a severe disease are candidates for Entyvio. But the question is, will the therapy work? And I don't think we have an answer for that, but we're looking into data and doing studies, where maybe we can do a blood test or have a stool sample or a mucosal sample that could inform us whether this person is going to respond to anti-TNF or that person's going to respond to anti-integrin therapy.

But we're not there yet. Hopefully, we'll get there soon. But yes, I think Entyvio is a great drug. It just depends on the person that I'd use it on. So, for someone who has severe disease, heading for surgery, I probably wouldn't use it. But if their disease is on the more moderate side, then, yes, I would.

Daniel Stein, Salina Faidhalla

Do you see any differences in the ways you manage IBD from the way gastroenterologists in the community do? Are there any general recommendations you would make?

Yes, there are a few. First, we see too much use of mesalamine in patients with Crohn's disease. Second, we find that community practitioners are occasionally too conservative with their treatment. Part of this may be an under-recognition of the severity of the disease. In addition, community practitioners tend to be hesitant to use advanced therapies. Although there are some risks with the use of advanced therapies the risk/benefit ratio remains quite low. Biologics, including the small molecules, should be strongly considered in patients with IBD who have moderate to severe disease.

We also see many UC patients treated with adalimumab, which is usually not a first choice for us; we prefer infliximab.

And, finally, we think there is some under-recognition of primary nonresponse, defined as no significant improvement without the aid of steroids. Too often patients are continued on agents for long periods of time despite being ineffective or requiring repeated doses of steroids.

References

1. Torres J, Boyapati RK, Kennedy NA, Louis E, Colombel JF, Satsangi J. Systematic review of effects of withdrawal of immunomodulators or biologic agents from patients with inflammatory bowel disease. Gastroenterology. 2015;149(7):1716–30. https://doi.org/10.1053/j.gastro.2015.08.055. Epub 2015 Sep 14.
2. Steenholdt C, Molazahi A, Ainsworth MA, Brynskov J, Østergaard Thomsen O, Seidelin JB. Outcome after discontinuation of infliximab in patients with inflammatory bowel disease in clinical remission: an observational Danish single center study. Scand J Gastroenterol. 2012;47(5):518–27. https://doi.org/10.3109/00365521.2012.660541. Epub 2012 Mar 1.
3. Waugh AW, Garg S, Matic K, Gramlich L, Wong C, Sadowski DC, Millan M, Bailey R, Todoruk D, Cherry R, Teshima CW. Maintenance of clinical benefit in Crohn's disease patients after discontinuation of infliximab: long-term follow-up of a single Centre cohort. Aliment Pharmacol Ther. 2010;32(9):1129–34.
4. Matsumoto T, Motoya S, Watanabe K, Hisamatsu T, Nakase H, Yoshimura N, Ishida T, Kato S, Nakagawa T, Esaki M, Nagahori M. Adalimumab monotherapy and a combination with azathioprine for Crohn's disease: a prospective, randomized trial. J Crohn's Colitis. 2016;10(11):1259–66.

Part III
Disorders of Gut–Brain Interaction

Chapter 51
Introduction to Disorders of Gut-Brain Interaction

W. Harley Sobin

The challenges of treating IBS-D, IBS-C, functional constipation, functional dyspepsia, bloating, and functional abdominal pain are discussed in multiple case presentations. A thorough review of medications, dietary therapy, and the interplay between anxiety, depression, and severity of symptoms is presented.

The use of eluxadoline, alosetron, rifaximin, IBgard, linaclotide, lubiprostone, prucalopride, buspirone, mirtazapine, and other drugs is reviewed. Tests involved in the diagnosis of these functional syndromes are discussed. Bloating, distension, and the interplay with the viscerosomatic reflex are explained. Tips for managing painful gas are outlined as well as the use of antidepressants in treating these patients and how to manage abdominal cramping.

Other issues covered in these case discussions include the following: Is it necessary to perform a colonoscopy to diagnose IBS-D? What other tests should be ordered in the patient with presumed IBS-D? What tests may be helpful in a patient with severe constipation? How best to manage constipation in a patient on chronic opiates, or a patient with possible outlet dysfunction. How to manage functional dyspepsia both postprandial distress syndrome (PDS) and epigastric pain syndrome (EPS) and how to treat abdominal wall pain.

Multiple causes of bloating are discussed along with potential therapies. The use of central neuromodulators in treating patients with hard-to-manage disorders of gut-brain interaction is discussed at length.

W. H. Sobin (✉)
Division of Gastroenterology and Hepatology, Department of Medicine, Medical College of Wisconsin, Milwaukee, WI, USA
e-mail: hsobin@mcw.edu

© The Author(s), under exclusive license to Springer Nature Switzerland AG 2023
W. H. Sobin et al. (eds.), *Managing Complex Cases in Gastroenterology*,
https://doi.org/10.1007/978-3-031-48949-5_51

Chapter 52
IBS-D

W. Harley Sobin and Patrick Sanvanson

Case 1 *A 32-year-old female presents with a history of weekly recurrent loose bowel movements over the past year, along with associated abdominal cramps. She works as a paralegal in a high-pressure law firm. She is on no medicines. Her frequent bathroom trips during the work day are now embarrassing her, so she sees her primary care physician. Her exam is unremarkable. Labs reveal a normal CBC, CRP, TSH, iron panel/ferritin, and fecal calprotectin. Her primary care doctor thinks she has IBS-D but is worried she might have inflammatory bowel disease (IBD) and sends her for a second opinion, asking whether she should have a colonoscopy.*

Is a colonoscopy necessary to rule out IBD and diagnose IBS?

No, the normal lab results all weigh against the diagnosis of IBD. The history, physical exam, and labs are all consistent with the diagnosis of IBS-D. A colonoscopy is not necessary at this time to confirm this diagnosis.

Are there other labs necessary to evaluate the patient before treating her?

Celiac serology is indicated in the evaluation of patients with suspected IBS-D [1, 2]. On occasion, we will obtain an abdominal X-ray upon initial presentation to confirm there is not an excessive stool burden and that we are not dealing with an overflow diarrhea situation.

Celiac serology returns negative. Abdominal X-ray demonstrates no increased stool burden. You suggest dietary manipulations, including avoiding caffeine, lactose, artificial sweeteners, and processed meats, which does not help much. You discuss a low-FODMAP (fermentable oligosaccharides, disaccharides, monosaccharides, and polyols) diet, which she tries but also gets no benefit from this

W. H. Sobin (✉) · P. Sanvanson
Division of Gastroenterology and Hepatology, Department of Medicine, Medical College of Wisconsin, Milwaukee, WI, USA
e-mail: hsobin@mcw.edu; psanvans@mcw.edu

© The Author(s), under exclusive license to Springer Nature Switzerland AG 2023
W. H. Sobin et al. (eds.), *Managing Complex Cases in Gastroenterology*, https://doi.org/10.1007/978-3-031-48949-5_52

intervention. You have prescribed Imodium (loperamide), which helps a little bit with the diarrhea but not the cramping. She is worried about taking this on a chronic basis, even though you assure her that it is okay.

What other treatments can you consider?

We may try psyllium-based fiber to see if it helps with regulating stools. Antispasmodics, like dicyclomine and hyoscyamine, have been part of our general armamentarium for decades. However, studies proving their efficacy are limited. The latest ACG (American College of Gastroenterology) guidelines [1] did not support their use, although more recent AGA guidelines [3] did. In our practice, we continue to use antispasmodics in younger patients. We worry more about their anticholinergic side effects in the elderly and are reluctant to use them in those patients. Other drugs that we will try include eluxadoline (Viberzi) [4], peppermint oil in the form of IBgard [5], rifaximin [6], cholestyramine [7, 8], and alosetron [9–11].

Eluxadoline [4] works on opioid receptors to decrease bowel frequency and abdominal pain, and we find that it helps a few of our patients with IBS-D. It is contraindicated in patients who have had a cholecystectomy. If we have a patient with presumed IBS-D who has had a cholecystectomy, we will always try cholestyramine first or obtain a 48-h stool collection for bile acids. Many of these patients will have bile-salt-related diarrhea and respond to this treatment [7, 8]. However, if the patient has an intact gallbladder, no past history of pancreatitis, and is not a heavy drinker, we will try eluxadoline.

IBgard is another drug worth trying [5]; it is an OTC medication containing peppermint oil. Rifaximin [6] will work to relieve symptoms in some patients with IBS-D. This is particularly true if your patient has had reason to have a hydrogen breath test and the results were consistent with SIBO. A breath test is not required before trying rifaximin, but it is those patients with IBS-D and a positive breath test who are most likely to respond. However, rifaximin is quite expensive, requires repeat treatment, and is often not covered by insurance. When starting any new IBS therapy, we ask patients to give us an update in 2–4 weeks.

The patient tries dicyclomine, eluxadoline, IBgard, and even rifaximin without much benefit. She describes her frustration to you and expresses feelings of hopelessness and anxiety and says she is starting to feel depressed.

What is the association between anxiety, depression, and IBS, and how do you manage it?

For patients with debilitating IBS, we let them know that we do not think their physical symptoms are simply manifestations of depression. There are several points we emphasize. First, it is natural to experience feelings of anxiety and even depression when physical symptoms continue unabated. Second, as physical symptoms continue, they tend to get embedded in the patient's psyche and lead to somatization, where a patient becomes obsessed with those physical symptoms. It is also common for patients to catastrophize, thinking in terms of gloom and doom regarding their ailments. We will typically try getting these patients to see a mental health provider, who provides the tools to help with these unhelpful behavioral patterns.

Cognitive behavior therapy is particularly useful in many of these patients [12]. Learning that they can control their thought processes can also benefit the level of their IBS.

Will you ever prescribe antidepressants for these patients?

We are comfortable using tricyclics in patients with IBS-D [13] as central neuro-modulators, not as antidepressants. Using a relatively low dose of nortriptyline helps decrease diarrhea and abdominal pain [14]. The dose we're using is much less than the usual antidepressant dose. We usually don't prescribe an SSRI in IBS-D, because SSRIs tend to increase diarrhea (with the exception of paroxetine (Paxil), which is somewhat constipating but has a number of problems associated with its use). Our tricyclic of choice is nortriptyline. We think it is better tolerated than amitriptyline. But in patients with severe diarrhea, amitriptyline may be preferable.

When we prescribe these drugs, we tell the patient that we are not using them to treat depression; we are giving them to treat the brain-gut connection that is out of kilter in IBS. Prior to starting a tricyclic, an EKG is obtained to confirm the absence of baseline QTc prolongation and is subsequently monitored with dose adjustments.

The patient is placed on nortriptyline 25 mg at bedtime, which is then increased to 50 mg. Her symptoms do improve. She is pleased that she is feeling somewhat better but wonders if there are any other specific GI drugs that might benefit her.

One other medicine worth considering is alosetron [9–11]. This is approved only for females with IBS-D who have failed other therapies. We have had some great success using alosetron in women with intractable symptoms of IBS-D. We do review the background history of the drug with our patients. It was taken off the market years ago because of cases of severe constipation and cases of bowel ischemia. But, at that time, the drug was being given in higher doses and being used in older patients who probably should not have been receiving it in the first place. So, now, we use lower doses and avoid its use in anyone who is at increased risk of ischemic colitis.

After trying alosetron, at the dose of 0.5 mg twice daily, the patient quickly feels marked relief of her diarrhea and abdominal pain. After a month on the medicine, she feels back to normal. You gradually taper her off of the nortriptyline while maintaining on alosetron. After tapering nortriptyline off, she has some increased diarrhea that rapidly responds to an increase in alosetron to 1 mg bid.

Case 2 A 43-year-old female presents with increased abdominal cramps and diarrhea over the past 8 months. She gives a long history of frequent, somewhat soft, bowel movements since she was in her 20 s. The fact that she moved her bowels 2–3 times a day never bothered her. One year ago, she divorced her husband of 22 years after learning of an affair he was having. Since then, she has been having increased abdominal cramps, along with even looser stools. There is no blood in her stool. She takes no medications. She has no surgical or other past medical history. On the physical exam, she winces when you press on her abdomen, but you think it is abdominal wall pain. Indeed, you do a Carnett test and it is positive. Her exam is otherwise negative. You decide to order a CBC, CRP, fecal calprotectin, iron panel/ferritin, and celiac panel. These tests all return negative.

How would you manage her abdominal wall pain?

We have tried lidocaine patches in many, gabapentin in a few, and have even sent a couple of patients to anesthesia pain specialists for local nerve root injections for presumed anterior cutaneous nerve entrapment [15].

The patient's abdominal wall pain improves after you explain its benign nature and after starting lidocaine patches. However, her abdominal cramping increases, generally accompanying her loose bowel movements.

How would you manage her loose stools and abdominal cramps?

This patient has a long history of frequent bowel movements, and now they are associated with increased cramping, which started at the time of her divorce. The history is very consistent with IBS-D. Many patients have long-standing symptoms of IBS and never see a physician, because they are not particularly alarmed or bothered by them. Those who do, however, often have associated anxiety or depression, and a life-altering stress can often precipitate an exacerbation of symptoms. Mental health counseling can really benefit a lot of patients.

Other things that could cause these symptoms include IBD, but the normal CBC, CRP, iron studies, and fecal calprotectin make that unlikely. You could potentially have normal labs with microscopic colitis, but she is young for this diagnosis and is not taking medications that might precipitate microscopic colitis. However, microscopic colitis may be considered, if she fails to respond to management of IBS-D.

So how would we manage her IBS-D? We might start with psyllium-fiber-based products [1, 3, 8]. If these are not totally effective, we might next try dicyclomine [3]. There is less concern about anticholinergic side effects in younger patients. Besides helping with cramps, dicyclomine can slow diarrhea. We like to start with 10 mg before meals and at bedtime, although many recommend 20 mg. We find the 10 mg dose to be much better tolerated and will occasionally titrate up to 20 mg if needed.

Loperamide is another option. In some people, loperamide will not only decrease stool frequency but also decrease abdominal cramping. We start slowly with loperamide because occasional patients may have severe constipation with even one dose.

The patient is started on dicyclomine but stops it because of side effects, such as dry mouth, and worry about altered vision. You have her try loperamide, which she finds slows her bowel frequency but does nothing for her cramping.

What would you try next?

We like to try eluxadoline [4] in those with an intact gallbladder and cholestyramine [7, 8] in those without. We will also have them try IBgard [5]. Occasionally, we will order rifaximin [6], particularly in those who might be predisposed to having small bowel bacterial overgrowth. We have had more problems getting rifaximin approved and, because of its expense, do not order it that often. Occasionally, we will try cholestyramine in someone with an intact gallbladder. Some patients may have a defective bile salt transporter in their terminal ileum [8]. But patients with an intact gallbladder are much less likely to benefit from cholestyramine than those who have had a cholecystectomy.

Unfortunately, response to any one medication can be unpredictable, and trial and error is required. As mentioned above, alosetron is our go-to in women who do not respond to other remedies.

The patient fails to improve with eluxadoline and IBgard. Rifaximin is not tried because it is not covered and is too expensive. She refuses to try alosetron because of fears of ischemic colitis even after being reassured that it is extremely uncommon. Her bowel frequency is reasonable with use of loperamide, and her main complaint is severe cramping. The cramping is now worse whenever she moves her bowels, whenever she feels stressed by things like deadlines, and whenever she feels like crying.

How would you manage her pain?

If she would agree to it, we would give her a trial of the SNRI (serotonin and norepinephrine reuptake inhibitor) duloxetine. Duloxetine has been found helpful in treating functional abdominal pain, and the fact that it is mildly constipating would benefit her IBS-D [14, 16]. We would educate her about the gut-brain connection and the possibility that she is suffering from a disorder of gut-brain interaction. The use of central neuromodulators has been found useful in patients with IBS, even with those who do not suffer from depression or anxiety, although this patient probably does.

In using drugs like SNRIs, TCAs, or SSRIs, it is necessary to explain to patients that it generally takes a month for them to be truly operational, but unfortunately, side effects may occur immediately [14]. We start with a lower dose and then titrate up to the desired dose. We also strongly recommend that the patient see a mental health specialist for cognitive behavioral or other therapy as an adjunct in treating her.

She agrees to take duloxetine, starting at 30 mg a day and then, after 2 weeks, going up to 60 mg a day. After 6 weeks, she is feeling better, and as a result, her mood is also improved. But she is still having some breakthrough pain and complains of insomnia.

She is doing better, but do you have other recommendations at this point?

An excellent augmenting drug, added to duloxetine, would be low-dose quetiapine (Seroquel) [17]. A nighttime dose of 100 mg works to help decrease pain and almost always reverses insomnia.

She adds quetiapine to duloxetine and feels great. She is seeing a counselor and feels the best she has in years. She is also ready to start dating again.

References

1. Lacy BE, Pimentel M, Brenner DM, Chey WD, Keefer LA, Long MD, Moshiree B. ACG clinical guideline: management of irritable bowel syndrome. Off J Am Coll Gastroenterol. 2021;116(1):17–44.
2. Smalley W, Falck-Ytter C, Carrasco-Labra A, Wani S, Lytvyn L, Falck-Ytter Y. AGA clinical practice guidelines on the laboratory evaluation of functional diarrhea and diarrhea-predominant irritable bowel syndrome in adults (IBS-D). Gastroenterology. 2019;157(3):851–4.
3. Lembo A, Sultan S, Chang L, Heidelbaugh JJ, Smalley W, Verne GN. AGA clinical practice guideline on the pharmacological management of irritable bowel syndrome with diarrhea. Gastroenterology. 2022;163(1):137–51.
4. Lembo AJ, Lacy BE, Zuckerman MJ, Schey R, Dove LS, Andrae DA, Davenport JM, McIntyre G, Lopez R, Turner L, Covington PS. Eluxadoline for irritable bowel syndrome with diarrhea. N Engl J Med. 2016;374(3):242–53.

5. Cash B. Novel peppermint oil formulation for dietary management of irritable bowel syndrome. Gastroenterol Hepatol. 2015;11(9):631.
6. Pimentel M, Lembo A, Chey WD, Zakko S, Ringel Y, Yu J, Mareya SM, Shaw AL, Bortey E, Forbes WP. Rifaximin therapy for patients with irritable bowel syndrome without constipation. N Engl J Med. 2011;364(1):22–32.
7. Wedlake L, A'hern R, Russell D, Thomas K, Walters JR, Andreyev HJ. Systematic review: the prevalence of idiopathic bile acid malabsorption as diagnosed by SeHCAT scanning in patients with diarrhoea-predominant irritable bowe syndrome. Aliment Pharmacol Ther. 2009;30(7):707–17.
8. Camilleri M. Diagnosis and treatment of irritable bowel syndrome: a review. JAMA. 2021;325(9):865–77.
9. Bardhan, Bodemar, Geldof, Schütz, Heath, Mills, Jacques. A double-blind, randomized, placebo-controlled dose-ranging study to evaluate the efficacy of alosetron in the treatment of irritable bowel syndrome. Aliment Pharmacol Ther. 2000;14(1):23–34.
10. Camilleri M, Chey WY, Mayer EA, Northcutt AR, Heath A, Dukes GE, McSorley D, Mangel AM. A randomized controlled clinical trial of the serotonin type 3 receptor antagonist alosetron in women with diarrhea-predominant irritable bowel syndrome. Arch Intern Med. 2001;161(14):1733–40.
11. Krause R, Ameen V, Gordon SH, West M, Heath AT, Perschy T, Carter EG. A randomized, double-blind, placebo-controlled study to assess efficacy and safety of 0.5 mg and 1 mg alosetron in women with severe diarrhea-predominant IBS. Off J Am Coll Gastroenterol. 2007;102(8):1709–19.
12. Everitt HA, Landau S, O'Reilly G, Sibelli A, Hughes S, Windgassen S, Holland R, Little P, McCrone P, Bishop FL, Goldsmith K. Cognitive behavioural therapy for irritable bowel syndrome: 24-month follow-up of participants in the ACTIB randomised trial. Lancet Gastroenterol Hepatol. 2019;4(11):863–72.
13. Ford AC, Lacy BE, Harris LA, Quigley EM, Moayyedi P. Effect of antidepressants and psychological therapies in irritable bowel syndrome: an updated systematic review and meta-analysis. Off J Am Coll Gastroenterol. 2019;114(1):21–39.
14. Sobin HW, Heinrich TW, Drossman DA. Central neuromodulators for treating functional GI disorders: a primer. Off J Am Coll Gastroenterol. 2017;112(5):693–702.
15. Srinivasan R, Greenbaum DS. Chronic abdominal wall pain: a frequently overlooked problem: practical approach to diagnosis and management. Am J Gastroenterol. 2002;97(4):824–30.
16. Drossman DA, Tack J, Ford AC, Szigethy E, Törnblom H, Van Oudenhove L. Neuromodulators for functional gastrointestinal disorders (disorders of gut– brain interaction): a Rome foundation working team report. Gastroenterology. 2018;154(4):1140–71.
17. Grover M, Dorn SD, Weinland SR, Dalton CB, Gaynes BN, Drossman DA. Atypical antipsychotic quetiapine in the management of severe refractory functional gastrointestinal disorders. Dig Dis Sci. 2009;54:1284–91.

Chapter 53
IBS-C

W. Harley Sobin and Patrick Sanvanson

Case 1 *A 32-year-old female presents for worsening constipation and abdominal pain. She has a long history of constipation since her menarche, at about age 12. She takes a tablespoon of Metamucil on a daily basis as well as MiraLAX several times a week to manage to have a bowel movement, about every other day, generally hard pellets (Bristol score 1–2). Over the past 6–9 months, she is also experiencing abdominal cramping that is generally relieved with a bowel movement. She has no family history of colon cancer. Her physical exam and basic lab panel are normal.*

Do you think a colonoscopy is warranted to rule out organic pathology, in a case like this?

Indications for colonoscopy would be if the patient was 45 or older or if there were any alarm features, like blood mixed with stool, unintentional weight loss, and iron deficiency anemia. In a case like this, the diagnosis of IBS-C is likely, and doing a colonoscopy to rule out organic pathology does not seem indicated. We would go ahead with managing the patient's symptoms after providing education to the patient about her disorder and reassurance that her symptoms can be managed.

How beneficial is fiber for patients like this?

We find the response to fiber is very variable. It seems to work well in about a third of our patients with IBS-C; in another third, there is a neutral response, and another third note worsened constipation or pain after taking fiber. But if fiber therapy works, we think that is the best approach.

In this case, where the patient continues to have hard stools despite taking a fiber supplement, we drill down on the importance of drinking more water. First, we would encourage more liquid intake. If the patient does not have a great response,

W. H. Sobin (✉) · P. Sanvanson
Division of Gastroenterology and Hepatology, Department of Medicine, Medical College of Wisconsin, Milwaukee, WI, USA
e-mail: hsobin@mcw.edu; psanvans@mcw.edu

© The Author(s), under exclusive license to Springer Nature Switzerland AG 2023
W. H. Sobin et al. (eds.), *Managing Complex Cases in Gastroenterology*, https://doi.org/10.1007/978-3-031-48949-5_53

we might have her try to increase the amount of fiber she is taking along with even more fluid. In a number of cases, this will work to enhance the bulk of the stool and may relieve cramping. Patients with IBS-C should be educated on soluble fiber intake, as insoluble fiber may increase abdominal bloating. Soluble fiber including psyllium-based products have been shown to improve both constipation and IBS symptoms. If the patient tries to increase fiber intake and does not improve, we would go on to other measures.

Is it safe to use MiraLAX on a long-term basis? Should the dose be increased?

It is safe to use MiraLAX (polyethylene glycol) on a chronic basis and the dose should be increased. We would certainly go to daily use of MiraLAX. If there is a limited response, we would increase the dose to twice daily. If we overshoot and start getting diarrhea, we would titrate the dose down. The only potential problem from using MiraLAX is if excessive doses are used and diarrhea ensues. Patients should be educated on how to titrate the dose of MiraLAX as needed.

Do you believe that MiraLAX works simply to relieve constipation or does it decrease pain as well?

In studies, MiraLAX improves constipation, but its benefit on abdominal pain is not statistically significant. However, in practice, we find that simply relieving constipation does improve underlying pain in many patients.

The patient does not benefit from increased fluid or fiber and doesn't tolerate the increased dosing of MiraLAX, complaining of increased bloating and gas.

What other regimens might you turn to?

We are looking for something to use on a chronic basis (at least in the near term). We turn first to the laxatives that increase small bowel secretion [1] by their action on the guanylate cyclase receptor (linaclotide or plecanatide) or the chloride channel receptor (lubiprostone). We usually start with linaclotide (Linzess) [2, 3] because it is well tolerated, works well, and is available in three different doses (72 mcg, 145 mcg, and 290 mcg), which offers very useful flexibility. Once patients start on this, it is usually taken daily. If a patient develops diarrhea after trying the lowest dose of linaclotide, then it would be reasonable to trial lubiprostone.

Does linaclotide work primarily to relieve constipation or does it work on pain as well?

Linaclotide works quickly to relieve constipation, but it also works to relieve abdominal cramping. However, the full effect on pain relief takes longer to kick in; it may take a month for the full benefit to be seen.

For patients who do not respond to the secretagogues like linaclotide or find it insufficient, what other medications are you using?

Another class of drugs is the 5-HT4 receptor agonists, which act as promotility agents. Prucalopride (Motegrity) [4] is the one we would try first. The combination of a secretagogue and a promotility agent can be efficacious. Prucalopride has also been found helpful in treating gastroparesis, although it's not yet approved for this indication. If we have a constipated patient with delayed gastric emptying, we will turn to prucalopride earlier. Tegaserod is another 5HT4 agonist, which is approved in women under age 65. If prucalopride is not approved or tolerated, we might try this.

Another drug that we occasionally add-on is misoprostol. This is a prostaglandin analogue, which we will use off-label because it is known to cause diarrhea. Used in constipated patients on a chronic basis, we have found it helpful in some of our refractory patients. Of course, it cannot be given to females of reproductive age without appropriate contraception as it is an abortifacient.

This patient is started on linaclotide starting at 145mcg a day and then goes up to 290 mcg a day. She gets marked relief but still feels like she is not emptying normally. After adding prucalopride to the linaclotide, she feels that she is emptying better.

Case 2 A 67-year-old female with severe osteoarthritis is seen in the ER because of *severe abdominal pain and constipation. She is on chronic opiates for arthritis pain. She has not had a bowel movement in about 10 days. On exam, her abdomen is protuberant, and X-ray confirms a large amount of stool throughout the colon. On the rectal exam, she has a large stool impaction.*

How would you manage this?

First, you need to evacuate the colon. If necessary, we would start out with a rectal disimpaction. Since this is often very painful, we may give an IV sedative at the bedside just prior to disimpaction. Following that, we would give the patient a bowel lavage. If possible, we would have the patient take a gallon of GoLYTELY (polyethylene glycol-3350) over a number of hours. If the patient cannot tolerate GoLYTELY, we would try to get them to at least take a bottle of magnesium citrate or a MiraLAX purge. After that, you will have addressed the acute constipation, but now it is a matter of addressing the chronic constipation. Obviously, you would like to get the patient off opiates, but that is often not possible. We do have regimens for managing constipation in chronic opioid users. The PAMORAs (peripherally acting mu-opioid receptor antagonists) were designed for patients on chronic opiates. We have used naloxegol (Movantik), which is an oral agent, and methylnaltrexone (Relistor) is something we have given subcutaneously in the hospital, although it is now available in oral form. Linaclotide has also been found effective in treating constipation from chronic opioid use, and it may be easier to access and potentially as effective.

Case 3 A 27-year-old female comes in with a history of constipation that started *within the last year. The constipation began after she started a new office job that requires a lengthier commute. She is very rushed getting out of the house in the morning. She does not have time to eat breakfast and then go to the bathroom to defecate before work, which was her normal pattern. Her workplace has many employees, and there are always women in adjacent stalls when she tries to defecate at work. Now, when she tries, she cannot relax enough to allow her bowels to "open up" and empty normally. She has been working for 3 months and things have not improved. Even on weekends or when she tries to go in the evening, she finds that she cannot evacuate normally. There is a lot of struggling and straining with only small amounts coming out and a continued sensation of incomplete evacuation. The mechanics of moving her bowels are feeling totally foreign to her.*

In taking a history, what questions do you ask to evaluate for outlet dysfunction?

For an assessment of outlet dysfunction, we tend to focus on obtaining a history that includes the following: "Do you strain with trying to have a bowel movement?" "Do you feel empty after having a bowel movement?" "Do you spend a lot of time on the toilet to have a bowel movement, how long on average?" "Do you have the urge/sensation when you want to have a bowel movement?" "Do you have to wipe excessively to get clean when you have a bowel movement?" "Any maneuvers on the toilet that help you have a bowel movement (elevating your legs, digital extraction of stool)?" "Do you have to press against the vagina and/or the space between the vagina and rectum to have a bowel movement?" "Do you have to return to the bathroom in a short time frame to have another bowel movement?" [5]

How would you approach this patient's outlet dysfunction?

We would take two different approaches here. First, we would suggest seeing a psychotherapist with an approach to relaxation exercises and cognitive behavior therapy. But if she doesn't respond to that and the constipation continues, we would send her for anorectal manometry. We suspect the patient now has dyssynergic defecation. If this is confirmed on anorectal manometry, she might do well with biofeedback therapy.

Case 4 A 35-year-old woman travels frequently to Europe and Asia for her work. She experiences bouts of constipation repeatedly during these excursions. She has mild constipation at home, which responds to a dose of MiraLAX taken as needed. She takes packets of MiraLAX with her on these trips but is afraid to take anything before her flight, fearing possible diarrhea on the airplane.

What is your approach to the occasional use of different laxatives for people with intermittent constipation?

The one we recommend most frequently is MiraLAX. It is safe and flexible, and you can titrate the dose. Patients need to know that MiraLAX usually does not work immediately; it may take hours to kick in. While patients can take more than one dose in a day, we warn them that the full effect may not demonstrate itself for 24 h (although in some, it can work in just a couple of hours), so they need to give the first dose some time to work before they take more.

For patients who want a more acute purge, we do like bisacodyl (Dulcolax) or senna tabs or bisacodyl suppositories. Some patients prefer the "kick" of a stimulant laxative, particularly those who experience more colonic inertia. Patients should be aware of the potential for abdominal cramping with use of stimulant laxatives.

Another agent some patients prefer is milk of magnesia, which has a gentler effect, and some do well taking this on a chronic basis. We do not suggest the use of docusate, as we do not think there is much benefit, particularly if used as a sole agent.

Case 5 A 46-year-old female presents with a history of chronic constipation. She had a recent screening colonoscopy that was negative, except for mild diverticulosis. She is already taking fiber and occasional MiraLAX. You suggest daily MiraLAX, but her response is limited. You order linaclotide, but she doesn't like it. You switch to lubiprostone (Amitiza), which she tolerates, and it gives her some relief, but the response is still incomplete.

Are there any other tests you will run to evaluate constipation?

In this case, the patient had a colonoscopy for screening purposes. We do not see any need to repeat the colonoscopy. Another simple test we like is a Sitzmarks study [6]. The patient swallows a capsule in the office that contains a number of tiny radiopaque markers, and then, we follow up with an abdominal X-ray 5 days afterward. Most, if not all, of the markers should be gone by day 5 (>80% of markers being passed on day 5 is considered a normal study). If the abdominal X-ray shows increased markers, it can be useful information. If there is a diffuse pattern of retained markers throughout the colon, it suggests general colon inertia. If they are all retained in the rectum it suggests more of an outlet problem and, possibly, dyssynergic defecation. If dyssynergic defecation is being considered, anorectal manometry is ordered. The Sitzmarks study may be performed on or off the patient's current bowel regimen, depending on the clinical situation: performed on regimen to determine efficacy of treatment while performed off regimen to determine diagnosis. We frequently use abdominal X-rays and Sitzmarks studies to objectively assess the degree of constipation and the response to therapy. This is especially helpful when patients state that they have tried and failed numerous therapies.

You end up ordering anorectal manometry, which is normal. A Sitzmarks test reveals increased markers throughout the colon – suggestive of generalized colon inertia. You try prucalopride with no response.

What other strategies might you add?

We might add tegaserod to enhance colon motility, but since she did not respond to prucalopride, another 5HT4 agonist, we would not be too optimistic. Tenapanor [7] is a sodium hydrogen exchange (NH3E) inhibitor that works in IBS-C and chronic constipation and may be considered.

Something that we have found useful in a number of patients is the off-label use of misoprostol as an add-on to a secretagogue. We always warn patients not to use misoprostol, which is an abortifacient, if they are intending to get pregnant, and not to share it with others.

The patient is on oral contraceptive pills and not intending to get pregnant. Misoprostol is added to lubiprostone, starting at 200 mcg bid and then increased to 400 mcg bid. She has an excellent response to combined lubiprostone and misoprostol.

References

1. Chang L, Sultan S, Lembo A, Verne GN, Smalley W, Heidelbaugh JJ. AGA clinical practice guideline on the pharmacological management of irritable bowel syndrome with constipation. Gastroenterology. 2022;163(1):118–36.
2. Videlock EJ, Cheng V, Cremonini F. Effects of linaclotide in patients with irritable bowel syndrome with constipation or chronic constipation: a meta-analysis. Clin Gastroenterol Hepatol. 2013;11(9):1084–92.
3. Chey WD, Lembo AJ, Lavins BJ, Shiff SJ, Kurtz CB, Currie MG, MacDougall JE, Jia XD, Shao JZ, Fitch DA, Baird MJ. Linaclotide for irritable bowel syndrome with constipation: a 26-week, randomized, double-blind, placebo-controlled trial to evaluate efficacy and safety. Off J Am Coll Gastroenterol. 2012;107(11):1702–12.

4. Sajid MS, Hebbar M, Baig MK, Li A, Philipose Z. Use of prucalopride for chronic constipation: a systematic review and meta-analysis of published randomized, controlled trials. J
   Neurogastroenterol Motil. 2016;22(3):412.
5. Rao SS, Patcharatrakul T. Diagnosis and treatment of dyssynergic defecation. J
   Neurogastroenterol Motil. 2016;22(3):423.
6. Metcalf AM, Phillips SF, Zinsmeister AR, MacCarty RL, Beart RW, Wolff BG. Simplified
   assessment of segmental colonic transit. Gastroenterology. 1987;92(1):40–7.
7. Chey WD, Lembo AJ, Rosenbaum DP. Efficacy of tenapanor in treating patients with irritable
   bowel syndrome with constipation: a 12-week, placebo-controlled phase 3 trial (T3MPO-1).
   Am J Gastroenterol. 2020;115(2):281.

Chapter 54
Functional Dyspepsia

W. Harley Sobin and Patrick Sanvanson

Case 1 *A 34-year-old female complains of feeling full about 10 min after starting a meal. She has begun to eat very slowly and will quit eating earlier to avoid feeling sick. These symptoms have been going on for over 6 months. They started after having a meal at a Mexican restaurant. Both she and her husband got sick with some sort of gastroenteritis. After that, her stomach never felt better. She has no other medical problems and no history of diabetes. She has come to loathe that full feeling and avoids eating to prevent feeling nauseated. Her family doctor saw her several months ago and started her on omeprazole, which initially helped her but then quit helping, and she subsequently stopped it. Her community gastroenterologist then sent off a stool test for H. pylori, which returned negative. He did an EGD, which was unremarkable with no evidence of gastritis, no ulcers, and no retained food. Biopsies of the stomach were negative for H. pylori and eosinophilic gastroenteritis. Duodenal biopsies were negative for celiac disease. He ordered gastric scintigraphy, which showed mild delayed gastric emptying at 4 h. He ordered metoclopramide for the patient, but she developed dystonia with the very first dose, leading to an ER visit to reverse the side effects of the metoclopramide. Because of her weight loss, he also ordered a CT scan of the abdomen and pelvis to rule out other organic pathology, which returned negative. He is sending the patient to you for a second opinion.*

What is your diagnosis and how would you manage the patient?

With this patient's postprandial fullness going on for more than 6 months, the diagnosis appears to be functional dyspepsia-postprandial distress type. Considering

---

W. H. Sobin (✉) · P. Sanvanson
Division of Gastroenterology and Hepatology, Department of Medicine, Medical College of Wisconsin, Milwaukee, WI, USA
e-mail: hsobin@mcw.edu; psanvans@mcw.edu

© The Author(s), under exclusive license to Springer Nature Switzerland AG 2023
W. H. Sobin et al. (eds.), *Managing Complex Cases in Gastroenterology*,
https://doi.org/10.1007/978-3-031-48949-5_54

267

the diagnosis of functional dyspepsia, it is important to rule out *H. pylori* [1], which was done here. A trial of PPIs is usually initiated [2], which was ultimately unsuccessful here.

Left with a patient who is still quite symptomatic, with the diagnosis of FD-postprandial distress type, we like to try buspirone [3], which has been found to increase gastric accommodation in these patients. What we tell the patient is that the stomach is overly stiff and doesn't expand appropriately to allow more food. Buspirone allows for better relaxation and expansion. We start with 5 mg TID before meals and then go up to 10 mg before meals if needed.

Doesn't the finding of delayed gastric emptying dissuade you against the diagnosis of FD, and isn't this more likely gastroparesis?

No, delayed gastric emptying is common in FD, present in about a third of patients. The two diagnoses are quite similar and may coexist or be indistinguishable in some [4]. However, the diagnosis of gastroparesis does not require symptoms to be present for 6 months, as they do in FD. Also, buspirone is generally not considered in gastroparesis, which is generally considered a disorder of delayed gastric emptying rather than decreased gastric accommodation. Promotility drugs have been tried in FD and may be effective; however in the USA, we do not have promotility agents that are safe to use long term.

Isn't buspirone used as an antianxiety drug? Doesn't it lead to sedation, tolerance, and addiction?

Some patients may find buspirone slightly sedating, but unlike the antianxiety benzodiazepines, buspirone does not cause tolerance or addiction and can be abruptly discontinued without withdrawal symptoms.

What would you use if the patient doesn't tolerate buspirone or it isn't effective?

We have tried STW-5 [4] (Iberogast), an OTC herbal preparation, which has been beneficial in a couple of cases. FDgard [5] is another OTC preparation. Others have used Rikkunshito [6], a Japanese herbal product.

If her symptoms and weight loss were to continue in spite of these measures, we would try mirtazapine [7] or olanzapine [8], which are two central neuromodulators that we generally reserve for patients with chronic nausea and vomiting. We generally try mirtazapine first at 15 mg at bedtime. While some people start with 7.5 mg first, it is reported that the likelihood of side effects is the same at 7.5 mg or 15 mg, but the efficacy is lower with the 7.5 mg dose.

Mirtazapine acts to decrease nausea and increase appetite, mostly through anti-5-HT3 blockade, and these are the reasons we would try it. It also happens to be an antianxiety medication that is a safe antidepressant. We have found this drug to be particularly effective in older patients, in their 50 s, 60 s, and 70 s, with chronic nausea and vomiting. Psychiatrists [8] think mirtazapine is one of the safer antidepressants to use in the elderly, and it also has the benefit of not causing sexual side effects. However, we have found that younger patients, like this 32-year-old, are more likely to find the side effects of daytime sleepiness and increased appetite problematic. In spite of this, we would try mirtazapine first. Prior to starting mirtazapine, we would recommend monitoring for evidence of QTc prolongation and monitoring QTc about 4 weeks after starting mirtazapine.

If she doesn't tolerate mirtazapine, then we would try olanzapine [8]. This is an atypical antipsychotic that has shown a lot of efficacy in patients with chronic nausea and anorexia. The drug works via both 5-HT3 and D2 blockade. We would start with 5 mg at bedtime. This drug may be better tolerated than mirtazapine in some patients.

If she fails these drugs, we would also entertain getting a psychologist involved. From the history, it sounds as if the patient may be experiencing a restrictive eating disorder that might benefit from psychotherapy [9].

What about the use of cannabinoids?

We have not used these and are concerned about the development of cannabinoid hyperemesis syndrome (CHS) [10] or further delay in gastric emptying with chronic use. We do have a lot of experience managing CHS, where we always instruct complete cessation of cannabinoids.

Case 2 A 35-year-old female has daily abdominal burning pain that has been going on for 7 months. There are no exacerbating or relieving factors. She has been avoiding spicy food, alcohol, and caffeine for months. She is not taking any aspirin or NSAIDs. There has been no weight loss, and there are no alarm features. Her MD sends off a stool H. pylori antigen, which returns negative. She takes omeprazole for 2 months without relief.

How would you manage this patient?

In a young patient like this, the risk of a GI malignancy is low, and the likelihood of finding anything on endoscopy, particularly after taking PPIs for 2 months, is very low. It is important that the stool for *H. pylori* was sent off prior to initiating PPI therapy, since PPIs could lead to a false-negative *H. pylori*. In a young patient who does not take NSAIDs, *H. pylori* is a more common cause of organic disease that would lead to chronic abdominal burning pain.

In this patient, it is likely that we are dealing with functional dyspepsia-epigastric pain syndrome type. In many patients, symptoms are relieved with PPIs. But if they are not, we would try central neuromodulators. Nicholas Talley [11] demonstrated that amitriptyline benefitted patients with FD-EPS type. We prefer the use of nortriptyline, which has fewer anticholinergic side effects, particularly less constipation. We would start with nortriptyline 25 mg at bedtime for 1 month and then go up to 50 mg at bedtime if tolerated. For patients who are more anxious, we might start with 10 mg at bedtime for a week before going up to 25 mg. In using the tricyclics, we explain to patients that it takes at least a month to see clinical efficacy, but side effects will commence right away. Prior to starting tricyclics, we would recommend monitoring for evidence of QTc prolongation and monitoring QTc about 4 weeks after starting tricyclics.

For patients who do not respond to any of these therapies, we will perform an EGD to rule out something like a PPI-resistant peptic ulcer, gastroduodenal Crohn's, or eosinophilic gastroenteritis. However, the likelihood of finding anything in these young patients is low.

In addition, we generally suggest working closely with a dietician to help understand patients' dietary patterns and what or when they eat, maintaining a food diary to assess for food triggers, and considering tailoring a diet that minimizes symptoms.

References

1. Ford AC, Mahadeva S, Carbone MF, Lacy BE, Talley NJ. Functional dyspepsia. Lancet. 2020;396(10263):1689–702.
2. Moayyedi PM, Lacy BE, Andrews CN, Enns RA, Howden CW, Vakil N. ACG and CAG clinical guideline: management of dyspepsia. Off J Am Coll Gastroenterol. 2017;112(7):988–1013.
3. Tack J, Janssen P, Masaoka T, Farré R, Van Oudenhove L. Efficacy of buspirone, a fundus-relaxing drug, in patients with functional dyspepsia. Clin Gastroenterol Hepatol. 2012;10(11):1239–45.
4. Von Arnim U, Peitz U, Vinson B, Gundermann KJ, Malfertheiner P. STW 5, a phytopharmacon for patients with functional dyspepsia: results of a multicenter, placebo-controlled double-blind study. Off J Am Coll Gastroenterol. 2007;102(6):1268–75.
5. Lacy BE, Chey WD, Epstein MS, Shah SM, Corsino P, Zeitzoff LR, Cash BD. A novel duodenal-release formulation of caraway oil and L-menthol is a safe, effective and well tolerated therapy for functional dyspepsia. BMC Gastroenterol. 2022;22(1):1–9.
6. Suzuki H, Matsuzaki J, Fukushima Y, Suzaki F, Kasugai K, Nishizawa T, Naito Y, Hayakawa T, Kamiya T, Andoh T, Yoshida H. Randomized clinical trial: rikkunshito in the treatment of functional dyspepsia—a multicenter, double-blind, randomized, placebo-controlled study. Neurogastroenterol Motil. 2014;26(7):950–61.
7. Ly HG, Carbone F, Holvoet L, Bisschops R, Caenepeel P, Arts J, Boeckxstaens G, Van Oudenhove L, Tack J. Mirtazapine improves early satiation, nutrient intake, weight recovery and quality of life in functional dyspepsia with weight loss: a double-blind, randomized, placebo-controlled pilot study. Gastroenterology. 2013;144(5):S.
8. Sobin HW, Heinrich TW, Drossman DA. Central neuromodulators for treating functional GI disorders: a primer. Off J Am Coll Gastroenterol. 2017;112(5):693–702.
9. Orive M, Barrio I, Orive VM, Matellanes B, Padierna JA, Cabriada J, Orive A, Escobar A, Quintana JM. A randomized controlled trial of a 10-week group psychotherapeutic treatment added to standard medical treatment in patients with functional dyspepsia. J Psychosom Res. 2015;78(6):563–8.
10. Allen JH, de Moore GD, Heddle R, Twartz J. Cannabinoid hyperemesis: cyclical hyperemesis in association with chronic cannabis abuse. Gut. 2004;53(11):1566–70.
11. Talley NJ, Locke GR, Saito YA, Almazar AE, Bouras EP, Howden CW, Lacy BE, DiBaise JK, Prather CM, Abraham BP, El-Serag HB. Effect of amitriptyline and escitalopram on functional dyspepsia: a multicenter, randomized controlled study. Gastroenterology. 2015;149(2):340–9.

Chapter 55
Bloating

W. Harley Sobin and Patrick Sanvanson

Case 1 *A 35-year-old female complains of abdominal bloating and distension. When she wakes up, she feels fine, but as the day proceeds, her belly pouches out, and toward the end of the day, she feels like she is 7 months pregnant. These symptoms have been present for at least 10 months. She feels progressively more distended and uncomfortable, and her clothes feel tighter. Her bowel movements are relatively normal, more on the harder side.*

In cases like this, do patients usually have increased gaseous retention?

No, usually most patients do not retain excess gas. What is more common is visceral hypersensitivity, increased sensitivity to normal levels of gas [1]. But another thing that might be going on is an abnormal viscerosomatic reflex [2]. Normally, when we eat, the diaphragm rises and the abdominal muscles contract. This is the viscerosomatic reflex, which prevents our stomachs from pouching out after meals. Some patients have an abnormal reflex, where the diaphragm drops and abdominal muscles don't contract. These patients have increased abdominal girth after meals when measured on MRI. There is actually an increase in abdominal diameter, although the amount of measured gas is the same. We think this may be going on with this patient.

She says that the gas is really painful and asks for something to alleviate the pain. Are there any tips you have found helpful?

We've counseled countless patients about gas pain through the years. First, we would prescribe a low-FODMAP (fermentable oligosaccharides, disaccharides, monosaccharides, and polyols) diet [3], which should result in less fermentation. Avoid raw fruits and raw vegetables. Stay away from carbonated beverages. Watch

W. H. Sobin (✉) · P. Sanvanson
Division of Gastroenterology and Hepatology, Department of Medicine, Medical College of Wisconsin, Milwaukee, WI, USA
e-mail: hsobin@mcw.edu; psanvans@mcw.edu

W. H. Sobin et al. (eds.), *Managing Complex Cases in Gastroenterology*, https://doi.org/10.1007/978-3-031-48949-5_55

out for lactose sensitivity. Avoid artificially sweetened candies with sorbitol, xylitol, or mannitol, all of which can produce a lot of gas.

In prescribing a low-FODMAP diet, we often have the patient work with a dietician to educate about the diet and also plan the reintroduction of food components to identify triggers. Giving a complete low-FODMAP diet for an indefinite period is usually not sustainable.

In terms of over-the-counter remedies, patients often try one of the products that contains simethicone (Mylicon, Phazyme, Gas-X). This is in spite of the fact that controlled studies have not shown a benefit from simethicone [4]. The results evidently are more lackluster than when we instill it during colonoscopies, to help dissolve gas bubbles. We have, on occasion, had patients try charcoal tables [5] to help absorb gas (some patients praise the effects of eating burnt toast). Beano [6] has been found effective in decreasing gas from beans and some other vegetables. Pepto-Bismol [7] has been used to decrease hydrogen sulfide production, which is helpful in the management of flatulence.

Once again, most of these patients do not really have increased gas, just an increased sensitivity to the gas that is present. For patients who are very symptomatic, we will occasionally prescribe central neuromodulators [8]. We particularly like the tricyclic nortriptyline to decrease painful bloating. Compared to the popular tricyclic amitriptyline, nortriptyline is less constipating, and constipation can certainly exacerbate bloating. We generally start nortriptyline at 25 mg at bedtime and after a couple of weeks go up to 50 mg at bedtime. We tell patients that side effects (dry eyes, dry mouth, occasionally sexual side effects) will start right away, but that full efficacy, with decreased visceral hypersensitivity, might take a month or so.

The SSRIs are not constipating (with the exception of paroxetine), but they don't have much effect on decreasing pain. The SNRIs are effective in decreasing pain and tend to be less constipating than the TCAs. Of the SNRIs, we generally prefer duloxetine [8]. We like to start with 30 mg at bedtime and then consider going up to 60 mg at bedtime after a couple of weeks.

In patients with underlying constipation who complain of bloating, we like to use Linzess (linaclotide) [9]. Linzess relieves constipation quickly, but it also has an effect on decreasing discomfort and bloating. However, it may take a month for this neuromodulatory benefit to fully kick in.

Case 2 *A 40-year-old female complains of painful abdominal distension. She has a history of Raynaud's. She has no clinical signs of systemic sclerosis. She is on diltiazem for the Raynaud's and has mild constipation, for which she has tried MiraLAX (polyethylene glycol). However, MiraLAX seems to exacerbate her bloating. On the exam, her abdomen is tympanitic, but bowel sounds are normal. The abdomen is mildly tender without guarding. Her doctor ordered a lactulose breath test to see whether she might have small intestinal bacterial overgrowth (SIBO). The breath test showed a baseline methane level of 25 and hydrogen of 10. Over the next 60 min, the methane rose to 50 and the hydrogen increased to 45. This was interpreted as a positive breath test.*

How would you interpret these findings and manage her bloating?

Constipation may be an exacerbating factor in anyone with bloating, and controlling constipation is always part of solving the bloating dilemma. While MiraLAX is our most commonly used laxative, occasional patients complain that it actually makes bloating worse.

Her history of Raynaud's does raise the possibility of altered small bowel motility, as one would see in full-fledged systemic sclerosis. The use of the hydrogen breath test (using lactulose or glucose) without synchronous scintigraphy has been questioned as a definitive test for SIBO [10]. When the hydrogen breath test is being considered, treatment of constipation prior to testing is essential.

So, the question is, does she really have SIBO and could this be causing bloating? The other interesting finding is the elevated methane level. There is some debate about whether everyone is capable of producing methane, but elevated methane levels have been associated with delayed colon motility, which can exacerbate bloating, as well as constipation [11].

If you wanted to treat this patient for SIBO, the treatment is more complicated because of the elevated methane. To knock out the methanogenic archaea along with the hydrogen producing bacteria, it is not sufficient to just use rifaximin. Generally, it requires the addition of neomycin to rifaximin. Therefore, the combination of rifaximin 550 TID and neomycin 500 mg BID for 2 weeks is indicated [12]. Metronidazole has been reported to inhibit growth of methanogenic archaea [13], and its use in place of neomycin has been considered.

Case 3 *A 33-year-old female was suffering from abdominal bloating and stomach upset and decided to start taking the probiotic, Align (bifidobacterium infantis). However, within a few weeks of starting Align, she started feeling lethargic and had the sensation of brain fog. In addition, her bloating seemed much worse. As a result, she stopped the Align, and her symptoms markedly improved.*

How do you interpret these findings?

There have been reports [14] of probiotic bacteria metabolizing carbohydrates into D-lactic acid. High levels of D-lactic acid have been associated with increased "brain fog," confusion, and bloating. If these patients stopped taking their probiotics, the brain fog and abdominal bloating improved. This has been reported with both lactobacillus and bifidobacterium species, which are both common components of probiotics. While most patients won't develop these problems from probiotics, it is important to be aware of the potential association. If your patient on probiotics develops worsened bloating and "brain fog," consider stopping the probiotic.

Case 4 *A 40-year-old female complains of abdominal bloating over the past month. She has a long history of constipation and started taking Metamucil on her own about 6 weeks earlier. She started on a low dose of Metamucil, mixing it with only a small amount of fluid because she doesn't like drinking fluids. She gradually increased the dose of Metamucil but avoided increasing the amount of fluid that she mixed it in. Because this caused increased cramping, she went to her family doctor, who started her on dicyclomine (Bentyl). Her bloating got worse, and she was referred to you.*

How would you manage this situation?

While fiber laxatives benefit a lot of people with constipation, they have to be taken with large amounts of fluid. We would say that these agents probably help about 1/3 of our constipated patients, have a neutral effect on another third, and may worsen constipation [15] in the others, usually in those who do not drink enough fluid.

Metamucil certainly may be a cause of gassiness, and it is not surprising that this patient developed increased bloating. In addition, the use of dicyclomine can further slow gut motility and worsen bloating. Dicyclomine is more beneficial in patients with diarrhea.

In a patient like this, we would stop the dicyclomine and try switching from metamucil to linaclotide (Linzess). Linzess should help the constipation without causing increased gas. In addition, after about a month, Linzess [9] can help with visceral hypersensitivity. So, there is an immediate benefit of Linzess in treating constipation, but you may also see a decrease in bloating and cramps after about a month of use.

Case 5 A 27-year-old female is referred to you with intractable abdominal bloating. She feels bloated several hours after eating and has modified her diet without much success. She has avoided meat, gluten, and dairy and now simply tries not to eat at all to try to relieve her discomfort. She has lost 10 pounds over the past 2 months. She has tried Gas-X and peppermint oil without much benefit. In going over her history, you find that she seems mildly depressed. She notes that the bloating always occurs over the suprapubic/pelvic area. She says that she has seen a gynecologist to make sure that there was nothing wrong with her uterus or ovaries that is causing this discomfort. Her thyroid and basic CBC and chemistries have been normal. When you ask whether she might be willing to try a central neuromodulator to work on visceral hypersensitivity, she is quite reluctant. She says that when she was 15, she had a "nervous breakdown" and was on heavy duty antidepressants. The breakdown was precipitated by several episodes of sexual abuse by an uncle who was briefly living with the family.

How do you manage patients with a history like this?

Douglas Drossman and others have shown that there is a high incidence of abuse, both sexual and physical, in patients who have refractory GI functional symptoms [16]. A case like this reveals how GI symptoms like bloating may be associated with significant psychopathology, and relieving these symptoms will require collaboration with a mental health specialist.

But while a psychiatrist might get involved in a case like this, they are not necessarily tuned into the effect of psychiatric drugs on the GI tract. As gastroenterologists, we can occasionally advise psychiatrists, in order to benefit our patients.

Certain psychiatric agents can be used as central neuromodulators to decrease abdominal pain and bloating. We can utilize low- to medium-dose tricyclics and full-dose SNRIs for their analgesic benefit [8]. These drugs can promote analgesia by inhibiting norepinephrine reuptake (due to their action on the norepinephrine transporter—NET), thereby increasing levels of norepinephrine.

Some of the atypical antipsychotics that may be used on our patients—like aripiprazole, lurasidone, and ziprasidone—can cause undesirable GI side effects, primarily early satiety and nausea [8]. If our patients develop these adverse symptoms on these agents, we can advise the psychiatrist to consider switching to the atypical antipsychotics, like olanzapine or quetiapine, which are good treatments for nausea.

Case 6 *A 53-year-old female complains of persistent abdominal bloating and mild constipation. She has a history of type 2 diabetes of 10-year duration. Her diabetes is not tightly controlled. She is aware that she can't eat large portions at meals; otherwise, she will fill up. She can avoid feeling full if she eats multiple small meals, but, regardless, as the day progresses, she does tend to get more bloated.*

How would you evaluate and treat this patient?

In this case, disordered GI motility due to diabetes may be a contributing factor. Diabetic neuropathy could contribute to decreased gastric emptying of food, decreased small bowel emptying of gas, and increased colon retention [17]. While small bowel motility measurement may not be widely accessible, measuring gastric emptying with nuclear medicine testing and colon emptying with a Sitzmarks study [18] are both inexact but broadly available tools.

Improved glucose control and dietary change (restricting fat and fiber and multiple small meals) can benefit the patient. Prucalopride [19] may be prescribed to treat constipation while enhancing gastric motility at the same time.

Case 7 *A 77-year-old male presents with the chief complaint of severe abdominal bloating. This has been going on for months. He has mild constipation. He has a past history of abdominal surgery and radiation therapy for a non-Hodgkin lymphoma. On exam, his abdomen is quite tympanitic and mildly tender. Bowel sounds are high pitched.*

An abdominal series shows dilated loops of small bowel but no suggestion of obstruction.

How would you manage this patient's bloating?

In this case, we think the patient probably has delayed small bowel motility and is certainly predisposed to developing SIBO, so we would order a breath test. In community-based practices, lactulose breath tests are frequently used. At the Medical College of Wisconsin, Dr. Benson Massey is a proponent of the glucose hydrogen breath test, done in combination with scintigraphy [10]. And, as he likes to point out, we want to manage constipation before doing a breath test.

The patient is given laxatives to treat his constipation, and a glucose hydrogen breath test is done 1 week later. He is placed on a low-fiber diet prior to testing, and on arrival, he promises the lab nurse that he has absolutely adhered to the diet. In spite of this, the breath test shows a markedly elevated baseline hydrogen of 120. He is given glucose, and the hydrogen level rises to 180 over 30 min.

What do you make of the elevated baseline hydrogen?

Sometimes, we do not know whether a breath test is uninterpretable if the baseline hydrogen is elevated. Did the patient really adhere to the diet? But in this case, it is likely that the elevation is truly due to background fermentation related to marked bacterial overgrowth. We then see the level rise appropriately after giving the glucose load, confirming the impression of SIBO.

How would you manage this patient's bacterial overgrowth?

We would start antibiotics and generally continue them for a couple of weeks. If we can get rifaximin covered, that would be our first choice. Since there are often barriers to prescribing rifaximin, we would try trimethoprim/sulfamethoxazole (Bactrim), ciprofloxacin, or amoxicillin/clavulanic acid (Augmentin).

Do you expect that to cure the bloating?

I certainly think it can help. However, the patient will continue to have bowel dilation, and it's possible that the trapped air will contribute to the sensation of bloating. Also, the patient will undoubtedly develop a relapse of bacterial overgrowth in the future. Antibiotics will generally improve SIBO, but recurrence in 3–4 months is common.

References

1. Malagelada JR, Accarino A, Azpiroz F. Bloating and abdominal distension: old misconceptions and current knowledge. Official J Am Coll Gastroenterol ACG. 2017;112(8):1221–31.
2. Accarino A, Perez F, Azpiroz F, Quiroga S, Malagelada JR. Abdominal distention results from caudo-ventral redistribution of contents. Gastroenterology. 2009;136(5):1544–51.
3. Halmos EP, Power VA, Shepherd SJ, Gibson PR, Muir JG. A diet low in FODMAPs reduces symptoms of irritable bowel syndrome. Gastroenterology. 2014;146(1):67–75.
4. Friis H, Bode S, Rumessen JJ, Gudmand-Høyer E. Effect of simethicone on lactulose-induced H2 production and gastrointestinal symptoms. Digestion. 1991;49(4):227–30.
5. Hall RG Jr, Thompson H, Strother A. Effects of orally administered activated charcoal on intestinal gas. Am J Gastroenterol. 1981;75(3)
6. Ganiats TG, Norcross WA, Halverson AL, Burford PA, Palinkas LA. Does beano prevent gas? A double-blind crossover study of oral a-galactosidase to treat dietary oligosaccharide intolerance. J Fam Pract. 1994;39(5):441–5.
7. Suarez FL, Furne JK, Springfield J, Levitt MD. Bismuth subsalicylate markedly decreases hydrogen sulfide release in the human colon. Gastroenterology. 1998;114(5):923–9.
8. Sobin HW, Heinrich TW, Drossman DA. Central neuromodulators for treating functional GI disorders: a primer. Off J Am Coll Gastroenterol. 2017;112(5):693–702.
9. Rao SS, Quigley EM, Shiff SJ, Lavins BJ, Kurtz CB, MacDougall JE, Currie MG, Johnston JM. Effect of linaclotide on severe abdominal symptoms in patients with irritable bowel syndrome with constipation. Clin Gastroenterol Hepatol. 2014;12(4):616–23.
10. Massey BT, Wald A. Small intestinal bacterial overgrowth syndrome: a guide for the appropriate use of breath testing. Dig Dis Sci. 2021;66(2):338–47.
11. Chatterjee S, Park S, Low K, Kong Y, Pimentel M. The degree of breath methane production in IBS correlates with the severity of constipation. Off J Am Coll Gastroenterol. 2007;102(4):837–41.

12. Low K, Hwang L, Hua J, Zhu A, Morales W, Pimentel M. A combination of rifaximin and neomycin is most effective in treating irritable bowel syndrome patients with methane on lactulose breath test. J Clin Gastroenterol. 2010;44(8):547–50.
13. Khelaifia S, Drancourt M. Susceptibility of archaea to antimicrobial agents: applications to clinical microbiology. Clin Microbiol Infect. 2012;18(9):841–8.
14. Rao SS, Rehman A, Yu S, De Andino NM. Brain fogginess, gas and bloating: a link between SIBO, probiotics and metabolic acidosis. Clin Transl Gastroenterol. 2018;9(6):e162.
15. Ho KS, Tan CY, Daud MA, Seow-Choen F. Stopping or reducing dietary fiber intake reduces constipation and its associated symptoms. World J Gastroenterol: WJG. 2012;18(33):4593.
16. Drossman DA, Talley NJ, Leserman J, Olden KW, Barreiro MA. Sexual and physical abuse and gastrointestinal illness: review and recommendations. Ann Intern Med. 1995;123(10):782–94.
17. Prasad VG, Abraham P. Management of chronic constipation in patients with diabetes mellitus. Indian J Gastroenterol. 2017;36:11–22.
18. Alame AM, Bahna H. Evaluation of constipation. Clin Colon Rectal Surg. 2012;25(01):005–11.
19. Sajid MS, Hebbar M, Baig MK, Li A, Philipose Z. Use of prucalopride for chronic constipation: a systematic review and meta-analysis of published randomized, controlled trials. J Neurogastroenterol Motil. 2016;22(3):412.

Part IV
Hepatology Compendium

Chapter 56
Introduction to the Hepatology Compendium

W. Harley Sobin

We gastroenterologists deal with many patients with liver disease in the community setting. We get many requests to see patients for abnormal liver enzymes or for questions about NAFLD. Managing complications of cirrhosis continues to consume a lot of our time. Treating hepatitis C used to be burdensome, but since the development of DAA treatment, this is rarely a problem.

While community gastroenterologists continue to spend a lot of time dealing with liver issues, we frequently curbside our hepatology experts at the regional tertiary care center for help with our complicated patients. There are numerous management decisions in hepatology that are confusing or controversial. In the sections below, we highlight how our liver specialists deal with some of these problem cases.

Oftentimes, our hepatology dilemmas start with abnormal liver enzymes. The workup is usually launched with a battery of serologic tests. At MCW, the standard panel of tests for evaluation of abnormal liver enzymes includes a viral hepatitis panel, an autoimmune panel that includes ANA, ASMA, and AMA, as well as ceruloplasmin, Fe/TIBC, ferritin, alpha-1-antitrypsin level, and celiac panel (occasionally IgG4 and others). This panel is a good starting point.

While these results often lead us to a diagnosis, the results are sometimes unrevealing and other times confusing. In addition, liver enzymes may be normal in cases where patients are consuming a lot of alcohol, cases where ultrasound reveals extensive hepatic steatosis, or even in cases of clear-cut cirrhosis. If the workup for abnormal liver enzymes is negative, what should the next steps be? These and many more issues are discussed in the case presentations that follow.

W. H. Sobin (✉)
Division of Gastroenterology and Hepatology, Department of Medicine, Medical College of Wisconsin, Milwaukee, WI, USA
e-mail: hsobin@mcw.edu

Below, we encounter a case of suspected hemochromatosis, where the transferrin saturation and the ferritin are discordant. How should we proceed? And if hemochromatosis is diagnosed, what is the end goal for phlebotomy?

The importance of Wilson's disease is highlighted in two different cases. We never want to miss Wilson's, which can lead to severe liver disease and debilitating neurodegenerative disease. In a case of suspected Wilson's, how is the diagnosis confirmed? The serum ceruloplasmin is a starting point in making the diagnosis, which, if low, triggers investigations. But, what about a case where the ceruloplasmin is normal? And, if Wilson's is confirmed, how is it treated? In the community, we may see one or two patients with Wilson's throughout our career, but it is imperative that we remain vigilant. If Wilson's is diagnosed, we certainly need advice about management.

A patient with abnormal LFTs and apparent alpha-1 antitrypsin deficiency is discussed. Alpha-1 antitrypsin deficiency may be the primary cause of chronic liver damage, or it can be a secondary, exacerbating factor in other cases. It is easily missed, if not specifically investigated.

We are all familiar with patients with indirect hyperbilirubinemia who have Gilbert's. But a case is discussed where Gilbert's is suspected but the patient also has an elevated direct bilirubin. How is this interpreted?

Normally, the ALT > AST, except in cases of active alcohol abuse. How do we interpret cases where the AST > ALT and alcohol abuse is apparently absent? Several authors discuss this phenomenon.

A case of profound hyperbilirubinemia is presented. In cases where the bilirubin is >20, it is usually not due to obstruction alone. What other factors may be contributing?

Community gastroenterologists are seeing more and more referrals for managing NAFLD. This is a confusing and controversial area, and it may be difficult to know what course of action to take. Talking to the hepatologists, there are several recommendations they all agree upon, but different viewpoints exist, even among the experts. Below, we share various approaches from several advisors with different management styles.

While this textbook was in production, the terminology-NAFLD was accepted by consensus. But, just prior to printing, NAFLD was replaced by MASLD. As Dr. Sourianarayanane says, "MASLD is the current terminology for non-alcoholic fatty liver disease (NAFLD), which is an encompassing diagnosis of those with fatty liver with metabolic risks. Similarly, metabolic dysfunction-associated steatohepatitis (MASH) is the replacement term for prior non-alcoholic steatohepatitis (NASH)". Since most of our readers are more familiar with NAFLD and NASH, we have not gone back to edit these terms that are still present in the majority of the chapters.

There is a case where we discuss the increased susceptibility women have to alcohol-induced liver disease. In another case, we discuss management of acute alcoholic hepatitis. Community gastroenterologists have managed patients with alcoholic hepatitis through the decades. We have gone through periods where pentoxifylline was recommended and where steroids have been advocated. Now, even the possibility of transplant has been raised. We hear about the management of alcoholic hepatitis in the tertiary care setting.

Another problem we commonly deal with in the community is managing ascites. In the initial evaluation of ascites, we know to examine the ascites albumin and cell count. We measure the SAAG (serum albumin minus ascites albumin), expecting it to be >1.1 in most cases, consistent with portal hypertension. We know that a PMN count in fluid >250 requires treatment for infection. We discuss cases of low SAAG ascites, ascites in a patient without apparent cirrhosis, and ascites in a patient with cirrhosis of unclear etiology. There is also a case that explores the possible etiologies of worsening ascites in an apparently stable cirrhotic.

Another issue we deal with in the community is managing bleeding esophageal varices. But what is the best approach to dealing with bleeding from post-banding ulcers? The other problem that may lead to a tertiary center referral is management of gastric varices. In the segments below, we discuss both of these challenging scenarios.

In the community, we spend a lot of time managing the complications of cirrhosis. Unfortunately, our therapies are themselves fraught with multiple potential complications. We present one such case. Ultimately, many of these patients with end-stage liver disease require a liver transplant. However, as we highlight in our section on transplantation, getting a liver may be frustratingly slow.

Portal vein thrombosis (PVT) is a known complication of cirrhosis. Decisions on anticoagulation for patients with PVT, who may have varices, bleeding portal hypertensive gastropathy, or GAVE, can be challenging. This is discussed in one of the cases.

Another complication of cirrhosis that we need to screen for is hepatocellular carcinoma (HCC). In our community hospital, once HCC is detected, the patient usually gets referred to the tertiary care center, where specific therapies and potential liver transplant are available. There are several cases discussing management of HCC.

While most patients with HCC have underlying cirrhosis, it is well-known that you can develop HCC without having cirrhosis if there is underlying chronic hepatitis B or hemochromatosis. Now there are reports of HCC occurring in NASH patients who don't have cirrhosis. With the huge numbers of patients with NAFLD in the USA, this is potentially a huge problem. This is also discussed.

We see quite a lot of PBC in the community, patients who are referred with an asymptomatic elevation of alkaline phosphatase. Management is often uncomplicated, but sometimes questions arise. We see far fewer patients with advanced PBC in the community, and this generally warrants referral to the transplant center. How do they approach these patients? An extensive discussion of management follows.

In the following chapters, we have several hepatologists who discuss cases of autoimmune hepatitis, overlap syndromes, and PSC. In PSC, of course, we need to be vigilant in screening for cholangiocarcinoma and colon cancer.

Chronic hepatitis B is not commonly seen by most community GIs. It can be a confusing disease to understand and treat. There are cases discussing management of immune-tolerant and immune-active chronic HBV. Another reviews the situation where a patient with chronic HBV stops taking his antiviral medication and disease relapses.

The question posed in a different case asks whether a patient once infected with HBV will continue to have lifelong stigmata of the infection.

The management of an exacerbation of chronic HBV differs from the treatment of acute HBV. Sometimes, it is unclear which we are dealing with. What are some clues to making this distinction and managing this?

While long-term management of HCV used to take up a lot of our time, the development of DAAs has made management so easy that often gastroenterologists in the community are not even consulted. However, there are occasional confusing cases that are sent our way. One such case is presented.

Liver failure and liver transplant are explored in several cases. A previously healthy patient who presents with acute liver failure always necessitates an urgent call to the transplant center. Here are some insights into their management once transferred. In the community, we get consulted on patients with a recent Tylenol overdose, and their management is often straightforward. But how should we manage patients with a delayed presentation?

Deciding who to refer for a transplant can be confusing. Four different cases highlight the controversies that occur. And then, once a patient goes on the transplant list, it can still be very frustrating for the community gastroenterologist to have to manage the recurring complications while waiting for the transplant to happen. It seems like the wait for a liver goes on forever.

Finally, the transplant hepatologists are the ones who commonly deal with complications that may occur post-liver transplant. However, community gastroenterologists may be the first to encounter these problems and need to know what to be on the lookout for. This is discussed in our last case.

Chapter 57
Liver Enzyme Elevation-negative Work-up

Francisco Durazo

A 47-year-old female is referred for abnormal liver enzymes. She has a normal BMI, does not drink or take street drugs, and is on no medications. Her AST is 78, ALT is 90, Alk phos is 100 (nl < 80), and bilirubin is 1.4, in which the direct is 1.0. The US of the liver is unremarkable. ANA + 1:16, ASMA negative, AMA negative, celiac panel, ceruloplasmin, and alpha-1 Antitrypsin are all normal, and Fe/ TIBC is 24%.

How do you approach the case of a patient with elevated LFTs where workup is negative?

My first approach with this patient would be to corroborate the history and do a detailed physical exam.

Is there any more information that you need to know?

It is helpful to know the time that the liver tests became abnormal and for how long they have been abnormal. When was the last time that the patient had normal liver tests? If we know this information, we can focus the interrogatory around that time and look for events that may be related. Is the patient symptomatic? Any changes in bowel habits that would suggest inflammatory bowel disease with primary sclerosing cholangitis or celiac sprue? Does the patient have itching that would suggest cholestasis? Any symptoms that would suggest heart failure such as paroxysmal nocturnal dyspnea or dyspnea on exertion? Any joint swelling and hyperpigmentation suggesting hemochromatosis? Does the patient have upper abdominal pain that would indicate biliary tract disease?

F. Durazo (✉)
Division of Gastroenterology and Hepatology, Department of Medicine,
Medical College of Wisconsin, Milwaukee, WI, USA
e-mail: fdurazo@mcw.edu

© The Author(s), under exclusive license to Springer Nature
Switzerland AG 2023
W. H. Sobin et al. (eds.), *Managing Complex Cases in Gastroenterology*,
https://doi.org/10.1007/978-3-031-48949-5_57

I would check for risk factors for viral hepatitis: recent travel to endemic areas, parenteral exposure, tattoos, blood transfusions before 1992, and eating under-cooked pork (hepatitis E).

Other important information that is frequently not disclosed accurately is the use of alcohol and illicit drugs. This patient apparently does not drink alcohol, but did she drink heavily in the past? She can have alcohol-related liver disease from previous drinking. The same with street drugs. Did she take street drugs in the past? Even if she did once, that's enough to acquire viral hepatitis. We saw this in the baby boomers that experimented with intravenous drugs in the 1970s and acquired hepatitis C. Many denied using intravenous drugs, but when asked more specifically, they confessed. Many street drugs can cause liver test abnormalities, hepatitis, and acute liver failure.

Frequently, patients do not offer the information we are looking for. Up to two thirds of patients taking supplements do not disclose this information to their physician. Others don't mention them when interviewed because they do not consider supplements to be part of their medications. Drug-induced liver injury is a frequent cause of liver test abnormalities. This patient was not taking medications at the time she was seen, but a thorough history of medications can be the culprit. Some medications can cause drug-induced liver injury with liver test abnormalities that persist even months after stopping them (intrahepatic cholestasis, i.e., amoxicillin/clavulanic acid, estrogens, anabolic steroids).

A detailed physical exam is most helpful. A good exam can narrow or even give you the diagnosis you are looking for. Does this patient have stigmata of chronic liver disease, such as palmar erythema or vascular spiders? Does she have a palpable liver? Is the liver firm and nodular? Is there a hepatic bruit suggesting alcoholic hepatitis or hepatocellular carcinoma? Is there a venous hum present (Cruveilhier-Baumgarten murmur, which is highly suggestive of portal hypertension)?

Are there other labs you would order?

I would like to rule out chronic viral hepatitis with hepatitis B surface antigen, hepatitis B core antibody, and hepatitis C antibody. I would also like to check her for type 2 and 3 autoimmune hepatitis with a liver-kidney microsomal antibody and a soluble liver antigen. Thyroid disease can affect the liver tests, especially hyperthyroidism. A thyroid panel with thyroid stimulating hormone is another test I would order.

A platelet count is helpful to assess for the presence of significant fibrosis. The AST to platelet ratio index (APRI score) or the Fib-4 score can be obtained with simple routine laboratory tests. They have good ability to differentiate patients with significant fibrosis (F2 to F4) from those without significant fibrosis (F0 to F1).

Would you do FibroScan®? If so, how would it help you?

A FibroScan® can be used as the first-line assessment for the severity of liver fibrosis in patients with chronic hepatitis. It performs best with regard to the ruling out of cirrhosis. It is primarily used as an alternative to liver biopsy for the assessment of hepatic fibrosis. It can also be used to predict complications in patients with cirrhosis. However, in this patient, I would be more interested in finding out the etiology of her liver test abnormalities. Depending on this information, I may or may not request a FibroScan® and may or may not proceed with a liver biopsy.

In considering a liver biopsy, what are you looking for? What might it show, and what are you hoping to rule out?

Doing a liver biopsy in a patient with a negative serologic workup is tempting. However, a liver biopsy doesn't always give you the answer. Pathologists base, to some extent, their histologic interpretation on the clinical history and the results of the serologic workup. If the work up is noncontributory, the histologic interpretation of the biopsy will be less specific. A liver biopsy may help to definitively establish the final diagnosis in some patients. However, the results rarely change your presumptive diagnosis or influence the patient management. On the other hand, if the liver test abnormalities persist, then I would proceed with a percutaneous liver biopsy. Occasionally, the liver biopsy may reveal an unsuspected diagnosis or dictate a change in the patient management. In most of the cases, the liver biopsy will reassure the patient and physician that there is no advanced liver disease.

Any other management decisions?

In the case of this patient, I would check the results of the viral hepatitis serologies and a thyroid panel. If these are noncontributory, like the rest of the workup, I would repeat the liver tests in 1 month and look at the trend. If the liver test abnormalities continue to get worse, I would proceed with a percutaneous liver biopsy (not a transjugular liver biopsy). If the liver test abnormalities would get better, I would continue to follow up the patient until these normalize.

Chapter 58
Increased LFTs with Increased Iron

Jose Franco

A 35-year-old male is being elevated for abnormal LFTs: AST, 60; ALT, 78; and ALK PHOS,100 (nl < 80). Hepatitis panel and autoimmune panel are negative, and Fe/TIBC is 20% but ferritin is 800.

Do you think this is hemochromatosis?

The protocol that I follow is that if the transferrin saturation (TS) is > or equal to 45% and/or the ferritin is elevated, you should order a hemochromatosis genotype. So, in this case, the ferritin is elevated, although the transferrin saturation isn't. You need to order the genotype, because one of them is elevated. I don't think hemochromatosis is very likely, with the TS being normal, but you do have to go that next step. Of course, many chronic liver diseases, besides hemochromatosis, may be associated with elevated ferritin.

What if the iron saturation was 55% and the ferritin was 250? What if the blood draw was non-fasting?

Once again, if *either* the transferrin saturation *or* the ferritin is elevated, you need to order *a* hemochromatosis genotype. In this instance, I also think it is unlikely to be hemochromatosis, with a normal ferritin, but I would still check the genotype. In terms of the iron level, this should be drawn fasting. Presumably, there can be some artifactual rise in the iron level, if the draw is postprandial, although I've never been able to find a good reason why (except where the patient is ingesting iron).

In what cases are you seeing elevated ferritin in patients with liver disease who don't have hemochromatosis?

Fatty liver, alcohol, chronic viral hepatitis, chronic cholestatic diseases, pretty much any chronic liver disease. Back in the 1990s, there was actually a movement to consider phlebotomy in patients with chronic HCV who had elevated ferritin

J. Franco (✉)
Department of Medicine-Division of Gastroenterology and Hepatology, Medical College of Wisconsin, Milwaukee, WI, USA
e-mail: jfranco@mcw.edu

© The Author(s), under exclusive license to Springer Nature Switzerland AG 2023
W. H. Sobin et al. (eds.), *Managing Complex Cases in Gastroenterology*,
https://doi.org/10.1007/978-3-031-48949-5_58

prior to initiating interferon therapy. The ferritin is elevated in these diseases because of ongoing inflammation, and it is an acute phase reactant.

What if the iron saturation is 55%, ferritin is 750, and the hemochromatosis genotype is C282Y homozygote in this patient with elevated liver enzymes. Would you bother with a liver biopsy? What if the ferritin was above 1000, would you want a biopsy then?

In my practice, any patient who is a C282Y homozygote with a ferritin >1000 and/or elevated liver enzymes should have a liver biopsy. If the liver enzymes were normal and the ferritin was <1000, a liver biopsy would not be required. The 1000 cutoff relates to the fact that patients with hemochromatosis and a ferritin <1000 are unlikely to have cirrhosis. The main reason for doing a liver biopsy would be to document the presence of cirrhosis.

It is important to look at the age in patients with suspected hemochromatosis. If this were a 20-year-old male, he would be unlikely to have cirrhosis. At 35, it is much more likely.

When you start your phlebotomies, what would be your goal level for TS or ferritin? What are the numbers you aim for?

I like to follow the ferritin and I aim to get it down below 100. Some people go as low as 50. It takes you a while to get that low, even with frequent phlebotomies, and then once you do, you go into a maintenance phase, where the patient gets phlebotomies quarterly. Sometimes, you are limited by the hemoglobin in some patients who are anemic for some other reason, and then you can't be as aggressive.

Is there any significance to patients with NASH who have an elevated ferritin?

Once again, chronic inflammatory conditions seem to be the common thread here. We tend to do a full chronic liver disease workup in our patients with suspected NASH, even when we're close to a hundred percent confident of our diagnosis, so we are routinely getting iron studies.

We do find that some patients with NASH have secondary iron overload, that's how I describe it to patients. Secondary iron overload doesn't require phlebotomy. However, is it possible to have NASH and hemochromatosis coexist? Absolutely. You hate to miss a potentially treatable component, and so we always check ferritin levels in these patients, and, once again, NASH doesn't really have a serologic test. Even though I may be dealing with somebody with a BMI of 40 who's diabetic and has fatty liver on imaging, I still do the autoimmune markers, the viral markers, and the iron studies.

Chapter 59
Increased LFTs with Low Ceruloplasmin

Jose Franco

A 27-year-old male is referred for elevated liver enzymes. His only complaint is mild chronic fatigue and difficulty concentrating at work. His AST is 100, ALT is 120, Alk phos is 40, and bilirubin is 1.2. His Hbg is 12.2. and iron saturation is 25%. Hepatitis panel is negative, while ANA, AMA, and ASMA are all negative. Serum ceruloplasmin is 17 (normal 20–40). The diagnosis of Wilson's is considered. He is sent to an ophthalmologist, who does a slit lamp exam and does not see K-F rings.

How would you evaluate this patient further?

In this young male with elevated liver enzymes and a decreased ceruloplasmin, Wilson's disease is a consideration. The absence of K-F rings does not rule out Wilson's. The next step would be to do a 24-h urine copper. I don't think there is any value in getting a serum copper or a spot urine copper; these tests are not useful.

Whatever the result of the 24-h urine copper, we should do a liver biopsy. In Wilson's, the 24-h urine copper should be high, > 40 µg. If it is high, this is likely Wilson's, and we do the biopsy for quantification of copper in liver tissue. More than 250 µg of copper/g dry weight is diagnostic for Wilson's. If, for some reason, the level is lower, between 50 and 250 µg/g dry weight, then molecular/genetic testing is indicated. If the 24-h urine copper is not elevated, I would do a liver biopsy for histology, and if significant copper is present, do quantitative copper levels. When you send quantitative copper studies, you need to send tissue in a dry tube to an institution capable of performing this test.

One interesting thing in this case is the low alkaline phosphatase. No one seems to know why this is low in Wilson's, but the only condition you ever really see a low alkaline phosphatase is in Wilson's disease.

J. Franco (✉)
Department of Medicine-Division of Gastroenterology and Hepatology, Medical College of Wisconsin, Milwaukee, WI, USA
e-mail: jfranco@mcw.edu

© The Author(s), under exclusive license to Springer Nature Switzerland AG 2023
W. H. Sobin et al. (eds.), *Managing Complex Cases in Gastroenterology*,
https://doi.org/10.1007/978-3-031-48949-5_59

If Wilson's is present, would you do further neuropsychiatric evaluation?

I'm not sure that doing further neuropsychiatric evaluation would help if the patient is already reporting difficulty concentrating at work. He's 27, and, obviously, this is a genetic disorder, so he has already had a couple of decades worth of disease, and I would attribute those symptoms to Wilson's disease. I don't know what further neuropsychiatric evaluation would tell me, and it's not going to alter my treatment, which is, of course, to treat the condition.

If Wilson's is diagnosed, how would you treat the patient?

Historically, penicillamine was the agent we used the most, but today, it is hardly ever used because there are less toxic options. Trientine is another agent that works like penicillamine, helping to increase the urinary excretion of copper. But my agent of choice is zinc, which has lower toxicity than both penicillamine and trientine. Zinc works to prevent absorption of copper from the GI tract. It is usually well tolerated. Occasionally, I'll use a combination of zinc and trientine because they work via different mechanisms.

How do you monitor their response to therapy?

I mostly follow their liver enzymes, but you can also monitor their 24-h urine copper. We tend to do that once a year. The urine copper should be low if the zinc is doing its job. Some also follow the non-ceruloplasmin-bound copper (or "free copper"), which can be calculated by subtracting ceruloplasmin-bound copper (3.15 × ceruloplasmin in mg/L equals the amount of ceruloplasmin-bound copper in μg/L) from the total serum copper concentration (in μg/L; serum copper in μmol/L × 63.5 equals serum copper in μg/L). In order to simplify this, you can use the following: total serum copper (in μg/L) − (3 × ceruloplasmin in mg/L) = non-ceruloplasmin-bound copper (to be more accurate, you can use 3.15). This can be cumbersome, and it is difficult when results return without specific numerical values (e.g., serum copper <3).

How many cases of Wilson's would you say you've seen over the years?

I would say 40–50, but right now, I'm following three quite actively.

Chapter 60
Normal Ceruloplasmin-Suspected Wilson's

Jose Franco

A 37-year-old male is referred for elevated LFTs; AST is 120, ALT is 150, Alk phos is 50, and Bili is 1.2.

The patient has had increased fatigue for the past 1 month. ANA, ASMA, AMA, celiac, alpha-1-AT, and Fe/TIBC are all normal. Ceruloplasmin is 20. Slit lamp exam is positive, and 24-h urine copper is elevated.

Can you comment on the finding of a normal ceruloplasmin in a case of likely Wilson's?

In this case, KF rings are present but ceruloplasmin is normal. It is important to remember that ceruloplasmin is an acute phase reactant. The elevated urinary copper level confirms the diagnosis of Wilson's. If the 24-h urine is normal or only mildly elevated, a liver biopsy is indicated.

J. Franco (✉)
Department of Medicine-Division of Gastroenterology and Hepatology, Medical College of Wisconsin, Milwaukee, WI, USA
e-mail: jfranco@mcw.edu

© The Author(s), under exclusive license to Springer Nature Switzerland AG 2023
W. H. Sobin et al. (eds.), *Managing Complex Cases in Gastroenterology*,
https://doi.org/10.1007/978-3-031-48949-5_60

Chapter 61
Increased LFTs-Alpha 1 Antitrypsin Deficiency

Jose Franco

A 49-year-old female is seen for a history of elevated liver enzymes. Her AST is 55 and ALT is 80; alk phos and bilirubin are normal. Also, she is mildly obese. She notes a family history of cirrhosis in her father and uncle, neither of whom were smokers or drinkers, but both also suffered from lung disease, presumed COPD. She has not had pulmonary problems. Because of the family history, alpha-1 antitrypsin levels and genotype were sent off. She was found to have mild AAT deficiency with ZZ genotype.

What manifestations of A1AT have you seen in your liver patients?

I have seen symptoms of liver involvement including liver failure, more in the pediatric patients. I have had one adult present with advanced liver disease requiring liver transplant.

Do you find it more as a primary disorder or a contributing disorder to some other underlying liver disease?

I would say it is more commonly a contributing factor in a patient with some other underlying liver disease.

Any treatments you have used?

While there is treatment for lung disease due to alpha-1 antitrypsin deficiency, there is none for liver disease. This is because of the different pathogenesis of the two. The lung disease of alpha-1 antitrypsin deficiency is due to proteolytic damage from PMNs, which is usually inhibited by alpha-1 antitrypsin. Synthetic alpha-1 antitrypsin is available to prevent this damage. The liver disease, on the other hand, is due to the retention of abnormal A1AT-Z molecules in the hepatocyte leading to cell damage. Synthetic alpha-1 antitrypsin is of no benefit here. Therefore, there is no treatment for liver disease except transplant when end-stage complications have developed.

J. Franco (✉)
Department of Medicine-Division of Gastroenterology and Hepatology, Medical College of Wisconsin, Milwaukee, WI, USA
e-mail: jfranco@mcw.edu

© The Author(s), under exclusive license to Springer Nature Switzerland AG 2023
W. H. Sobin et al. (eds.), *Managing Complex Cases in Gastroenterology*,
https://doi.org/10.1007/978-3-031-48949-5_61

295

Chapter 62
Suspected Gilbert's

Jose Franco

A 37-year-old male is seen because of an elevated bilirubin. He is asymptomatic. His total bilirubin ranges from 2.2 to 2.9 with a direct of 0.4–1.0 over the last 3 months. Physical exam is normal. An US of the liver with Doppler is normal. Hepatitis panel, autoimmune markers, iron saturation, ceruloplasmin, and alpha-1 antitrypsin are all normal. His reticulocyte count and LDH are normal.

Would you diagnose this as Gilbert's? How do you approach cases of suspected Gilbert's, where the direct bilirubin is higher than expected?

In this case, where you have an elevated unconjugated bilirubin, I think you're either dealing with Gilbert's or hemolysis, and you never want to miss hemolysis. I check the reticulocyte count and haptoglobin and have them look at the red blood cells on the smear to make sure there is no hemolysis.

Here, the elevated bilirubin is mostly unconjugated and ranges from 2.2 to 2.9. But, from personal experience, I will tell you that it can go into the mid-three range. I know this because I have Gilbert's, and I'll frequently be in that 3.5 range when they have me go for blood tests. They'll always call me back with a critical lab value, and I have to explain it to them. The unconjugated bilirubin is worsened with physiologic stress, and when you're fasting. My wife can look at me when I get home and tell whether I have skipped lunch, seeing whether I look jaundiced. But if you are under the weather, if you have any viral syndrome, many things will increase it. You're supposed to check the bilirubin in a fasting state.

Now in this case, there is a mild elevation of the conjugated bilirubin. In cases where it is predominantly conjugated bilirubin, rather than unconjugated, you may be looking at those rare disorders—Rotor and Dubin-Johnson. In these two disorders, the basic defect is in the transporter that gets the conjugated bilirubin out

J. Franco (✉)
Department of Medicine-Division of Gastroenterology and Hepatology, Medical College of Wisconsin, Milwaukee, WI, USA
e-mail: jfranco@mcw.edu

© The Author(s), under exclusive license to Springer Nature Switzerland AG 2023
W. H. Sobin et al. (eds.), *Managing Complex Cases in Gastroenterology*,
https://doi.org/10.1007/978-3-031-48949-5_62

of the hepatocyte, into the bile duct. These conditions are very rare, Gilbert's on the other hand is very common, 6–7% of the population. But in a case like this, where the vast majority is unconjugated, I think the mild elevation of the direct bilirubin is probably a red herring.

There are certainly cases where you can have other underlying liver disease in association with Gilbert's, but then you usually see a rise in the AST and ALT or alkaline phosphatase, in addition to the bilirubin. If it's just a rise in bilirubin and it's mostly indirect with a slight elevation of the direct, it's usually going to be Gilbert's.

Chapter 63
The Significance of AST > ALT

Francisco Durazo

A 42-year-old female is referred for abnormal liver enzymes with an AST of 52 and ALT of 38. She has a normal BMI but mildly increased waist circumference. She has two glasses of wine a night. An US shows some steatosis but is otherwise negative.

Does the AST > ALT send off any alarm bells?

Yes, we wonder if she is actually drinking more than two glasses of wine a day; is alcohol-induced liver injury responsible for these numbers? The normal pattern for transaminases is ALT > AST, which also holds true for most liver diseases, including viral hepatitis, autoimmune hepatitis, and even fatty liver disease. But we tend to see AST > ALT in patients with alcoholic liver disease, and we see it in patients who have gone on to develop cirrhosis. In cirrhosis, the production of ALT is decreased and so the AST > ALT. Therefore, in this patient, what is the explanation for the AST > ALT? Is it coming from alcohol or from occult cirrhosis, or might the elevated AST be coming from muscle damage or hemolysis?

We also note that the ultrasound shows steatosis. Anyone with fatty liver deserves a workup for chronic hepatitis, which includes serology for hepatitis B, hepatitis C, autoimmune hepatitis, Wilson's disease (in the right age cohort), alpha-1 antitrypsin deficiency, and celiac disease.

If the workup for chronic hepatitis returns negative, would you pursue a liver biopsy?

If all those labs return negative, we suspect the patient has alcoholic steatohepatitis. The only way to make this diagnosis is with liver biopsy. We would discuss liver biopsy with the patient, elaborating on how it could alter management and help with determining prognosis. In the meantime, we would suggest the patient stop

F. Durazo (✉)
Division of Gastroenterology and Hepatology, Department of Medicine,
Medical College of Wisconsin, Milwaukee, WI, USA
e-mail: fdurazo@mcw.edu

© The Author(s), under exclusive license to Springer Nature
Switzerland AG 2023
W. H. Sobin et al. (eds.), *Managing Complex Cases in Gastroenterology*,
https://doi.org/10.1007/978-3-031-48949-5_63

drinking and recheck liver enzymes after 3 months. If the labs normalize, we would probably cancel the biopsy. If they remain abnormal, we would proceed with biopsy. An important pearl is that the biopsy appearance of NASH is identical to that of alcoholic steatohepatitis, and the only way of distinguishing the two is by history. But, as noted, the fact that the AST is higher suggests alcohol is the culprit; usually in NASH, the ALT > AST, although the ratio has been noted to reverse in some cirrhotics with NASH.

Chapter 64
Marked Hyperbilirubinemia

Kia Saeian

A 75-year-old male presents to the ER with fever and elevated LFTs. An US shows a stone in the CBD, with a very high bilirubin. His alk phos was 480, his AST was 160, and his ALT was 200. His total bilirubin is >30, and direct bilirubin was >20. The patient had a normal bilirubin 1 month earlier. MRI of the liver shows multiple stones in the gallbladder, a common duct stone, and no suggestion of biliary stricture, hepatobiliary, or pancreatic neoplasm. PMH is positive for mild CHF and mild renal insufficiency.

His abdominal pain started about a week before coming to the ER. He is mildly hypotensive. His congestive heart failure is worsened. He is started on broad-spectrum antibiotics and has an urgent ERCP and stone extraction with clearing of the bile duct and pus. His blood cultures return positive, growing gram-negative rods. After the procedure, all his liver enzymes are improving except his bilirubin. He remains mildly hypotensive. Four days after the procedure, his bilirubin remains >30, although all the other liver enzymes are returning toward baseline.

How can you get such a high bilirubin in this setting?

A good rule of thumb that I use is that it is atypical to have a bilirubin over 20 and, particularly, a bilirubin of over 30 with pure bile duct obstruction. In these circumstances, I always consider other potential contributors that may lead to intrahepatic cholestasis and hemolysis. In this particular case, the history provides a number of clues to other potential contributors. The mild congestive heart failure can lead to cholestasis due to passive congestion. Renal insufficiency can result in more prolonged hyperbilirubinemia and slower clearance of the bilirubin. And, most importantly, the positive blood cultures with gram-negative rods can result in

K. Saeian (✉)
GI/Hepatology Division, Department of Medicine, Medical College of Wisconsin, Milwaukee, WI, USA
e-mail: ksaeian@mcw.edu

© The Author(s), under exclusive license to Springer Nature Switzerland AG 2023
W. H. Sobin et al. (eds.), *Managing Complex Cases in Gastroenterology*,
https://doi.org/10.1007/978-3-031-48949-5_64

cholestasis of sepsis, which can develop from impairment of bile transport in the setting of sepsis. In this setting, continued hypoperfusion, either due to his low blood pressure or passive congestion from his heart failure, can further prolong this episode.

What are the different issues to keep in mind when you are confronted with hyperbilirubinemia (in the 20 s or 30 s range) in patients who are septic, have cardiac surgery, or have multisystem disease, often in an ICU setting?

By far, the most common scenario is due to infection or cholestasis of sepsis, which, again, is believed to be, at least in part, due to a defect in bile transport due to sepsis. The most severe form of this is cholangitis lenta, which has more commonly been reported in liver transplant patients and is commonly associated with a poor overall prognosis. Cholangitis lenta itself is a histologic diagnosis in which there is proliferation of dilated bile ductules and inspissated bile along with neutrophils and, on occasion, portal inflammation with a lymphoplasmacytic infiltrate. As many physicians know, it is common to see episodes of cholestasis of sepsis, but physicians rarely encounter cholangitis lenta because we rarely proceed with liver biopsy in such settings. This is often because these patients are so critically ill and the biopsy is not felt to alter management. This may also be why it is thought to be more common in liver transplant patients, since those patients are much more likely to undergo a liver biopsy when critically ill.

We already touched on a couple of scenarios outlined in the first question of this section that can result in hyperbilirubinemia, often with aminotransferase and alkaline phosphatase elevations. Entities that can result in more of an isolated hyperbilirubinemia with mild alteration of other liver enzymes, albeit not always in the 20–30 range, include heart failure/passive congestion, medications (ceftriaxone for instance is a common contributor), hemolysis (in the setting of indirect hyperbilirubinemia), and the effects of anesthesia. The latter is particularly an issue in patients with underlying cirrhosis. It is not uncommon for us to see patients without known prior liver disease who were subsequently diagnosed as having cirrhosis, because they developed hyperbilirubinemia in response to undergoing anesthesia, particularly for an abdominal or cardiac operation.

Chapter 65
Suspected NAFLD

James Esteban

A 35-year-old Latin female is being evaluated for elevated liver enzymes. She has an ALT of 160, AST of 120, Alk phos of 140 (nL up to 80), bilirubin of 1.2, platelet count of 180,000, and albumin of 3.8. She has no alcohol and no family history of liver disease. She is on no medications. Her BMI is 32, and her HbA1C is 6.2. Hepatitis panel is negative, autoimmune markers are negative, and ceruloplasmin and alpha-1 antitrypsin phenotype are normal.

How would you approach this patient?

She may have nonalcoholic fatty liver disease, or NAFLD, based on her risk factors of increased BMI and prediabetes. We need to get an abdominal or right upper quadrant ultrasound for confirmation that she has hepatic steatosis. It is important to test and exclude other causes of chronic liver diseases, such as chronic viral hepatitis; autoimmune liver diseases, like autoimmune hepatitis and primary biliary cholangitis; and inherited metabolic types of liver diseases, such as hemochromatosis, Wilson's disease, and alpha-1 antitrypsin deficiency. We should check that the patient is not receiving known steatogenic medications, such as methotrexate, amiodarone, or certain systemic chemotherapeutic agents.

Recognizing the primacy of metabolic risk factors on the pathogenesis of the disease and the exclusionary and potentially stigmatizing verbiage of the current nomenclature, an international expert panel recently published a consensus statement renaming NAFLD to metabolic dysfunction-associated steatotic liver disease, or MASLD [1].

Ultrasound shows steatosis without obvious signs of cirrhosis or portal hypertension.

J. Esteban (✉)
Division of Gastroenterology and Hepatology, Department of Medicine, Medical College of Wisconsin, Milwaukee, WI, USA
e-mail: jesteban@mcw.edu

© The Author(s), under exclusive license to Springer Nature Switzerland AG 2023
W. H. Sobin et al. (eds.), *Managing Complex Cases in Gastroenterology*, https://doi.org/10.1007/978-3-031-48949-5_65

What are your next steps?

First, I will stratify the patient's risk for significant fibrosis. Inflammation (or nonalcoholic steatohepatitis, NASH) and fibrosis are the most important predictors of hepatic decompensation, hepatocellular carcinoma, and mortality [2]. This can be done noninvasively through the use of serum biomarkers or through elastography or invasively with liver biopsy.

Biomarkers from standard lab tests can be used to calculate risk scores, such as NAFLD fibrosis score (NFS) or the Fibrosis-4 (FIB-4) index. Both are accessible from various publicly available websites. There are also proprietary serum biomarkers such as FibroMeter® (Echosens) and the Enhanced Liver Fibrosis or ELF™ score (Siemens). Proprietary biomarkers are slightly more accurate that nonproprietary biomarkers in diagnosing significant and advanced liver fibrosis.

On the other hand, elastography measures the stiffness of the liver and uses this as a surrogate for the stage of liver fibrosis. In the clinic, vibration-controlled transient elastography or FibroScan® (Echosens) is available and provides real-time results at the bedside. Radiologists are also able to measure liver stiffness through ultrasound elastography or magnetic resonance (MR) elastography.

Negative predictive values of these noninvasive markers are generally very good and, thus, "low" or "low risk" values, in general, excludes advanced liver disease. However, the positive predictive values of these tests for diagnosing significant stages of fibrosis (i.e., stage 2 and above), and cirrhosis, are not as good (although still reasonable). Patients with "indeterminate," "high," or "high risk" values on noninvasive testing may be offered a liver biopsy to clarify fibrosis staging and determine the presence of steatohepatitis. If the biopsy shows NASH and fibrosis, then the patient may benefit from off-label use of pharmacotherapies, such as pioglitazone and glucagon-like peptide-1 (GLP-1) receptor analogs, or from enrollment in a clinical trial.

Next, all patients with NAFLD/MASLD should be counseled on lifestyle interventions. We should counsel the patient to lose at least 5–7%, and ideally >10%, of their body weight. Weight loss of at least 5%, 7%, and 10% is associated with, respectively, reduction in hepatic steatosis, resolution of NASH, and stabilization and potential regression of liver fibrosis [3]. Other lifestyle interventions that can be recommended include:

- Reduce daily calories by 500–1000 kcal/day.
- Minimize saturated fats and refined carbohydrates.
- Avoid sugar-sweetened beverages.
- Mediterranean diet should be considered, although low-carb/low-fat diet and intermittent fasting both appear to have comparable efficacy.
- Regular physical activity equivalent to 150–300 min weekly of moderate intensity aerobic exercise.
- Some resistance and weight training should complement aerobic exercise.

While weight loss is very important, many of these other interventions can improve hepatic steatosis and steatohepatitis, even without significant weight loss, especially among patients with lean NAFLD/MASLD.

Patients always ask if they should avoid alcohol. Early data suggested that light alcohol may be protective in NAFLD or MASLD. However, more recent data from prospective studies indicate that "moderate" alcohol use reduces the likelihood of clearing NASH while increasing the risk of fibrosis [4].

You have a FibroScan® in your clinic, are you getting a FibroScan® on all patients like this? How accurate is the FibroScan® in NAFLD?

I routinely obtain a FibroScan® on all of my NAFLD/MASLD patients. FibroScan has >90% negative predictive value for ruling out advanced fibrosis in NAFLD/MASLD [5]. Thus, if liver stiffness on FibroScan® is low, or less than 7–8 kPa, I feel comfortable and confident in excluding advanced fibrosis. I reassure the patient, and we continue working on lifestyle interventions.

The positive predictive value for FibroScan® in diagnosing significant fibrosis and cirrhosis in NAFLD/MASLD patients is modest, ranging from 40 to 70% [6], especially if the patients are overweight and obese. The positive predictive value is better in those with lean NAFLD/MASLD. For these patients, I offer liver biopsy for staging purposes.

How do liver biopsies get done at your institution?

Liver biopsies can be done percutaneously, by a hepatologist or by a diagnostic radiologist, or transvenously, by an interventional radiologist. In percutaneous biopsies, the proceduralist may elect to do the procedure under direct ultrasound guidance (usually the radiologists) or "blindly" after identifying and marking suitable intercostal areas via bedside ultrasound (usually the hepatologists).

In transvenous or transjugular liver biopsy, the interventional radiologist passes a wire and needle through the internal jugular vein, down the vena cava, and into a hepatic vein (usually the right), from where they collect cores of liver tissue. The interventional radiologist can also measure free and wedged hepatic venous pressures during the same procedure, which provides valuable information in diagnosing portal hypertension.

References

1. Rinella ME, Lazarus JV, Ratziu V, Francque SM, Sanyal AJ, Kanwal F, et al. A multisociety Delphi consensus statement on new fatty liver disease nomenclature. Hepatology. 2023;29(1):101133.
2. Sanyal AJ, Van Natta ML, Clark J, Neuschwander-Tetri BA, Diehl A, Dasarathy S, et al. Prospective study of outcomes in adults with nonalcoholic fatty liver disease. N Engl J Med. 2021;385(17):1559–69.
3. Vilar-Gomez E, Martinez-Perez Y, Calzadilla-Bertot L, Torres-Gonzalez A, Gra-Oramas B, Gonzalez-Fabian L, et al. Weight loss through lifestyle modification significantly reduces features of nonalcoholic steatohepatitis. Gastroenterology. 2015;149(2):367–78.

4. Ajmera V, Belt P, Wilson LA, Gill RM, Loomba R, Kleiner DE, et al. Among patients with nonalcoholic fatty liver disease, modest alcohol use is associated with less improvement in histologic steatosis and steatohepatitis. Clin Gastroenterol Hepatol. 2018;16(9):1511–20.
5. Mózes FE, Lee JA, Selvaraj EA, Jayaswal ANA, Trauner M, Boursier J, et al. Diagnostic accuracy of non-invasive tests for advanced fibrosis in patients with NAFLD: an individual patient data meta-analysis. Gut. 2022;71(5):1006–19.
6. Xiao G, Zhu S, Xiao X, Yan L, Yang J, Wu G. Comparison of laboratory tests, ultrasound, or magnetic resonance elastography to detect fibrosis in patients with nonalcoholic fatty liver disease: a meta-analysis. Hepatology. 2017;66(5):1486–501.

Chapter 66
Treatment of NAFLD

Francisco Durazo

An obese nondiabetic male, age 39 with a BMI of 34, is referred with an ultrasound showing steatosis. He has one or two drinks each weekend. His platelet count is 170 K. His ALT is 75, AST is 48, and alk phos is 150. His hepatitis panel, ANA, ASMA, alpha-1-antitrypsin, ceruloplasmin, and celiac panel are all normal.

How would you manage this patient?

We explain that this is not purely a liver disease but rather a systemic inflammatory condition. Many people with fatty liver and normal glucose have insulin resistance. Therefore, just having a fatty liver should be a red flag for insulin resistance, present in as many as 95% of people with fatty liver.

Treatment is not aimed specifically at the liver but rather at the entire body. The first thing we recommend is exercise. Studies have shown that consistent exercise over a 2-year period significantly improves steatosis and fibrosis on liver biopsy. We recommend a Mediterranean diet, avoiding fructose and avoiding alcohol. We recommend drinking 2–3 cups of regular coffee daily.

We recommend weight loss. Evidence shows that weight loss of 10% of total weight leads to dramatic improvement in liver histology. In a patient who weighs 240, a 10% loss in weight requires only losing 1 pound a week over 6 months.

For patients who are diabetic, pioglitazone is beneficial. It is certainly a far better choice than insulin for patients with NAFLD. We offer vitamin E to patients with biopsy proven NASH. We prefer to use it in women because vitamin E may increase the rate of prostate cancer.

F. Durazo (✉)
Division of Gastroenterology and Hepatology, Department of Medicine,
Medical College of Wisconsin, Milwaukee, WI, USA
e-mail: fdurazo@mcw.edu

© The Author(s), under exclusive license to Springer Nature
Switzerland AG 2023
W. H. Sobin et al. (eds.), *Managing Complex Cases in Gastroenterology*,
https://doi.org/10.1007/978-3-031-48949-5_66

We recommend bariatric surgery for those patients with NAFLD and a BMI >40, who can't lose weight by other means, or in patients with a BMI >35, who have other comorbidities, like obstructive sleep apnea, diabetes that is hard to control, or severe hyperlipidemia.

Can you predict which patients with NAFLD will have a more ominous clinical course?

Yes, we think the NAFLD fibrosis score is a good noninvasive predictor.

Chapter 67
Treatment of MASLD

Achutan Sourianarayanane

A 43-year-old female with a BMI of 31 is seen by her primary care doctor and found to have an AST of 60 and an ALT of 90. She is prediabetic and has one or two drinks on weekends. Alkaline phosphatase and bilirubin are normal. Other labs are sent off, including hepatitis panel, autoimmune panel, ceruloplasmin, A1AT, and Fe/TIBC, which return normal. Ultrasound shows steatosis. The doctor tells her to abstain completely from alcohol and try to lose 20 lbs. over the next 3 months. If her liver enzymes don't improve, he says, he will refer her to a hepatologist, and she might end up needing a liver biopsy.

1. Is this initial strategy of weight loss and abstention and then waiting and seeing reasonable?

Her imaging suggests the presence of hepatic steatosis. Based on the pattern of liver chemistry, along with the presence of metabolic risks and the absence of excess alcohol intake, her fatty liver is secondary to metabolic dysfunction-associated steatotic liver disease (MASLD). MASLD is the current terminology for nonalcoholic fatty liver disease (NAFLD), which is an encompassing diagnosis of those with fatty liver with metabolic risks. Similarly, metabolic dysfunction-associated steatohepatitis (MASH) is the replacement term for prior nonalcoholic steatohepatitis (NASH). Lifestyle changes are the most important components for the management of this condition and should be incorporated in every patient with MASLD. Although she does not consume excess alcohol, reduction or abstinence from alcohol will facilitate improvement in her liver disorder. Hence, the recommendation for abstinence is appropriate within the current guidelines. Studies recommend lifestyle changes that result in sustained weight loss of 5–7%, which has been found to be beneficial to patients with MASLD. It also helps many patients with prediabetes improve their

A. Sourianarayanane (✉)
Division of Gastroenterology and Hepatology, Department of Medicine, Medical College of Wisconsin, Milwaukee, WI, USA
e-mail: asourianar@mcw.edu

© The Author(s), under exclusive license to Springer Nature Switzerland AG 2023
W. H. Sobin et al. (eds.), *Managing Complex Cases in Gastroenterology*,
https://doi.org/10.1007/978-3-031-48949-5_67

overall health and the metabolic risk associated with MASLD. Although a target weight loss of 5–7% is considered appropriate, it may be difficult for most patients to achieve consistently. Improvement in metabolic risks has been noticed, with consistent lifestyle changes, including diet and exercise, even in the absence of weight loss. This may need to be considered in subsequent clinical visits and recommendations [1–3].

2. If the numbers were reversed and the AST was 90 and ALT 60, would that raise any alarm bells?

A liver chemistry pattern with an AST higher than ALT can suggest more than one clinical possibility in this patient. The occurrence of AST higher than ALT in patients with MASLD could raise concerns about advanced fibrosis or even the presence of cirrhosis. However, her AST was 1.5 higher than her ALT. This could also raise concerns about other causes, such as a relatively higher level of alcohol consumption than could be safely metabolized by her liver. Her alcohol usage is well within liver societies' and the American Dietary Association's recommendations. It is possible a person's perception of the standard unit of alcohol measure differs from those recommendations; besides, the effect of a given amount of alcohol may vary in an individual [2, 4].

She is only able to lose 5 lbs., and her repeat LFTs 3 months later are essentially unchanged. She is referred to you, the hepatologist.

3. Is there any role for FibroScan®? Would you order one? What would be the considerations in deciding on this or using any other noninvasive measure for the presence of fibrosis or potentially classifying her as having steatohepatitis versus simple fatty liver?

Liver chemistries, commonly called liver function tests, do not reflect the severity of liver disease. She could have hepatic steatosis with an ongoing inflammatory process and fibrosis. The MASLD fibrosis score and FIB-4 are commonly used noninvasive biomarkers based on clinical and biochemical parameters. These biomarkers stratify patients into a low, intermediate, or advanced stage of MASLD. These tests are easily available and less costly to administer. Although these biomarkers are sensitive enough to detect an advanced stage of the disease, they are less specific in diagnosing them. Hence, a second test, such as FibroScan®, should be used to confirm the diagnosis, when available [5, 6].

The duration of the disease was not known in this patient. She also has a metabolic risk and elevated aminotransferases. As MASLD is a "silent disease" with minimal or no symptoms until the onset of decompensated cirrhosis, assessing the severity of the disease is appropriate. An evaluation by FibroScan® is appropriate.

4. How accurate is FibroScan® when evaluating fatty liver? Do you rely on the CAP score?

FibroScan® can diagnose the presence of fat in the liver if it is more than 11%. Following a FibroScan® (also called vibration-controlled transient elastography®), two sets of results are obtained. One is a controlled attenuation parameter (CAP), which correlates with the presence of hepatic steatosis or a fatty liver. It requires the presence of hepatic steatosis of >11% to be detected and quantified by this method.

Studies have shown that the CAP value correlates with the histological grade of steatosis. The cutoff ranges used to differentiate various histological grades of steatosis may vary due to patient characteristics, such as BMI. The other value obtained from FibroScan® is transient elastography measured in kilopascals, which indicates the fibrosis stage of liver disease in MASLD. The elastography results may be less reliable in patients with a BMI of >35 [7, 8].

The SAF score (steatosis, activity, and fibrosis) is a histological scoring system for patients with MASH. It is used mostly in Europe and in MASLD research. A similar histological scoring system called NAFLD activity score (NAS) proposed by the NASH Clinical Research Network (CRN), which is often referred to as the NASH-CRN, is used commonly in the United States.

5. Would you do a liver biopsy? Which patients do you think should have a liver biopsy?

A liver biopsy to diagnose or stratify a patient with MASLD is becoming less common. The use of liver biopsy is usually considered for patients in whom there is a concern for an advanced stage of fibrosis. Noninvasive tests are recommended to stratify MASLD patients initially as a screening test. These tests, such as the MASLD fibrosis score, FIB-4, etc., are based on clinical and biochemical parameters. These tests have a high sensitivity for detecting patients with an advanced stage of MASLD. Individuals who are found to have a low probability of advanced MASLD do not require further testing. A second test with higher specificity, such as elastography (FibroScan®), is performed on patients with an intermediate or advanced stage on initial screening tests. Patients who cannot be categorized and are considered to have intermediate risk will benefit from liver biopsy staging. A liver biopsy is also required if the patient is considered for a clinical trial [5].

If this patient has a BMI of less than 35, the FibroScan® test results could be considered reliable. If FibroScan® elastography does not suggest advanced fibrosis (<10 kPa), a liver biopsy is not recommended. A liver biopsy could be considered otherwise [8].

6. Other than avoiding alcohol and weight loss, are there any other secondary, behavioral, or dietary measures that can be helpful? Would you have done any other serologic or other testing at this point? Do you routinely check all your patients for alcohol use even if they claim to drink minimally, such as in this patient?

Significant sustained weight loss has been shown to improve many histological parameters seen in MASLD. A 5–7% weight loss has been associated with a reduction in steatosis. With additional weight loss, other histological features, such as inflammation and fibrosis reduction, have been documented. A weight loss of >15% has been shown to improve fibrosis stages on histology. Avoidance of alcohol is an important factor among those who have histological improvements with weight loss. Significant and sustained weight loss is not easily achievable by most patients. Other lifestyle changes, such as regular exercise outside work, improve the overall health of the liver. Some of the biochemical parameters and insulin sensitivity have improved with this measure, even in the absence of weight loss [2, 3].

Different diets have been suggested for the management of patients with MASLD. These include diet modification based on the reduction of macronutrients, such as fat, and carbohydrates, including fructose, either individually or in combination and along with a variation in the time of meal consumption. These modifications have resulted in weight loss and an improvement in their body weight, metabolic risks, and liver aminotransferases. Many of these modifications are difficult to maintain, and a long-term benefit is less often achieved. A portion- and calorie-controlled Mediterranean diet (without alcohol use) is beneficial in MASLD and is also easier to adhere to in the long term. Studies have also found that caffeine intake is associated with a reduced progression of MASH.

Some providers routinely recommend tests such as phosphatidylethanol (PEth) to measure alcohol in patients with a presumed diagnosis of MASLD to corroborate the role of alcohol in their disease. This is considered, because an individual's perception of the standard unit of alcohol measure may differ from the guidelines of liver societies and the American Dietary Association. Additionally, many people underestimate their alcohol use. Patients with MAFLD can include those with alcohol usage or viral infection. This is a move away from the use of MASLD, which is a diagnosis of exclusion in those with an absence of other causes.

Scenario 1 Liver biopsy shows steatosis without any changes of steatohepatitis or any fibrosis.

7. Is steatosis without steatohepatitis a benign entity? Is the prognosis that much better? Do you have thoughts on what proportion of these patients progress to more severe liver injury? Does this depend on the risk factors?

Our initial understanding of the minimal or nonprogressive form of MASLD patients with simple steatosis was mainly from retrospective studies. These studies found that patients with hepatic steatosis without MASH had a benign course and did not progress to MASH. Newer studies suggest that a portion of patients with steatosis alone without MASH on initial biopsy had findings of MASH on subsequent histological evaluation. The proportion of patients with initial simple steatosis who progress to advanced disease is unknown. Some studies suggest that nearly 25% of these patients may progress to MASH or may even have fibrosis later. Insulin resistance plays a significant role in progressive disease. Among all the factors, the presence of fibrosis is significant and associated with poor outcomes in patients with MASLD [9].

8. In this scenario, are there any medications that you would consider or would initiate at this point?

Currently, there are no FDA-approved medications for patients with simple steatosis. The only approved medication is vitamin E, which is considered for patients with biopsy-proven MASH without type II diabetes. This patient has diabetes and does not have MASH; hence, lifestyle changes without additional pharmacological agents is appropriate for her [10, 11].

Scenario 2 Same patient but now the liver biopsy shows changes of steatohepatitis, including ballooning without any fibrosis.

9. What does it take to turn steatosis into steatohepatitis? Are there any causative factors you can identify, modify, or even prevent?

Multiple pathophysiological processes are now considered to contribute to the progression of MASLD. Type II diabetes, or insulin resistance, is an important factor associated with the progression of the disease. An inflammatory process secondary to lipid accumulation and a dysfunctional oxidative process, called lipotoxicity, occur. Different chemicals are released because of these inflammatory processes. This creates a subsequent event that results in neutrophil and lymphocyte accumulation, altered cell death, fibrosis deposition by macrophages, and the progression of the disease to steatohepatitis. Lifestyle changes that result in a consistent reduction of metabolic risks, such as excess body weight, insulin resistance, and other modifiable factors, reduce the progression to steatohepatitis [2, 3, 10].

10. Once you've developed steatohepatitis, is this fully reversible? What is the chance of sampling error on the biopsy?

Fortunately, this patient does not have fibrosis. It may be easier to reverse the inflammatory process and steatosis in the absence of fibrosis. Both steatosis and steatohepatitis reversal are possible with significant weight loss (possibly 7–10%), along with metabolic risk reduction. However, complete improvement may not occur in all patients. A liver biopsy is a reliable way to diagnose MASLD and stage accurately, although it samples only 1/50,000 or 1/100,000th of the entire liver organ. It has been suggested that there could be errors due to this. Studies have shown variations between two samples taken on the same day and from different lobes of the liver. Despite these variations, liver biopsy is the current gold standard for the diagnosis of this condition.

11. Do you think you can "save" many of these patients from developing advanced fibrosis?

Active research and clinical trials are being conducted to mitigate MASLD and its progression. As more than one pathophysiological process is involved, a combination of medications is administered to reduce fibrosis formation and progression. Lifestyle changes remain a consistent and valuable component of this disease's management. If possible, a combined holistic approach would be the key to improvement for most of these patients.

12. What medications, if any, would you initiate in this particular case based on the biopsy? Any other secondary measures?

Studies have shown that a sustained weight loss of 7–10% could reverse the inflammatory process. With this weight loss, there is an associated improvement in metabolic risks, such as insulin resistance, hypertension, and lipid profile, which contribute to an overall improvement in MASLD patients. This could be achieved through consistent lifestyle changes, such as dietary and exercise modifications. There are also a few pharmacological agents being considered.

Vitamin E is used in patients without diabetes and has shown improvement in steatohepatitis. Incretins, such as GLP-1 agonists (liraglutide and semaglutide), are beneficial for MASLD patients with and without diabetes. Studies have shown improvement in liver aminotransferase levels, improvement of steatohepatitis, and weight loss, and lowering of HbA1c among diabetes patients is seen with GLP-1 agonists. Obeticholic acid is another agent that modifies bile acid synthesis; it reduces inflammation in the liver and fibrosis in MASH patients because of this. These agents are in the final stages of clinical trials for MASH. Many newer pharmacological agents are undergoing clinical trials, either alone or in combination; they modify different metabolic processes involved in MASLD. These agents include those modifying lipid synthesis, the oxidative process, cell death, and fibrosis formation. Bariatric surgery is another important and valid consideration in appropriate patients with MASH [10–12].

Scenario 3 Liver biopsy shows steatohepatitis and stage 3 fibrosis.

13. How often would you expect to detect patients with fatty liver who are already in stages of advanced fibrosis/cirrhosis?

Most patients with MASLD do not have symptoms; hence, many are diagnosed incidentally on abdominal imaging for other reasons. A portion of this diagnosis can occur in their late stages of the disease. It is estimated that <5% of patients with MASLD may progress to cirrhosis; therefore, we can expect that <5% of MASLD patients may have advanced fibrosis at the time of detection.

14. How reversible is this stage of liver disease? With what measures?

Fibrosis is less likely to reverse with lifestyle changes and with currently approved pharmacological agents. A weight loss of >15% may be required for improvement in fibrosis. Bariatric surgery is one option, especially for patients with advanced fibrosis. A reduction in the fibrosis stage has been observed many years after successful bariatric surgery. Newer pharmacological agents that modify collagen synthesis and deposition are being considered. If these agents are successful, they may also alter the course of this disease [10–12].

15. Assuming that you implement screening for esophageal varices and considering HCC surveillance, are there other measures you would implement now?

Esophageal varices screening and HCC surveillance are usually considered for patients with cirrhosis. Liver societies do not recommend routine screening for varices or HCC in patients without cirrhosis. As this patient has advanced fibrosis, she will benefit from periodic evaluation for fibrosis progression and the onset of cirrhosis with FibroScan® or transient elastography. Elastography, as measured in kilopascals, correlates with portal pressure and decompensated liver disease. If there is an increase in kilopascals and a significant reduction in platelets (<180), the above screenings should be considered. When performing ultrasound-based elastography, the results may be less reliable if the patient has a high BMI. Due to a similar reason, ultrasound is less reliable in detecting liver lesions in subjects with high BMI. Some consider an MRI (which is costly) or a CT scan (which could be a concern in patients with renal dysfunction), alternating with ultrasound imaging for HCC screening [2, 8].

16. Any medications you would start in this case?

In this patient, with the suggestions of steatohepatitis and the absence of overt diabetes, adding 800 units of vitamin E to her medication regimen is appropriate. Semaglutide, a GLP-1 agonist, or a similar agent can also be considered after appropriately educating the patient about the side effects and how to use it. This can improve her body weight, insulin sensitivity, and liver aminotransferases. If she has hyperlipidemia, a statin to reduce it would also be appropriate [10, 11].

17. Do you believe that patients with MASH truly progress to HCC without developing cirrhosis first? Why is this, and do you screen any/all of your patients with MASH for HCC?

About 10% of patients who have HCC with a diagnosis of MASLD do not have cirrhosis. Many of the risk factors related to MASLD, such as a high BMI and diabetes, are also associated with malignancy, including HCC. However, no definitive pathway has been found in MASH patients. Many of our screening protocols are based on the costs involved in diagnosing a treatable condition and the quality of life rendered to society as a result of it. This is based on the prevalence of the disease and the incidence of HCC in a specific population. The current consensus guidelines do not recommend screening for patients with MASH without cirrhosis for HCC, unlike in patients with hemochromatosis or hepatitis B infection, where it is recommended even in the absence of cirrhosis [2].

18. When would you refer this patient for a liver transplant? What would be the chance of recurrence of MASH post-transplant?

MASH patients should be evaluated for liver transplantation in the appropriate clinical setting, like any other patient. This would be in patients who have decompensated liver disease or those with a relatively high model for end-stage liver disease (MELD). The referrals and transplantations for patients with MASLD are usually no different from those for other chronic liver disorders. Many MASLD patients also have other comorbidities that could be a concern during the perioperative and postoperative phases. These should be evaluated to reduce morbidity or mortality posttransplant through a multidisciplinary approach.

Following liver transplantation, the recurrence of hepatic steatosis among patients with a pretransplant diagnosis of MASH is high. Hepatic steatosis occurs in patients who have undergone liver transplantation for more than one reason [13]. Immunosuppressive agents required for the maintenance of the transplanted liver are associated with many metabolic factors and increase the risks for hepatic steatosis posttransplantation. However, not all post-liver transplant patients with hepatic steatosis develop MASH.

General Questions

1. Which patients with MASLD/MASH should consider having bariatric surgery?

Any patient who could otherwise benefit from a bariatric procedure for their health will also benefit if they have MASLD. Patients with MASH with advanced fibrosis would benefit from significant weight loss following a bariatric procedure. A weight loss of >15% occurs frequently following a bariatric procedure. A reduction or clearance of steatosis and inflammation, including ballooning cells, is found following a successful bariatric procedure. Stabilization or even a reduction of fibrosis is seen after many years (>5 years). Patients with decompensated cirrhosis, however, do not do well following bariatric surgery and are not generally recommended to undergo this procedure [12].

2. How do patients with MASLD and fibrosis/cirrhosis compare to patients with ALD in the same stage of disease? Assuming the alcoholic has stopped drinking, which has the worse prognosis? Who will have a better outcome after a liver transplant?

A direct comparison of outcomes between patients with ALD and MASLD is not easy. Patients with MASLD may continue to have metabolic risks and may have gradual MASLD progression over time. However, many patients with ALD may improve or may not progress if their consumption of alcohol is discontinued entirely. The patient outcomes in these two groups could also be affected by their age and comorbidity, in addition to their liver disease-related outcomes. Many patients with MASLD are older and have comorbidities due to the presence of metabolic risk (i.e., high BMI, diabetes, and hyperlipidemia), such as cardiovascular, cerebrovascular, and renal disorders. These could contribute to reduced overall outcomes following liver transplantation.

3. Is liver transplant restricted for any of the MASLD patients?

It is possible that MASLD patients have significant cardiovascular or other comorbidities. As in any other patient, these risk factors have a bearing on perioperative and postoperative complications and may restrict those undergoing liver transplantation. The body habitus of the patient may also cause some restrictions on undergoing liver transplantations. Retrospective and large database studies suggest that patients with a BMI >50 do not do as well as those with a BMI <50 following liver transplantation. With the increasing technology and training of surgeons, many patients with a higher BMI are undergoing liver transplantation with a good outcome [14].

4. In which MASLD patients do you like to use vitamin E, pioglitazone, and GLP-1 agonists?

Currently, the FDA recommends pharmacological intervention for patients with a histological diagnosis of MASH. Vitamin E has been found to be beneficial in MASH patients with improvement of inflammation and balloon cells on histology among patients without diabetes. In patients with diabetes, vitamin E has not proven to be beneficial. Some researchers recommend a combination of pioglitazone and vitamin E for patients with diabetes and MASH. Others feel that the benefit observed with this combination therapy is from pioglitazone alone and that the use of vitamin E may not be required. Pioglitazone causes a reduction in hepatic steatosis. They also have an increase in subcutaneous fat and overall weight gain. Hence, it is not considered a preferred treatment for most patients. GLP-1 agonists can be used in all patients with MASH, especially those with type II diabetes. They have also been considered for the management of obesity. These patients should be educated about potential hypoglycemic episodes when a GLP-1 agonist is used [10, 11].

5. Are any other drugs you like to use today in MASLD patients?

Statins have been found to benefit patients across the spectrum of MASLD. They have been associated with a reduction in the progression of the disease. Statins also benefit patients with hyperlipidemia, which is an important metabolic risk factor in MASLD.

6. Are there any other drugs that are promising that you anticipate being available in the next 5 years?

There are many drugs undergoing clinical trials in various phases that could be used for the treatment of MASH. Obeticholic acid, an FXR agonist, has been promising. It reduces the inflammatory process in addition to fibrosis reduction in MASH patients. A variation of this agent (Cilofexor) with fewer side effects is also being considered. Cenicriviroc, a chemokine antagonist, reduced fibrosis in MASH patients. Aramchol, an acetyl-co A inhibitor, and resmetirom, a thyroid hormone receptor (β) agonist, reduced hepatic steatosis among MASLD patients. Elafibranor, lanifibranor, and other peroxisome proliferator-activated receptor agonists reduce inflammation in MASH. Agents that directly act on collagen and elastin cross-linkage (e.g., simtuzumab), reduce cell death and apoptosis (e.g., selonsertib), and reduce fibrosis may also be available. These drugs could be used either alone or in combination for an overall effective management of MASH in the future [10, 11].

References

1. Rinella ME, Lazarus JV, Ratziu V, et al. A multi-society Delphi consensus statement on new fatty liver disease nomenclature. Hepatology. 2023;29(1):101133. https://doi.org/10.1097/HEP.0000000000000520.
2. Chalasani N, Younossi Z, Lavine JE, et al. The diagnosis and management of nonalcoholic fatty liver disease: practice guidance from the American Association for the Study of Liver Diseases. Hepatology. 2018;67:328–57.
3. Sourianarayanane A, Pagadala MR, Kirwan JP. Management of non-alcoholic fatty liver disease. Minerva Gastroenterol Dietol. 2013;59(1):69–87.
4. Services. USDoAaUSDoHaH. Dietary Guidelines for Americans, 2020–2025. 2020; 9th Edition.
5. Sourianarayanane A, McCullough AJ. Accuracy of steatosis and fibrosis NAFLD scores in relation to vibration controlled transient elastography: an NHANES analysis. Clin Res Hepatol Gastroenterol. 2022;46(7):101997.
6. Sumida Y, Yoneda M, Tokushige K, Kawanaka M, Fujii H, Yoneda M, Imajo K, Takahashi H, Eguchi Y, Ono M, Nozaki Y, Hyogo H, Koseki M, Yoshida Y, Kawaguchi T, Kamada Y, Okanoue T, Nakajima A, Japan Study Group Of Nafld Jsg-Nafld. FIB-4 first in the diagnostic algorithm of metabolic-dysfunction-associated fatty liver disease in the era of the global metabodemic. Life (Basel). 2021;11(2):143.
7. Sasso M, Miette V, Sandrin L, Beaugrand M. The controlled attenuation parameter (CAP): a novel tool for the non-invasive evaluation of steatosis using Fibroscan. Clin Res Hepatol Gastroenterol. 2012;36(1):13–20.
8. Caussy C, Chen J, Alquiraish MH, Cepin S, Nguyen P, Hernandez C, Yin M, Bettencourt R, Cachay ER, Jayakumar S, Fortney L, Hooker J, Sy E, Valasek MA, Rizo E, Richards L,

Brenner DA, Sirlin CB, Ehman RL, Loomba R. Association between obesity and discordance in fibrosis stage determination by magnetic resonance vs transient elastography in patients with nonalcoholic liver disease. Clin Gastroenterol Hepatol. 2018;16(12):1974–1982.e7.

9. Angulo P, Kleiner DE, Dam-Larsen S, Adams LA, Bjornsson ES, Charatcharoenwitthaya P, Mills PR, Keach JC, Lafferty HD, Stahler A, Haflidadottir S, Bendtsen F. Liver fibrosis, but no other histologic features, is associated with long-term outcomes of patients with nonalcoholic fatty liver disease. Gastroenterology. 2015;149(2):389–97.

10. Sourianarayanane A, Challa SR. Non-alcoholic fatty liver: current management and future trends. Gut Gastroenterol. 2020;3:001–17.

11. Oseini AM, Sanyal AJ. Therapies in non-alcoholic steatohepatitis (NASH). Liver Int. 2017;37(Suppl 1):97–103. https://doi.org/10.1111/liv.13302.

12. Sasaki A, Nitta H, Otsuka K, Umemura A, Baba S, Obuchi T, Wakabayashi G. Bariatric surgery and non-alcoholic fatty liver disease: current and potential future treatments. Front Endocrinol (Lausanne). 2014;5:164.

13. Sourianarayanane A, Arikapudi S, McCullough AJ, Humar A. Nonalcoholic steatohepatitis recurrence and rate of fibrosis progression following liver transplantation. Eur J Gastroenterol Hepatol. 2017;29(4):481–7.

14. Alvarez J, Mei X, Daily M, Shah M, Grigorian A, Berger J, Marti F, Gedaly R. Tipping the scales: liver transplant outcomes of the super obese. J Gastrointest Surg. 2016;20(9):1628–35.

Chapter 68
Alcohol and Liver Disease in Women

Veronica Loy

A 60-year-old female is referred for elevated liver enzymes. She and her husband enjoy drinking wine with dinner and have it most evenings. They generally each have two glasses of wine, finishing off about 2/3 of the bottle.

Her physical exam is unremarkable. Her BMI is 20. Her AST is 90, ALT is 70, Alk phos is 80, and bilirubin is 1.0. Hepatitis panel, autoimmune panel, ceruloplasmin, and alpha-1 antitrypsin are all unremarkable. An US of the liver shows mild steatosis and no nodularity.

She is surprised because her husband recently had his annual physical exam and his liver enzymes were normal.

What is your interpretation of these findings, and can you describe the increased susceptibility women have to alcoholic liver disease?

It looks to me like this woman has some mild alcohol-related steatohepatitis. Thankfully, her synthetic function is intact with that normal bilirubin. Her ultrasound does not show nodularity, so there is no obvious cirrhosis, but that doesn't necessarily mean that she doesn't have some fibrosis, because that is difficult to assess by ultrasound alone. She does appear to have some mild alcohol-related steatohepatitis.

Why would she have this and her husband doesn't? I think that in every individual, their own risk for developing steatohepatitis and ultimately cirrhosis of the liver is multifactorial. One of those factors is gender. There are certainly a lot of other factors. I don't know other health differences between her and her husband, but gender alone is a driving factor in the risk of developing fibrosis, cirrhosis, or just alcohol-related steatohepatitis.

V. Loy (✉)
Division Gastroenterology and Hepatology, Department of Medicine, Medical College of Wisconsin, Milwaukee, WI, USA
e-mail: vloy@mcw.edu

© The Author(s), under exclusive license to Springer Nature Switzerland AG 2023
W. H. Sobin et al. (eds.), *Managing Complex Cases in Gastroenterology*,
https://doi.org/10.1007/978-3-031-48949-5_68

There are many reasons for gender differences in liver disease. First, we know that female patients metabolize alcohol differently than males. As a result, females have a higher rate of steatosis and inflammation and cytokine release at a much lower level of alcohol intake than males. Over the years, two to three glasses of wine a night, for a decade, for a female, is enough to put someone at risk for cirrhosis. Whereas in a male, it would be more like four to six a night. There is a very big difference in the way the body metabolizes alcohol at a lower level, which presents a higher risk to these people. It also relates to body size and body mass. A smaller stature person is going to have a lower threshold for damage from alcohol and generally women are smaller than men.

Most women are not aware of this distinction. Most of the women I see say that they're not drinking any more than their peers and they're not drinking more than their husband. They are astonished to end up in this situation. I really don't think there is enough awareness of the increased risk females have with alcohol consumption.

We also know that in the primary care setting and the ER setting, women are far less likely to be screened for alcohol use disorder. Even if female patients are screened, they are far less likely to be referred for counseling or medical therapies. We are really just not doing a good job of awareness in the medical community to help these people prevent alcohol related liver damage.

What do you make of the AST > ALT?

Briefly, the AST, being greater than the ALT, is thought to be predictive of alcohol-related liver disease. The one caveat to that is once someone is cirrhotic, regardless of the cause of cirrhosis, typically the AST is going to be higher than the ALT.

I often see patients where their medical team is grilling them and accusing them of drinking, because their AST is higher than their ALT. And they're not drinking, but they're cirrhotic and that's just what happens once someone is cirrhotic.

Would you simply advise the patient to stop drinking and follow the enzyme levels over the next 3–6 months, or would you do further investigations (i.e., FibroScan®, biopsy, etc.).

As far as what to do next, I would probably advise her to work on minimizing or stopping alcohol and repeat the enzymes in 3–6 months. The reason that I would not advocate for a FibroScan® or a biopsy is that, first of all, FibroScan® is not validated in people who are actively using alcohol. We tend to see an overestimate of the level of fibrosis on FibroScan® in someone who's using alcohol. It's just not accurate in my opinion. Similarly, with biopsy, if a biopsy is obtained on someone when there is a lot of active inflammation, it's very challenging for the pathologist to estimate the amount of fibrosis. Finally, there is a really good chance in this woman that with complete abstinence from alcohol the liver has a great chance to heal and regenerate. Therefore, what you see on a biopsy today may be very different from what you see after 6 months of abstinence, during which you give the body the tools it needs to repair itself. If she's willing to stop, I think you'll get a more accurate assessment after waiting 6 months. Unfortunately, many people aren't willing to stop. Without alcohol cessation, I would move on to a biopsy, not a FibroScan®. If they're not going to stop alcohol, the FibroScan® isn't something I offer them.

Chapter 69
Alcoholic Hepatitis

Francisco Durazo

A 52-year-old executive is fired from his job. Prior to that he would have two hard drinks a day after work. After being fired, he goes on a drinking binge for a month. He finally gets dragged in to see the doctor by his wife when he becomes jaundiced. His PT is 17, INR is 2.1, bilirubin is 12, AST is 80, ALT is 50, Alk phos is 120, creatinine is 1.2, Hgb is 11.8, and Maddrey score is 34.

How would you manage this patient with presumed acute alcoholic hepatitis?

These days, acute alcoholic hepatitis is overdiagnosed. It seems like everyone who is drinking and presents with jaundice is immediately diagnosed with alcoholic hepatitis. As a result, we see many patients placed on steroids and getting infections, where steroids weren't needed in the first place.

So, the first thing is to make sure this really is acute alcoholic hepatitis. On physical exam, we need to see an enlarged liver with a bruit. If we examine the patient and there is not an enlarged liver, then it is probably alcoholic cirrhosis we are dealing with.

The benefit of steroids is limited. Even in the studies where acute alcoholic hepatitis was appropriately diagnosed and steroids given according to protocol, there were a lot of complications, and the benefit of steroids was quite modest. Therefore, we refrain from using steroids, unless a patient presents with florid alcoholic hepatitis, where the diagnosis is obvious. Steroids are approved if the Maddrey score is >32 (I prefer to hold out for an even higher Maddrey score). In that case, we will give prednisolone for up to 28 days.

F. Durazo (✉)
Division of Gastroenterology and Hepatology, Department of Medicine,
Medical College of Wisconsin, Milwaukee, WI, USA
e-mail: fdurazo@mcw.edu

There has been a recent push for transplanting patients with acute alcoholic hepatitis. What are your thoughts?

Those studies were done in France, where there is a national healthcare program and patients got close follow-up and rehabilitation for their alcoholism. In those studies, the results of transplant were excellent and alcohol recidivism low.

However, in this country, we are not good at treating the major disease, which is alcoholism. We may be good at treating liver problems, but our approach to alcohol rehabilitation is poor.

In centers in the USA, where transplant for acute alcoholic hepatitis has been more successful, there have been four qualifiers that are essential: (1) this is the first episode of acute alcoholic hepatitis, (2) the patient has no history of relapse from sobriety, (3) there is strong family support, and (4) the patient has no history of psychological problems. Under these conditions, there is a much higher likelihood of success without relapse.

Chapter 70
Fatty Liver on Ultrasound with Normal LFTs

Francisco Durazo

A 43-year-old male was having mid-abdominal pain, and an ultrasound was obtained to rule out gallbladder disease. This showed a normal gallbladder but some fatty steatosis. The patient drinks two glasses of wine a week. His liver enzymes are totally normal. His BMI is 26.

In this case, does the finding of steatosis with normal liver enzymes merit further workup?

All patients with fatty liver deserve a workup for chronic hepatitis. Some patients with autoimmune hepatitis will present with fatty liver, some patients with Wilson's disease will present with fatty liver, and some patients with hepatitis C, particularly those with genotype 3, will present with fatty liver. We also want to look for signs of metabolic syndrome.

It would be appropriate to send off labs but not necessarily to perform liver biopsy. In terms of liver biopsy, there is not enough manpower to do liver biopsies on the huge number of people with fatty liver. We want to select those patients who are most at risk of having NASH, those patients who demonstrate more components of the metabolic syndrome. I personally use the NAFLD fibrosis score to help me decide whether to perform a liver biopsy in these patients.

F. Durazo (✉)
Division of Gastroenterology and Hepatology, Department of Medicine,
Medical College of Wisconsin, Milwaukee, WI, USA
e-mail: fdurazo@mcw.edu

© The Author(s), under exclusive license to Springer Nature
Switzerland AG 2023
W. H. Sobin et al. (eds.), *Managing Complex Cases in Gastroenterology*,
https://doi.org/10.1007/978-3-031-48949-5_70

325

Chapter 71
Evaluation for Liver Damage from Chronic ETOH Use

Francisco Durazo

A 52-year-old male is concerned about his drinking history. He has 3–4 glasses of wine or 2–3 hard drinks a day. He is concerned that this could be causing liver damage. His liver enzymes are normal as is his ultrasound.

Is there any role for FibroScan®? Has FibroScan® become a basic component of the exam and evaluation of most patients with liver problems?

The jury is still out on how useful the FibroScan® is. Some practitioners find it very useful while others believe that a good history, physical exam, and a basic ultrasound will give you the same information. They point out that FibroScan® is most accurate in detecting extremes – full-blown cirrhosis or a normal liver. These clinicians feel that the basic workup will yield the same information. For those in-between cases, they believe there is too much discrepancy between the FibroScan® results and liver biopsy, or MR elastography.

What are some factors that can confound FibroScan® results?

Factors that can blur FibroScan® results include hepatic congestion, biliary obstruction, and obesity. Some believe that FibroScan® is very unreliable in patients with NAFLD; it is most accurate in patients with viral hepatitis.

F. Durazo (✉)
Division of Gastroenterology and Hepatology, Department of Medicine,
Medical College of Wisconsin, Milwaukee, WI, USA
e-mail: fdurazo@mcw.edu

© The Author(s), under exclusive license to Springer Nature
Switzerland AG 2023
W. H. Sobin et al. (eds.), *Managing Complex Cases in Gastroenterology*,
https://doi.org/10.1007/978-3-031-48949-5_71

Chapter 72
Ascites in a Patient Without Obvious Cirrhosis

Jose Franco

The patient is a 60-year-old male who presents with a complaint of abdominal distension. There is no history of heavy alcohol abuse; he has 1–2 drinks a day on weekends only. The patient does have a strong family history of heart disease. He has very mild dyspnea on exertion. On exam, there is moderate abdominal ascites; his liver is not palpable. There is mild peripheral edema. Lungs are clear. There is no S3. However, he has a BNP of 400. His albumin is 3.2, AST is 30, ALT is 45, alk phos is 140 (Nl < 80), INR is 1.2, Hgb is 12.8, and platelet count is 140,000. Hepatitis serology, autoimmune markers, and Fe/TIBC are all negative. An ultrasound of the liver does not show any liver nodularity, but there is some dilation of the IVC and hepatic vein, and moderate ascites is present. EF is 30% on echocardiogram. The patient is started on diuretics for mild peripheral edema, and a paracentesis is performed to evaluate the ascites. The SAAG is 1.2 with ascites albumin of 2.0 and ascites total protein of 3.2. Cytology and AFB are negative. Cell count is 20 PMNs. FibroScan® shows 8 kPa.

What is your differential diagnosis for patients who present with ascites but do not have obvious cirrhosis?

I always tell students that cirrhosis is the leading cause of ascites, but it's certainly not the only cause. When we do a paracentesis, we send an ascites albumin and serum albumin to determine the SAAG (serum albumin-ascites albumin gradient) as well as an ascites total protein (TP). These results help us determine the etiology of the ascites.

We break the findings into four categories:

Category 1: SAAG >1.1 g/dL and ascites TP < 2.5 g/dL. Most cases of cirrhosis, also seen in fulminant liver disease.

J. Franco (✉)
Department of Medicine-Division of Gastroenterology and Hepatology, Medical College of Wisconsin, Milwaukee, WI, USA
e-mail: jfranco@mcw.edu

© The Author(s), under exclusive license to Springer Nature Switzerland AG 2023
W. H. Sobin et al. (eds.), *Managing Complex Cases in Gastroenterology*,
https://doi.org/10.1007/978-3-031-48949-5_72

329

Category 2: SAAG >1.1 g/dL and TP > 2.5 g/dL. Patients with CHF, constrictive pericarditis, Budd-Chiari, and veno-occlusive disease.

Category 3: SAAG <1.1 g/dL and TP < 2.5 g/dL. Patients with nephrotic syndrome, peritoneal carcinomatosis (where the TP is usually high but on occasion low).

Category 4: SAAG <1.1 g/dL and TP > 2.5 g/dL. Patients with peritoneal carcinomatosis, TB, pancreatic ascites, and chylous ascites.

This patient has a SAAG of 1.2. The high SAAG indicates portal hypertension. If we look at the differential diagnosis for high SAAG ascites fluid, we have cirrhosis, fulminant liver disease, CHF, constrictive pericarditis, Budd-Chiari syndrome, and veno-occlusive disease (VOD) or sinusoidal obstruction syndrome (SOS). Occasionally, in advanced CHF, you will see a low SAAG. In a patient like this with mild CHF, you would expect to see a high SAAG.

This patient has an elevated ascites fluid total protein of 3.2, which is usually not seen in cirrhosis by itself. It is seen in cases of CHF, constrictive pericarditis and Budd-Chiari. The reason for the high total protein in these cases is that hepatic synthetic function is usually preserved. In this case, the patient's serum albumin of 3.2 and INR of 1.2 demonstrates good functional reserve. This is quite different from the cirrhotic patient who presents with a serum albumin of 2.3 or 2.5. It is more similar to patients with portal vein thrombosis, who have preserved synthetic function and a high total ascites protein.

This patient received some diuretics prior to paracentesis. Will this have any effect on the SAAG or total protein?

Usually, you don't see any change but occasionally the total protein will increase due to volume contraction.

In cases where ascites is due to CHF, how often do they have cardiac cirrhosis?

Most patients with ascites due to heart failure do not have cirrhosis. Most of the time, they have congestive hepatopathy, with associated portal hypertension. This congestion is verified by the finding of a dilated IVC and hepatic veins on ultrasound. Patients who have severe, long-standing CHF, however, may get end-stage cardiac cirrhosis after many years of complications.

Is there any role for doing an EGD looking for varices in a patient like this?

Yes, to me, this is no different than evaluating a patient with portal vein thrombosis. These patients can get esophageal and gastric varices from non-cirrhotic portal hypertension. If you ask what the most feared complication is in a patient like this it is bleeding varices. Ascites fluid could get infected, but the highest mortality would be bleeding varices, and you don't want to miss these. So, you do need to do an EGD.

Another thing we look at in deciding whether to do an EGD is the platelet count. If the platelet count is <150,000, they are more likely to have varices. In this case, it is 140,000.

Chapter 73
Ascites in Cirrhosis of Unclear Etiology with Increased Mononuclear Cells

Jose Franco

A 57-year-old female with a normal BMI is found to have marked ascites. There is no history of significant alcohol use. Ultrasound shows a mildly nodular liver. The AST is 34, ALT is 47, Alk phos is 90, bilirubin 1.3, and albumin is 2.9. Hepatitis panel and autoimmune markers – including ANA, ASMA, and AMA – are negative. A paracentesis is performed, which reveals 300 wbc/hpf, and 80% are mononuclear cells. The Aa gradient is 1.0.

There is no obvious cause for her apparently cirrhotic liver, what are some possible etiologies for this?

You've ruled out viral hepatitis. PBC is unlikely with the normal alkaline phosphatase and negative AMA. The patient could have late-stage PSC – but there is no history of IBD here. I always check for alpha-1 antitrypsin deficiency and Wilson's. You know, alpha-1 antitrypsin deficiency is the leading indication for metabolic liver transplant, in the pediatric population. But while we always check for alpha-1 and Wilson's, it would be very unusual for the first presentation to be at age 57.

Another consideration is hemochromatosis. A 57-year-old female is now postmenopausal. It is possible for hemochromatosis to first manifest itself at this age in a woman. Remember, men will present much earlier than women. Women tend to present when they are 50, 60, and 70. When they are younger, they are autophlebotomizing through menstruation. So, it is a diagnosis worth considering.

The most common cause of cirrhosis, however, in a 57-year-old female would be nonalcoholic fatty liver disease. Patients don't have to be obese; they just have to have insulin resistance and/or elevated triglycerides, those by themselves are risk

J. Franco (✉)

Department of Medicine-Division of Gastroenterology and Hepatology, Medical College of Wisconsin, Milwaukee, WI, USA

e-mail: jfranco@mcw.edu

© The Author(s), under exclusive license to Springer Nature Switzerland AG 2023
W. H. Sobin et al. (eds.), *Managing Complex Cases in Gastroenterology*,
https://doi.org/10.1007/978-3-031-48949-5_73

factors. Obviously, there are no blood tests to diagnose nonalcoholic fatty liver disease; you diagnose it by ruling out other possible causes, and then, consider doing a liver biopsy. So that's how I would approach it.

In this case, the tests are all negative, yet I know she has cirrhosis. If my serologic workup remains negative, I would consider doing a liver biopsy to see if it helps me establish an etiology.

What would be causing the increase in mononuclear cells?

An increase in mononuclear cells on paracentesis is not something we commonly see. You have to think about atypical things, like fungal infections or tuberculosis. But it is also possible that they might represent cancer cells. Could the patient have peritoneal carcinomatosis? If the fluid looked milky, we'd consider chylous ascites, which could involve the lymphatics leading to ascites fluid with increased lymphocytes.

Chapter 74
Low SAAG Ascites

Jose Franco

A 67-year-old male who drinks alcohol on a daily basis is being seen for moderate ascites. He has anorexia and has lost 20 lbs. over the past month. Ultrasound shows a nodular liver, with marked ascites and no obvious masses. His AST is 40, ALT is 25, alk phos is 120, and bilirubin is 1.4. A paracentesis is performed and reveals an Aa gradient of 0.8. The ascites total protein is 2.3. Fluid cell count is 20 wbc. Cytology is negative. UA is negative for protein. Because the patient's creatinine is 1.8, you are reluctant to do a contrast-enhanced CT scan. An MR abdomen shows no obvious cancer.

Normally, if it were just alcoholic cirrhosis, you would expect a high Aa gradient. What might be causing a low gradient here? What further investigations would you do?

So, the patient has a nodular liver and normally you would expect to see a high SAAG, but here it is low. Let's review our categories again:

Category 1: SAAG >1.1 g/dL and ascites TP < 2.5 g/dL. Most cases of cirrhosis, also seen in fulminant liver disease.

Category 2: SAAG >1.1 g/dL and TP > 2.5 g/dL. Patients with CHF, constrictive pericarditis, Budd-Chiari, and veno-occlusive disease.

Category 3: SAAG <1.1 g/dL and TP < 2.5 g/dL. Patients with nephrotic syndrome, peritoneal carcinomatosis (in which the TP is usually high but on occasion low).

Category 4: SAAG <1.1 g/dL and TP > 2.5 g/dL. Patients with TB, pancreatic ascites, and chylous ascites.

J. Franco (✉)
Department of Medicine-Division of Gastroenterology and Hepatology, Medical College of Wisconsin, Milwaukee, WI, USA
e-mail: jfranco@mcw.edu

© The Author(s), under exclusive license to Springer Nature Switzerland AG 2023
W. H. Sobin et al. (eds.), *Managing Complex Cases in Gastroenterology*,
https://doi.org/10.1007/978-3-031-48949-5_74

In this case, I am concerned that the low SAAG may represent peritoneal carcinomatosis. The negative cytology does not rule this out. That's because cytology of ascites fluid is a poor test, less than a quarter of cases will actually be positive. It's great for diagnosing infection, but if you're trying to find malignant cells, it is not a very good test.

I believe that this patient has cancer, and we just haven't found it. In terms of the other diagnoses for a low SAAG ascites, I don't think he has pancreatic ascites, because you would've seen something on an MRI. He doesn't have chylous ascites, because you obviously would have seen milky-looking fluid. There's nothing to suggest nephrotic syndrome or TB. So, to me, this patient has a primary with peritoneal metastases causing ascites, and we just haven't found the primary. So, he might need a laparoscopy, to look at what is going on in his peritoneal lining.

Chapter 75
Banding Esophageal Varices

Kia Saeian

A 43-year-old male with a long history of alcoholism presented to your ER a week earlier. One of the newer gastroenterologists on staff did an EGD and found grade 3 esophageal varices with stigmata of prior hemorrhage but were not actively bleeding. He placed a total of 10 bands on the varices. The patient was discharged and now presents again to the ER with torrential UGI bleeding. Endoscopy reveals several post-banding ulcers, one of which is actively bleeding.

How do you stop bleeding from these ulcers? Can it be done endoscopically or do you need IR?

In general, we think that banding ulcers resulting in bleeding occur in less than 5% of the cases, and while most of these bleeding episodes are minor, some of them can be significant, and fatal cases have been reported. Ulceration itself is almost universal and typically occurs 3–7 days after the banding with healing expected within the first 2–3 weeks. While the thought is that it is often the perforating veins as opposed to the main varix that is bleeding in the setting of post-banding ulceration resulting in lower volume bleeding, they are often very difficult to control if they bleed significantly.

It may seem flippant to answer in this way, but the short answer is that you pretty much do whatever it takes to stop the bleeding. There are reports of attempting almost anything you can think of to try to stop them from bleeding, including repeat band ligation, cyanoacrylate glue injection, proceeding with TIPS or other portal decompressive procedures, or even esophageal stents and Hemospray®. In my experience, I start with band ligation and then in a couple of cases have used glue

K. Saeian (✉)
Division of Gastroenterology & Hepatology, Medical College of Wisconsin, Milwaukee, WI, USA
e-mail: ksaeian@mcw.edu

W. H. Sobin et al. (eds.), *Managing Complex Cases in Gastroenterology*, https://doi.org/10.1007/978-3-031-48949-5_75

injection (This is not FDA-approved in the United States and is costly). I have not had to resort to TIPS or other modalities as a primary measure but have considered TIPS more actively after stopping the bleeding if the TIPS is otherwise not contraindicated for the particular patient. Temporizing with an esophageal stent or using balloon tamponade seem reasonable as a bridge to TIPS.

What are your tips for initial banding of varices to best initiate control of varices and also avoid complications?

In the setting of active bleeding initially, I do start as close to the GE junction as possible and band in a preferably spiral fashion upward until I gain control. As with standard band ligation of esophageal varices, I limit my banding to the distal 5 cm of the esophagus as this is the culprit region in the vast majority, and banding more proximally is less likely to be effective but can precipitate ulceration and bleeding that's much more difficult to control. Without much data to support my practice, I do routinely avoid placing a lot more bands if I have gained control of the bleeding and I administer sucralfate slurry 1 g four times daily for at least 7 days and in some patients for 14 days. While many follow the recommendation to bring the patient back within the first 2–4 weeks for repeat band ligation, if there is ulceration still present, which there often is if you bring the patient back in 2 weeks, I do not band in the presence of any suggestion of ulceration. My practice has changed over the years, and I typically bring the patients back closer to 4 weeks to avoid putting the patient through an extra unnecessary endoscopy.

Chapter 76
Gastric Varices

Kia Saeian

A 54-year-old male presents with a history of hematemesis, which stops after initiation of octreotide and PPI. He has a long history of alcohol abuse. On exam, there are multiple stigmata of cirrhosis. The Hbg is 8, his platelet count is 90,000, and INR is 2.3. EGD reveals small esophageal varices and large gastric varices in the fundus and body not felt to be an extension of esophageal varices. It is your impression that bleeding occurred from gastric varices but has stopped for the time being.

What are the scenarios in which you most commonly encounter significant gastric varices, either isolated or in association with esophageal varices?

When I see a patient with significant gastric varices, I always suspect they may have thrombosis. We sometimes see isolated gastric varices in patients with chronic pancreatitis who have developed thrombosis of their splenic vein. In cirrhotics, we sometimes see gastric varices in the setting of thrombosis of the portal and/or mesenteric veins. We see occasional patients with myeloproliferative disorders who develop thromboses in the portal system and can develop pretty large gastric varices.

I would want cross-sectional imaging in this case.

Cross-sectional imaging reveals portal vein thrombosis in a cirrhotic liver with significant splenorenal shunting and large gastric varices.

How would you manage this situation?

From a management standpoint, the presence of the thrombus creates an extra layer of complexity, especially if it is chronic, because this may take TIPS out of the equation.

If you do think the bleeding is from a gastric varix, particularly if there is an erosion or a red mark present, I think you have to evaluate whether you have the option

K. Saeian (✉)
Division of Gastroenterology & Hepatology, Medical College of Wisconsin,
Milwaukee, WI, USA
e-mail: ksaeian@mcw.edu

© The Author(s), under exclusive license to Springer Nature
Switzerland AG 2023
W. H. Sobin et al. (eds.), *Managing Complex Cases in Gastroenterology*,
https://doi.org/10.1007/978-3-031-48949-5_76

of performing TIPS or BRTO. BRTO is balloon occluded retrograde transvenous obliteration of the varices. This procedure is becoming more and more common.

Another option is to perform an EGD with cyanoacrylate glue injection of gastric varices. Glue injection of varices is not yet FDA-approved in the United States, but it is widely used in other countries around the world. However, we are getting much more experience using it, off-label and it should be considered when BRTO is not an option.

In the acute setting, of course, you do the standard things including infusing a vasoactive substance, which in this country is usually octreotide and in other countries tends to be terlipressin. Terlipressin has recently been approved in the United States for the treatment of hepatorenal syndrome and may soon replace octreotide as the vasoactive agent of choice. We also start antibiotics, typically ceftriaxone.

After that, you need to make a decision about which of the more robust treatments for gastric varices you want to attempt. At our institution, more and more frequently it means going to BRTO. Our interventional radiologists have a lot of experience with BRTO, but there are a couple of caveats you need to know about. The first is that BRTO can actually worsen ascites, and another is that it can lead to enlargement and possibly bleeding from esophageal varices if they are present. So, in those patients who have esophageal varices as well as gastric varices and either could be the source of bleeding, we prefer to go with TIPS placement. However, in some patients with severe thrombosis, TIPS is not a feasible option, and therefore BRTO is performed. You really want to get good cross-sectional imaging to allow the radiologist to evaluate the anatomy to see if he is a good candidate for BRTO. They can look at the imaging and see if there is a splenorenal shunt or some other systemic-portal venous shunt that would allow you to do the BRTO.

How is BRTO performed?

The interventional radiologist usually inserts a catheter via a transfemoral approach and advances the catheter into the splenic vein (or another vein) injects contrast and gets opacification. Once they get filling of the gastric varix, they will advance the balloon occlusion catheter and position it in the descending portion of the veins that are draining the varix. Then, they inflate the balloon to prevent injected material from escaping the system. They usually inject ethanolamine oleate (EO), which acts similarly to our use of cyanoacrylate glue to help occlude the varix. However, thanks to the balloon occlusion, their glue remains in contact with the varix for a longer interval, and they can inject a larger volume of EO. As a result, there is usually a better result from BRTO than endoscopic glue injection of gastric varices. In theory, it works in a similar manner to our variceal glue injections.

Why might BRTO lead to enlargement and possible bleeding from esophageal varices?

If the occluded gastric varix is in continuity with esophageal varices, you have now occluded the drainage system of the esophageal varices. The portal hypertension then gets transmitted back into the esophageal varices, leading to enlargement and possible bleeding. This is the result of occluding one of the escape channels for the elevated portal pressures.

A couple of our patients who received BRTO developed such prominent enlargement of esophageal varices that the interventional radiologist asked us to scope the patient and consider banding the esophageal varices. One of them had bleeding from the esophageal varices before we were able to do her endoscopy.

When you have your conference with the radiology department to evaluate the patient with portal vein thrombosis, how do you decide whether they are TIPS candidates or not?

If the portal vein thrombosis is not that extensive, sometimes the interventional radiologist can recanalize the vein and TIPS placement can be performed. Following TIPS placement, anticoagulation is started to prevent thrombosis and help maintain patency of the TIPS. However, if the thrombosis is very extensive, the standard TIPS approach may not be an option. Another option, in some of these cases, is DIPS (direct intrahepatic portosystemic shunt). While TIPS involves a transvenous approach to the portal system, DIPS involves a percutaneous approach to the portal vein and its branches. The patient has to have a large enough vein target for the percutaneous approach. The number of cases of DIPS performed is much lower than the number of TIPS at our institution.

Now, if neither TIPS nor DIPs are feasible, BRTO remains a promising option. The other group of patients in whom BRTO is preferred are those patients in whom TIPS is relatively contraindicated. This includes those with hepatic encephalopathy, pulmonary hypertension, or CHF. In these cases, TIPS may be off the table.

It is really important that the hepatologist uses good judgment. Whenever you decide between TIPS and BRTO, you want to consider whether there are secondary benefits from one approach over the other. Certainly, in patients with gastric varices who also have significant esophageal varices or ascites, the secondary benefits of TIPS are really attractive. In hepatic encephalopathy and CHF, BRTO is preferred.

Why is banding of gastric varices usually avoided, and why may there be some concern about banding esophageal varices when gastric varices are present?

Banding of large isolated gastric varices is avoided because patients can develop post-banding ulcers, and bleeding from those ulcers can be torrential. This doesn't apply to banding of GOV-1 varices, the proximal gastric varices that are in contiguity with esophageal varices. Banding for GOV-1 varices is widely accepted. It is the banding of GOV-2 and other gastric varices that should be avoided because that can lead to catastrophic consequences.

The concern about banding of esophageal varices, when gastric varices are present, is that after esophageal varices are banded, you will occasionally see enlargement of gastric varices, which might precipitate bleeding.

With the initial endoscopy, no intervention was done. While deciding which procedure to perform to definitively treat the gastric varices, the patient develops much more active bleeding. He is intubated and repeat endoscopy initiated; however, there is too much blood to see anything.

How do you manage the bleeding diathesis in cirrhotics with an elevated INR, and how do you manage the torrential bleeding at the time of endoscopy?

It is difficult to evaluate the degree of anticoagulation in many of our cirrhotic patients. Most of our experience demonstrates that the INR is not a good indicator of the bleeding propensity of these patients. Unfortunately, the thromboelastogram (TEG) is not a panacea either. Some of our literature supports checking fibrinogen levels, targeting a fibrinogen level between 170 and 200. We generally try to replenish fibrinogen using FFP, because it is cheaper than some of the other agents. Kcentra certainly works as well.

My preference in these cases is to improve the coagulopathy as rapidly as possible so we do not delay definitive therapy. We realize that it is generally impossible to totally correct the coagulopathy. So, in this case, where the patient is actively bleeding, I would try to correct things using FFP because it is more readily accessible in our center, and then we can proceed to the next step in management as quickly as we can.

With the patient bleeding so heavily, I might try to temporize things by inserting a Minnesota tube (we use these at our center rather than the Segnstaken-Blakemore tube). My approach to placing the tube is to do it blindly, and then, after placement, call for a C-arm and confirm the position radiographically. On occasion, I have placed a transnasal scope alongside the tube to confirm that the balloon is in the proper position. But generally, the use of the endoscope is unnecessary. We are usually comfortable relying on the radiographic confirmation alone. And when dealing with a bleeding gastric varix, we just need to inflate the gastric balloon; we do not need to inflate the esophageal balloon, which could risk esophageal pressure necrosis. Even in the setting of bleeding from esophageal varices, inflation of just the gastric balloon may suffice in stopping the bleeding.

Chapter 77
Increased Ascites in a Stable Cirrhotic

Kia Saeian

A 54-year-old male with alcoholic cirrhosis, diagnosed 6 months earlier, has been abstinent for 6 months following drinking heavily for about 30 years. He presents because of new-onset ascites. He has gynecomastia, palmar erythema, shifting dullness and a fluid wave, and palpable splenomegaly. His last ultrasound, done 6 months earlier, showed cirrhosis without any liver mass and an EGD was negative for varices at that time.

When a patient with alcoholic cirrhosis who is abstinent starts decompensating, what are your considerations?

With stable alcoholic cirrhotics who are abstinent, we expect their symptoms to get better not worse. This patient's turn for the worse is surprising, and I consider the possible decompensating events. First, I question whether the patient may have gone back to drinking, although this does not appear to be the case here. Second, I worry about portal vein thrombosis or any kind of venous thrombosis as a precipitant. And third, even though the ultrasound was okay previously, you always worry about malignancy. Those are the three things that are highest in the differential for me. Portal vein thrombosis is very common in our cirrhotic population so that is probably the most common explanation we encounter.

In terms of whether he has gone back to drinking, do you use the PEth (phosphatidylethanol) levels often?

We do, particularly in our transplant patients, but there are a couple of caveats to using the PEth that the reader has to be aware of. Patients can be abstinent and still have the PEth return positive, because you get a numerical result, and it can be dropping and takes a long time to return zero. It's more useful if you have a

K. Saeian (✉)
Division of Gastroenterology & Hepatology, Medical College of Wisconsin,
Milwaukee, WI, USA
e-mail: ksaeian@mcw.edu

© The Author(s), under exclusive license to Springer Nature
Switzerland AG 2023
W. H. Sobin et al. (eds.), *Managing Complex Cases in Gastroenterology*,
https://doi.org/10.1007/978-3-031-48949-5_77

baseline value taken when the patient was drinking. While the test is helpful, it does detect alcohol use for 30 days and perhaps up to 90 days. We have had cases where patients have claimed abstinence and a positive PEth result has led the patient to feel like they have been falsely accused of drinking. Patients need to know that the threshold of the test is so low that a positive result may simply be an indicator of prior alcohol use.

Another test we use is the serum ethanol glucuronide (EtG), which can detect alcohol use for 72–96 h. The advantage of this test (at our hospital) is that the turn-around on this test is much more rapid than the PEth. In the inpatient setting, the Peth test may take too long to return, and the patient gets discharged before you get the results back. So, if you are basing decision-making on these tests, the ethanol glucuronide may be preferable if you need quick results.

An US is performed and there is a 3-cm lesion, suggestive of hepatoma that was absent on the last US. Triple-phase CT scan confirms the likely diagnosis of HCC in the background of cirrhosis.

Are there any clues that make you suspect a patient may have developed hepatoma? Do you develop a sixth sense for who may develop a hepatoma?

I wish I had a sixth sense that would tell me who the patient is who will develop a hepatoma. But there are some patients who you suspect are at higher risk. We do not see as many hepatitis C patients with hepatomas as we used to, now that we are eradicating hepatitis C, but those patients with cirrhosis from alcohol and hepatitis C are at increased risk. Also, those patients with cirrhosis from hemochromatosis and alcohol are at greater risk, as are hepatitis B patients. For patients with these risk factors, we have a much lower threshold for being worried about HCC.

Another worrisome scenario is when a stable patient starts doing more poorly unexpectedly, for instance, a patient who develops anorexia, or starts losing a lot of muscle mass, or starts developing ascites, in spite of good control of their underlying liver disease. In cases like those I start worrying about HCC.

In terms of detecting bruits on auscultation and those sorts of things that have been advocated in the past for detecting hepatoma, honestly, now with the excellent imaging at our fingertips, we usually don't come across those secondary manifestations before we get back positive results from our radiology exams.

I would say in this particular patient, though, that once he developed ascites, I would have gone directly to CT imaging, or if I was going to do an ultrasound make it a Doppler ultrasound. Because I am worried that there could be a portal vein thrombus with or without HCC, I would get one of those examinations. Now, usually a 3-cm HCC is not going to cause this degree of ascites, so I would be worried that there could be a tumor thrombus.

Do you follow the AFP in surveillance of your cirrhotic patients?

I do, although I know the national guidelines from the AASLD have gone back and forth on this. The AASLD had removed alpha-fetoprotein a number of years ago from their guidelines but societies are now recommending it again. But in my surveillance of cirrhotics for HCC, I have found it to be a helpful tool. There have been cases where an elevated alpha-fetoprotein would jump-start me to order a CAT scan in a patient whose ultrasound was negative for a mass, and we've found some early HCCs this way. Occasionally, it's also useful to have a baseline alpha-fetoprotein because it helps you in terms of therapeutic decisions down the line, especially when the patients get liver-directed therapy.

What if this patient was not abstinent and could not quit drinking and asks you for help, are there meds you would prescribe to prevent alcohol relapse?

Yes, first we have been fortunate in that we have a transplant psychology team that we can use even in patients who we are not being evaluated for transplant. In that subset of patients, having our psychology team involved early is helpful in decreasing recidivism.

Personally, I have started a number of patients on baclofen. The original article in the Lancet [1] that used baclofen to decrease recidivism showed that it was promising; however, the study has not always been replicated. But if I am going to use something, I rely on baclofen. Some other people may use other agents like Suboxone. I am most comfortable with baclofen, and I have found that it helps patients with their cravings. It also gives the patient the sense that he is taking action to do something about his problem and makes him feel empowered that he has a shot at not going back to drinking. I will start at 5 mg bid and then go up to 10 mg and may go up to 15 mg, increasing the frequency to tid. We treat the patient for 6 weeks. More recently, there is now more and more experience with the use of both naltrexone and acomprosate. While many use naltrexone as first line, it should be avoided in acute alcoholic hepatitis or acute on chronic liver failure thus I tend to use acomprosate (666 mg three times daily with normal renal function) for my patients intolerant of baclofen. Acomprosate should be avoided in those with severe renal failure.

Another intervention to help protect patients from relapsing is to try to engage family and others to help the patient maintain his sobriety. It is particularly effective when patients have kids that are involved with their care, we find they are much more apt not to go back to alcohol.

Reference

1. Addolorato G, Leggio L, Ferrulli A, Cardone S, Vonghia L, Mirijello A, Abenavoli L, D'Angelo C, Caputo F, Zambon A, Haber PS. Effectiveness and safety of baclofen for maintenance of alcohol abstinence in alcohol-dependent patients with liver cirrhosis: randomized, double-blind controlled study. Lancet. 2007;370(9603):1915–22.

Chapter 78
Complications Related to Managing Ascites

James Esteban

A 46-year-old male with a history of heavy alcohol use presents for evaluation and management of ascites. On presentation, his creatinine is 1.1 mg/dL. A therapeutic and diagnostic paracentesis reveals straw-colored fluid that is a transudate, with low WBC and only 80 neutrophils per mm³. The serum albumin-ascitic fluid gradient is 1.5. You start furosemide 40 mg and spironolactone 100 mg once daily. One week later, the creatinine has increased to 1.4 mg/dL. His ascites is improved, though still present.

Would you change the dose of his diuretic? Do you monitor urine sodium in these patients?

I might decrease the dose while making sure that the patient follows a sodium-restricted diet (<2000 mg of sodium per day). The alternative is to maintain the patient on the current dose while closely monitoring the creatinine and electrolytes. I don't routinely check urine sodium, although this can be beneficial in determining whether persistent ascites is due to inadequate diuresis or nonadherence to sodium restriction [1].

Staying on the same diuretic dose, his creatinine increases to 1.7 mg/dL the following week.

Assuming the patient is adhering to sodium restriction, it looks like he is intolerant of diuretics. I would have to decrease his diuretic dosing, and in some patients, we may have to discontinue diuretics entirely. He would have to continue serial large volume paracentesis to manage his symptoms.

I would consider referring him to interventional radiology for transjugular intrahepatic portosystemic shunt, or TIPS, if he does not have contraindications. For

J. Esteban (✉)
Division of Gastroenterology and Hepatology, Department of Medicine, Medical College of Wisconsin, Milwaukee, WI, USA
e-mail: jesteban@mcw.edu

© The Author(s), under exclusive license to Springer Nature Switzerland AG 2023
W. H. Sobin et al. (eds.), *Managing Complex Cases in Gastroenterology*, https://doi.org/10.1007/978-3-031-48949-5_78

this, I would order an echocardiogram, to ensure cardiac function and pulmonary arterial pressure would tolerate TIPS, and contrast-enhanced CT or MRI of the abdomen (based on his kidney function), to check the vascular anatomy of the liver.

We have to calculate his model for end-stage liver disease or MELD score. If his MELD score is high enough, typically above 15, we should begin a liver transplant evaluation [2]. Many hepatologists would hesitate to insert a TIPS in a patient with a MELD score of 18–20 and above, although there is not necessarily a specific MELD cutoff for TIPS placement [3].

TIPS is performed, and ascites improves; however, the patient starts to develop increased lethargy and forgetfulness. You start lactulose and rifaximin. The patient improves, but a few weeks later he becomes markedly confused and is hospitalized frequently. You confirm that he is having 3–4 bowel movements daily with lactulose and takes rifaximin as prescribed.

How would you manage this?

Hepatic encephalopathy may occur in 20–30% of patients after TIPS insertion. In many cases, medical management with lactulose and rifaximin is sufficient to treat encephalopathy. However, in this patient, encephalopathy is significant and becomes difficult to treat medically. I would refer him back to interventional radiology to consider restricting, or narrowing, the TIPS stent. Unfortunately, restricting the stent may cause the return of ascites.

References

1. Biggins SW, Angeli P, Garcia-Tsao G, Ginès P, Ling SC, Nadim MK, Wong F, Kim WR. Diagnosis, evaluation, and management of ascites, spontaneous bacterial peritonitis and hepatorenal syndrome: 2021 practice guidance by the American Association for the Study of Liver Diseases. Hepatology. 2021;74(2):1014–48.
2. Brown RS, Lake JR. The survival impact of liver transplantation in the MELD era, and the future for organ allocation and distribution. Am J Transplant. 2005;5(2):203–4.
3. Boike JR, Thornburg BG, Asrani SK, Fallon MB, Fortune BE, Izzy MJ, Verna EC, Abraldes JG, Allegretti AS, Bajaj JS, Biggins SW. North American practice-based recommendations for transjugular intrahepatic portosystemic shunts in portal hypertension. Clin Gastroenterol Hepatol. 2022;20(8):1636–62.

Chapter 79
Portal Vein Thrombosis in Cirrhosis

James Esteban

A 56-year-old male was diagnosed with alcohol-associated cirrhosis 2 years ago and stopped drinking at that time. He has been undergoing abdominal ultrasound every 6 months for hepatocellular cancer screening. On his last ultrasound, a portal vein thrombus was seen. The last ultrasound 6 months ago did not show PVT.

Would you anticoagulate this patient?

Portal vein thrombosis (PVT) is a known complication of cirrhosis. It appears paradoxical that patients with cirrhosis, who often have prolonged prothrombin time and thrombocytopenia, would develop PVT. However, cirrhosis is a state of rebalanced hemostasis, where patients experience simultaneous changes in both pro- and anticoagulant factors [1]. Decisions on anticoagulation for patients with PVT, who may have varices, bleeding portal hypertensive gastropathy, or GAVE, can be challenging.

The first thing I would do is obtain contrast-enhanced CT or MRI, to confirm the PVT; determine the presence of collaterals (or cavernoma), which indicate chronicity, determine the extent of the clot, in terms of being partially or totally occlusive and extension into superior mesenteric vein (SMV) or splenic veins; and make sure it is not a malignant thrombus. My decision about anticoagulation will be based on chronicity of the clot, extent of the clot and the presence of symptoms of intestinal ischemia, and the patient's potential liver transplant candidacy [2, 3].

If the clot is chronic, with well-established collaterals and cavernoma, there is no established benefit with anticoagulation. We would be continuing medical management and surveillance of portal hypertension.

J. Esteban (✉)
Division of Gastroenterology and Hepatology, Department of Medicine, Medical College of Wisconsin, Milwaukee, WI, USA
e-mail: jesteban@mcw.edu

© The Author(s), under exclusive license to Springer Nature Switzerland AG 2023
W. H. Sobin et al. (eds.), *Managing Complex Cases in Gastroenterology*,
https://doi.org/10.1007/978-3-031-48949-5_79

If the clot is recent (<6 months) but involves only intrahepatic PV branches or only partially occludes the main PV, I would offer either anticoagulation or surveillance imaging with expectant management. It is reasonable to repeat abdominal imaging after 2–3 months, and anticoagulate only if the clot progresses.

If the clot is recent and extensive, which is to say that it totally occludes the main PV or extends into the SMV, particularly if the patient is a liver transplant candidate or has symptoms of intestinal ischemia, I would anticoagulate as soon as possible. I would go as far as discussing with interventional radiology and transplant surgery whether we should consider portal vein recanalization and transjugular intrahepatic portosystemic shunt (TIPS), especially if the patient has another indication for TIPS (e.g., ascites or variceal bleeding) or if clot extension threatens portal anastomosis during transplant.

In this case, the patient is felt to have a recent clot, which is totally occluding the main portal vein. He does not have abdominal pain or bloody diarrhea. The patient's last EGD was 2 years earlier, and at that time, there were no varices present. The decision is made to repeat EGD, and this reveals two grade 2 varices and one grade 3 varix, with a red mark.

How do you want to manage this?

Since the patient has high-risk esophageal varices and needs anticoagulation, I would pursue band ligation.

If you band, how long will you wait before starting anticoagulation?

It is debatable if anticoagulation should be delayed until varices are eradicated. I feel that cirrhotic patients with totally occlusive clots of the main PV and/or SMV should be anticoagulated without delay, while patients with less extensive clots may hold off anticoagulation until varices are banded or eradicated. Early anticoagulation of PVT is important for clot recanalization and prevention of clot progression [4, 5]. The AASLD does recommend initiating anticoagulation as soon as possible and not delaying until varices are eradicated [3]. Available data do not suggest higher risk of bleeding with this practice. Moreover, the data suggest that anticoagulation can continue uninterrupted through band ligation without risk of bleeding [6].

I treat patients with small and low-risk varices with nonselective beta-blockers such as carvedilol (my preference), propranolol, or nadolol instead of band ligation, with the goal of preventing the growth and rupture of varices. I prefer carvedilol over propranolol because studies show that it more effectively lowers portal pressure [7] as a result of its additional effect on alpha-1 adrenergic receptors, which reduce intrahepatic vascular resistance in addition to reducing portal blood flow.

I also use carvedilol in patients even after large varices are eradicated by band ligation because studies show that carvedilol not only reduces the risk of variceal bleeding but also hepatic decompensation events such as ascites [8].

What anticoagulant agents do you use and how long do you anticoagulate patients?

I have used warfarin and direct oral anticoagulants as first-line agents for anticoagulation in PVT. Warfarin probably has the most data on efficacy and safety, and it is also cheaper and more easily reversible if the patient develops a bleeding complication, but it requires normal baseline INR – which many cirrhotics don't have – and also frequent INR monitoring. Direct oral anticoagulants (DOAC) do not require INR monitoring and are thus easier to use. Many recent studies show DOAC's success in PVT, but it is unclear if they are safe to use in patients with more advanced stages of liver disease (i.e., Child's C). I would request hematology consultation in more complicated cases, such as patients with progressive clot despite anticoagulation or underlying thrombophilia.

I anticoagulate patients for at least 6 months. I obtain cross-sectional abdominal imaging after 2–3 months to check if the clot resolves, improves, or progresses. If the clot completely resolves, I will discontinue anticoagulation, but continue routine surveillance with doppler ultrasound or cross-sectional imaging every 6 months. If the clot progresses, assuming the patient is being adherent, my options are changing anticoagulants with the guidance of hematology or interventional radiology consultation for intravascular procedures or TIPS.

References

1. Lisman T, Caldwell SH, Intagliata NM. Haemostatic alterations and management of haemostasis in patients with cirrhosis. J Hepatol. 2022;76(6):1291–305.
2. De Franchis R, Bosch J, Garcia-Tsao G, Reiberger T, Ripoll C, Abraldes JG, Albillos A, Baiges A, Bajaj J, Bañares R, Barrufet M. Baveno VII–renewing consensus in portal hypertension. J Hepatol. 2022;76(4):959–74.
3. Northup PG, Garcia-Pagan JC, Garcia-Tsao G, Intagliata NM, Superina RA, Roberts LN, Lisman T, Valla DC. Vascular liver disorders, portal vein thrombosis, and procedural bleeding in patients with liver disease: 2020 practice guidance by the American Association for the Study of Liver Diseases. Hepatology. 2021;73(1):366–413.
4. Loffredo L, Pastori D, Farcomeni A, Violi F. Effects of anticoagulants in patients with cirrhosis and portal vein thrombosis: a systematic review and meta-analysis. Gastroenterology. 2017;153(2):480–7.
5. Delgado MG, Seijo S, Yepes I, Achécar L, Catalina MV, García-Criado Á, Abraldes JG, de la Peña J, Bañares R, Albillos A, Bosch J. Efficacy and safety of anticoagulation on patients with cirrhosis and portal vein thrombosis. Clin Gastroenterol Hepatol. 2012;10(7):776–83.
6. Guillaume M, Christol C, Plessier A, Corbic M, Péron JM, Sommet A, Rautou PE, Consigny Y, Vinel JP, Valla CD, Bureau C. Bleeding risk of variceal band ligation in extrahepatic portal vein obstruction is not increased by oral anticoagulation. Eur J Gastroenterol Hepatol. 2018;30(5):563–8.
7. Jachs M, Hartl L, Simbrunner B, Bauer D, Paternostro R, Balcar L, Hofer B, Pfisterer N, Schwarz M, Scheiner B, Stättermayer AF. Carvedilol achieves higher hemodynamic response and lower rebleeding rates than propranolol in secondary prophylaxis. Clin Gastroenterol Hepatol. 2022;21(9):2318–2326.e7.
8. Villanueva C, Albillos A, Genescà J, Garcia-Pagan JC, Calleja JL, Aracil C, Bañares R, Morillas RM, Poca M, Peñas B, Augustin S. β blockers to prevent decompensation of cirrhosis in patients with clinically significant portal hypertension (PREDESCI): a randomized, double-blind, placebo-controlled, multicentre trial. Lancet. 2019;393(10181):1597–608.

Chapter 80
PVT and Budd Chiari as a Complication of UC

Kia Saeian

The patient is a 28-year-old female with a history of ulcerative colitis that was well controlled on mesalamine. She presents with increased diarrhea and rectal bleeding but also has marked abdominal distension. An US of the abdomen confirms the presence of a large amount of ascites. There is no history of liver disease, alcohol use, etc. Her labs show AST of 120, ALT of 140, AP of 100, and bilirubin of 1.4. Hepatitis panel and autoimmune panel are negative. A CT is obtained, which shows thrombus in the hepatic vein, IVC, and portal vein. There is a suggestion of gastroesophageal varices. There is hepatomegaly but no suggestion of cirrhosis. She has a combined EGD/colon, and while on EGD there are grade 2 esophageal varices, on colon there is evidence for moderately severe ulcerative colitis. The patient is placed on IV steroids and beta-blockers. Anticoagulation is started (IV heparin), and the next day the patient starts having more active rectal bleeding. Her abdominal distension is getting worse. Heparin is put on hold.

How would you manage the presumed Budd-Chiari and portal vein thrombosis?

First, I'm not sure I would have started her on beta-blockers in the first place, particularly in the setting of a large amount of ascites, where the use of beta-blockers is controversial. And with grade 2 varices, I don't think you have to jump in and immediately do anything about her varices.

But, of course, we do have to address the thromboses. Here, it's a little unusual, it's not only Budd-Chiari, and it's also portal vein thrombosis and extension into the IVC, which makes it a pretty extensive thrombus. She's very young, so I'm not as concerned about malignancy. But while the IBD could be a trigger for her

K. Saeian (✉)
Division of Gastroenterology & Hepatology, Medical College of Wisconsin, Milwaukee, WI, USA
e-mail: ksaeian@mcw.edu

© The Author(s), under exclusive license to Springer Nature Switzerland AG 2023
W. H. Sobin et al. (eds.), *Managing Complex Cases in Gastroenterology*, https://doi.org/10.1007/978-3-031-48949-5_80

351

hypercoagulable state, it seems a little out of proportion. Since it's very extensive, I would look for other causes of hypercoagulable state, even though IBD might remain the sole explanation. I'd want to make sure that there is nothing else going on with her bone marrow. These days, it is almost mandatory, when you have someone who presents with Budd-Chiari, to rule out polycythemia vera, or some of the other myeloproliferative disorders that can certainly trigger this. That would be on my radar as well.

Looking at the bigger picture, we have to decide how to manage this very complex patient who is bleeding but needs treatment for thrombosis. In this setting, we have really discovered that TIPS is the way to go. I would get interventional radiology and transplant surgery involved. While TIPS is generally feasible in Budd-Chiari, the portal vein thrombus in this case presents an increased level of complexity for performing a successful TIPS. And, if you are successful in placing a TIPS, you want to anticoagulate afterward to prevent shunt thrombosis. So, in this case you should notify colorectal surgery as well, because even though I'm not recommending a colectomy at the time, that's where you may end up heading if rectal bleeding becomes intractable.

Even though she is young, I would get an echocardiogram, to see whether she has any pulmonary hypertension and whether she is a suitable candidate for TIPS, and get IR involved to see if it's feasible to place a TIPS and maintain its patency.

In most cases of Budd-Chiari, the thrombus is fairly new and the radiologist can get a wire through it. In this case, however, the clot is more extensive, and it goes into the IVC, and so the question is whether there are other channels that IR can get into. In some of these cases, it might require DIPS to be successful.

If you only have hepatic vein thrombosis, is stenting the vein ever an option?

You could consider it, but in almost all cases, the thrombus in Budd-Chiari involves multiple small venous tributaries, almost like a spider web configuration. If you have the classic Asian type of Budd-Chiari, where there is an IVC web, then a stent is a very good option for those patients. But in the patients we tend to see who have involvement of all the little venous radicals, you really do need TIPS decompression. There's good evidence that if you intervene early with TIPS, you can help prevent some of these patients from needing a liver transplant. But if you don't act quickly and aggressively, cirrhosis can develop pretty quickly.

Chapter 81
HCC Management, Solitary Lesion in a Child's A Cirrhosis

Francisco Durazo

A 63-year-old man with chronic HCV is sent to you with Child's A cirrhosis and a 3-cm mass in the liver with characteristics of an HCC. The patient's overall health is otherwise quite good.

Can you ever consider surgical resection of a hepatoma in a patient with cirrhosis? Is there anything that would make you want to put this patient on a transplant track?

Our current guidelines state that if a patient with Child's A cirrhosis has a single resectable lesion, surgery is the treatment of choice. There is a 50% chance of recurrence after surgical resection, but that means 50% of patients may be cured.

If, instead, you recommend liver transplant, the patient needs to undergo transplant evaluation, go on a waiting list, and will require locoregional therapy as a temporizing bridge to transplant. If he gets transplanted, the patient will be condemned to lifelong immunosuppression.

This patient is a male, and it should be noted that HCC is much more common in males; the management is the same in males and females.

F. Durazo (✉)
Division of Gastroenterology and Hepatology, Department of Medicine, Medical College of Wisconsin, Milwaukee, WI, USA
e-mail: fdurazo@mcw.edu

© The Author(s), under exclusive license to Springer Nature Switzerland AG 2023
W. H. Sobin et al. (eds.), *Managing Complex Cases in Gastroenterology*, https://doi.org/10.1007/978-3-031-48949-5_81

Chapter 82
Management of Unresectable HCC in a Cirrhotic

Francisco Durazo

A 59-year-old male with alcoholic cirrhosis has been abstinent for 5 years and presents with a 6 cm HCC and portal vein thrombosis. The AFP is 400. You had last seen him 3 years ago, at which time ultrasound showed no lesion in the liver. He was subsequently lost to follow-up, until now.

What do you recommend for HCC surveillance?

For patients with cirrhosis, we get an ultrasound and AFP every 6 months. If there is an abnormality on ultrasound, we order a CT or MRI.

Is AFP still recommended for surveillance?

Actually, the American Association for the Study of Liver Diseases (AASLD) "fired" the AFP a while back, but the 2018 recommendations had a soft reintroduction, with the recommendation of surveillance using ultrasound, with or without AFP, every 6 months. However, we still find the AFP to be helpful. There are occasional patients who have a normal ultrasound but an AFP of 1000, so we order an MRI. On MRI, we see the hepatoma that was missed on US. I think that most hepatologists still follow the AFP.

How would you manage this patient if there was no portal vein thrombosis?

We think about possible liver transplant to cure the HCC and cirrhosis, but according to Milan criteria the lesion is too large. Therefore, we would try to downsize the lesion. For lesions under 4 cm in size, ablation with radiofrequency or microwave is effective. For lesions larger than 4 cm, transarterial catheterization and chemoembolization (TACE) or radioembolization, with Yttrium 90 (TARE), are recommended for downsizing, with TARE causing fewer side effects than TACE, although the two modalities have not been compared head-to-head for efficacy.

F. Durazo (✉)
Division of Gastroenterology and Hepatology, Department of Medicine,
Medical College of Wisconsin, Milwaukee, WI, USA
e-mail: fdurazo@mcw.edu

© The Author(s), under exclusive license to Springer Nature
Switzerland AG 2023
W. H. Sobin et al. (eds.), *Managing Complex Cases in Gastroenterology*,
https://doi.org/10.1007/978-3-031-48949-5_82

355

Do you ever see cures with locoregional therapies?

Yes, the lesions may disappear and be absent in the liver explant. In spite of this, transplant is still recommended, because new tumors will form in the cirrhotic liver; you treat one tumor and a new one pops up.

This patient has portal vein thrombosis. In patients with HCC, are the portal vein thrombi assumed to be malignant?

No, benign portal vein thrombosis is common in cirrhotics. Malignant portal vein thrombi are generally easy to differentiate from benign PVT. They are usually contiguous with the HCC, and they take up contrast on CT and MRI, so usually they are easily discernible. The distinction between malignant and benign portal vein thrombosis is important because malignant PVT closes the door on transplant.

How do you manage benign PVT in a transplant candidate?

Some centers will anticoagulate these patients, usually with coumadin. Other centers will take the patient to transplant with a PVT and do thrombectomy at the time of transplant, as long as the PVT does not extend to the SMV (in which case anticoagulation is necessary).

This patient gets therapy with TACE and the lesion shrinks to 3 cm. AFP is 500.

Can you list the patient for transplant now?

Not yet. Once the lesion is downsized and the AFP is under 500, you then have to wait 6 months before giving exception points to the patient. It was found that delaying transplant leads to better outcomes by weeding out those tumors that have the most unfavorable biology. In addition, it was found that hepatomas with an AFP >1000 had a very unfavorable prognosis, leading to the requirement that patients had to have an AFP under 500 to be listed.

Chapter 83
HCC in NAFLD Without Cirrhosis

Francisco Durazo

A 57-year-old, obese female is seen in the community and referred for elevated LFTs and a mass in the liver. Her labs include ALT of 220, AST of 150, Alk phos of 170, and platelets of 180,000. US reveals diffuse steatosis and a 4-cm mass in the liver. All viral and autoimmune serology is negative. CT scan shows a lesion that has characteristic findings of hepatocellular carcinoma and no evidence of cirrhosis. There is no liver nodularity or enlarged spleen nor suggestion of varices.

Do some patients with NAFLD develop HCC without first having cirrhosis?

Over the past 10 years, there have been cases of HCC in patients with NASH without cirrhosis, although it remains uncommon. This is called steatohepatitic hepatocellular carcinoma, a kind of noncirrhotic HCC in patients with underlying fatty liver. Many of these patients have a single-nucleotide polymorphism. We've seen a couple of cases like this at our institution.

How should we be screening for this possibility?

In the absence of warning signals, we continue to screen patients with NAFLD and cirrhosis for HCC every 6 months, but now I am also screening patients with fatty liver without cirrhosis every 12 months with ultrasound and AFP. A number of our colleagues are doing the same thing, to help us all sleep better at night.

F. Durazo (✉)
Division of Gastroenterology and Hepatology, Department of Medicine, Medical College of Wisconsin, Milwaukee, WI, USA
e-mail: fdurazo@mcw.edu

© The Author(s), under exclusive license to Springer Nature Switzerland AG 2023
W. H. Sobin et al. (eds.), *Managing Complex Cases in Gastroenterology*,
https://doi.org/10.1007/978-3-031-48949-5_83

357

Chapter 84
Managing Primary Biliary Cholangitis

Juan Trivella

The patient is a 45-year-old female who's referred for abnormal liver enzymes. She has an alkaline phosphatase of 240 (nl < 80), and her AST is 25, ALT is 30, and bilirubin is 1.0. Her GGTP is three times normal. Her anti-mitochondrial antibody is positive at 1:80, ANA is negative, anti-smooth-muscle antibody is negative, albumin is 3.6, platelets are 210,000, and ultrasound of the liver is normal. The patient doesn't drink alcohol and is on no medications.

Are you comfortable making the diagnosis of primary biliary cholangitis? Do you need a liver biopsy?

Yes, I am comfortable making the diagnosis. This female patient has cholestasis and a clearly positive AMA, with no risk factors for other chronic liver disorders. No liver biopsy is needed in this case. If you are considering a superimposed diagnosis or are unable to stage the degree of fibrosis via noninvasive methods, then I would perform a liver biopsy [1].

It appears that the majority of patients with PBC are asymptomatic at the time of diagnosis. Is that your experience?

Yes, this has been my experience, and although most patients are asymptomatic at diagnosis, almost everyone with PBC will experience symptoms within two decades [2]. The presence or absence of symptoms at diagnosis or on follow-up does not correlate well with the stage of the disease and has shown no difference in survival outcomes.

J. Trivella (✉)
Division of Gastroenterology and Hepatology, Department of Medicine, Medical College of Wisconsin, Milwaukee, WI, USA
e-mail: jtrivella@mcw.edu

© The Author(s), under exclusive license to Springer Nature Switzerland AG 2023
W. H. Sobin et al. (eds.), *Managing Complex Cases in Gastroenterology*, https://doi.org/10.1007/978-3-031-48949-5_84

Primary care providers are more aware of the disease. In turn, patients with chronic cholestasis are referred earlier to the hepatology clinic, and treatment is started before decompensated cirrhosis has ensued. This is why clinical signs and symptoms of portal hypertension are a rather uncommon presentation in patients with PBC nowadays.

Now, we are most aware of PBC occurring in females. Are you seeing it in males, are they being diagnosed later? Is the course more severe in males?

PBC affects people of all sexes, races, and ethnicities. Earlier reports showed a median female-to-male ratio of 10:1, but these were case-finding studies and, therefore, subjected to numerous biases. Modern literature from epidemiologic studies—which, although not perfect, provide a more general vision of the actual number of cases—have shown that the female to male prevalence ratio is closer to 4–6:1 [3, 4].

PBC in males is often diagnosed at an older age once the disease is more advanced. It has also been associated with a lower biochemical response to ursodeoxycholic acid (UDCA), greater progression to cirrhosis, higher rates of liver-related death or transplantation, and higher risk for primary liver cancer [5].

It's important that we continue to create awareness among providers that PBC can affect people from all backgrounds. Being vigilant will lead to an earlier diagnosis, particularly in males and racial minorities, allowing for prompt treatment initiation, which will in turn slow down the rate of progression to cirrhosis.

If patients are diagnosed early with PBC and started on ursodeoxycholic acid immediately, do you find that the vast majority will do well for years, decades even?

Yes, the introduction of ursodeoxycholic acid in the mid-1990s has helped reshape the transplant-free survival in patients with PBC. Those treated with the medication have a survival rate of 90% at 5 years and 66% at 15 years. In the pre-ursodeoxycholic acid era, these percentages were significantly lower with a 79% transplant-free survival at 5 years and 32% at 15 years [6].

Why does ursodeoxycholic acid work so remarkably well for PBC?

Ursodeoxycholic acid is a hydrophilic bile acid that is normally present in human bile at a low concentration (around 3% of the total bile acid pool). When administered orally, only 30–60% is absorbed by the bowel. In the hepatocytes and biliary ducts, ursodeoxycholic acid has anti-inflammatory properties, solubilizes the bile, and stimulates bile flow [7].

When you see patients who are initially doing well but then take a turn for the worse, what sort of symptoms do they usually present with?

Symptoms do not correlate well with the degree of cholestasis or fibrosis, although, observationally, patients with more severe disease tend to have more symptoms.

Symptoms can appear at any point in the disease course, with fatigue being the most common one. It is experienced by about 80% of the patients, and it is very disabling. Fatigue is also very challenging to manage, with no effective medications currently approved for its treatment. The second most frequent symptom is pruritus. It is more intense in the limbs, particularly in the palms and soles, and has a circadian rhythm. It is more intense in the evening and overnight. Pruritus is associated with sleep deprivation, worsening fatigue, depression, social isolation, and self-mutilation, thus leading to significant impairment in quality of life [1].

Sicca complex symptoms, including dry mouth and dry eyes, are usually under reported by patients but are highly prevalent in PBC. Providers should proactively ask about them when following patients with PBC and treat them accordingly [1].

Right upper quadrant abdominal pain is present in about 25–30% of patients. This is a very nonspecific symptom, and other etiologies like gallbladder or pancreatic disease and abdominal/chest wall pathology would have to be excluded before attributing the pain solely to PBC [1].

How do you like to manage pruritus in PBC?

My initial approach consists of utilizing commercially available skin moisturizers, emollients, and topical agents with camphor or menthol. The only currently approved treatment for pruritus in PBC is cholestyramine. This is a bile acid binding resin. It is usually started at a dose of 4 g by mouth per day and can be increased to a maximum of 16 g per day. It is important to remember that cholestyramine can inadvertently bind other medications—particularly ursodeoxycholic acid—when taken at the same time, preventing their absorption. Therefore, it is recommended that cholestyramine should be taken 3–4 h before or after other prescribed drugs. A recent trial utilizing bezafibrate (400 mg by mouth per day) for the management of cholestatic itch showed a 50% reduction in the severity of pruritus in PBC patients treated with this fibrate. This medication can be considered an alternative to cholestyramine, where it is available. Rifampin (150–300 mg PO BID) enhances the rate of bile acid metabolism and increases the excretion of pruritogens. This medication works well in PBC, but its use is off-label, and although very rare, it has been associated with severe hepatitis.

Now, if you have a patient who doesn't tolerate cholestyramine, does colestipol work for pruritus?

Colestipol can be used for PBC since this is also a bile acid binding resin, but it has not been FDA-approved for this particular indication.

She is started on UDCA at a dose of 13–15 mg/kg per day.

When you start ursodeoxycholic acid, when do you want to recheck liver enzymes?

Liver chemistries should be rechecked every 3–6 months in patients treated with ursodeoxycholic acid. Alkaline phosphatase has a log linear association with the risk of liver transplant and death and can be used to monitor response to therapy. There are multiple other scores like the UK-PBC and the GLOBE score that are excellent at estimating outcomes and can be found online. In clinical practice, the goal should be to normalize or near normalize the ALP after 1 year of treatment with UDCA. This is only possible in about two thirds of the patients. Those who do not respond may require the combination of UDCA with other drugs, like obeticholic acid or fibrates, where it is available [8].

In this case, recheck of the alkaline phosphatase at 6 months returns 160 (nl < 80).

Would you change your management?

Although the ALP is still elevated, it is much improved in comparison to her baseline numbers. Since the patient has only been on UDCA for 6 months, I would keep her on this medication. I would make sure that the dose is appropriate to her weight and that she is being compliant with the medication. It is also important to assess for side effects like stomach upset, hair thinning, and weight gain each follow-up visit.

Will you go to a higher dose of ursodeoxycholic acid?

No, the dose of UDCA should range between 13 and 15 mg/kg per day, and higher doses have not shown any benefit in terms of biochemical response or mortality. I would only increase the dose of this medication if it has been miscalculated previously and the patient is being undertreated [9].

The patient remains on ursodeoxycholic acid, and at the end of 1 year, the alkaline phosphatase is 150.

Would you change your treatment?

This is a difficult question to answer since the patient responded well to the medication but did not completely normalize her ALP. Data supports that this near normalization of her ALP should decrease her rate of PBC progression, transplant-free survival, and overall mortality. I would have a discussion with the patient regarding her overall prognosis and pros and cons of starting obeticholic acid (OCA) and come up with a collaborative plan after [10].

Do patients tend to have problems tolerating ursodeoxycholic acid or tolerating obeticholic acid?

Patients usually tolerate ursodeoxycholic acid well. Some patients complain of hair thinning, stomach upset (particularly bloating and diarrhea), and weight gain. UDCA should be taken with food. If patients can't tolerate a single dose of the medication per day, then UDCA can be split into two doses.

OCA is a synthetic bile acid, which acts as a very potent farnesoid X receptor agonist. It was approved by the FDA for the management of PBC patients who respond inadequately to UDCA after 1 year of therapy. Although over 45% of patients achieve a significant ALP improvement with the concomitant use of OCA and UDCA, this medication is associated with pruritus in a dose-dependent fashion, leading to the discontinuation of the drug in up to 25% of patients. This is why OCA should be started at a dose of 5 mg per day and then slowly increase the dose up to 10 mg PO daily. OCA also decreases HDL cholesterol and increases LDL cholesterol independently of the dose. Providers should be aware that OCA is contraindicated in patients with cirrhosis with a Child-Pugh score of B or C and in those with a Child-Pugh score of A who have previous or current clinical evidence of portal hypertension [8].

Can you use it in a grade A cirrhosis?

Yes, you can use it in cirrhotic patients with a Child-Pugh score of A, as long as there is no evidence of portal hypertension. In these patients, the recommended maximum dose is 5 mg PO/daily.

Is it known why OCA might precipitate hepatic decompensation?

I don't think this has been fully clarified. The current black label warning is based on post-marketing reports.

In this case, the alkaline phosphatase drops down to 100 on the combination of OCA and ursodeoxycholic acid.

So, I assume you just continue the two medicines indefinitely?

Yes, I would continue both medications indefinitely.

Besides tracking liver enzymes, how are you following your PBC patients?

The holistic management of PBC should include four different aspects. The first one is the disease treatment per se, which includes the utilization of UDCA and monitoring liver chemistries for response every 3–6 months. The second important aspect is to stage the disease in terms of fibrosis status via elastography. Elastography should be performed every 2–3 years in those PBC patients without evidence of advanced fibrosis at baseline and on a yearly basis in those with evidence of advanced fibrosis at baseline or on follow-up. In general, a liver stiffness measurement below 6.5 kPa or above 11 kPa measured by transient elastography accurately discriminates between the absence or presence of advanced fibrosis respectively with high sensitivity and specificity. Surveillance for hepatocellular carcinoma and esophageal varices should follow the same guideline recommendations that apply for cirrhotic patients from other etiologies. A third important aspect is to address and manage symptoms directly derived from PBC like pruritus, fatigue, and sicca complex. Lastly, patients with cholestasis should be screened and treated for bone disease, dyslipidemia, and liposoluble vitamin deficiencies, particularly if jaundice has ensued [8].

References

1. Lindor KD, Bowlus CL, Boyer J, Levy C, Mayo M. Primary biliary cholangitis: 2018 practice guidance from the American Association for the Study of Liver Diseases. Hepatology. 2019;69(1):394–419.
2. Prince MI, Chetwynd A, Craig WL, Metcalf JV, James OF. Asymptomatic primary biliary cirrhosis: clinical features, prognosis, and symptom progression in a large population based cohort. Gut. 2004;53(6):865–70.
3. Lu M, Zhou Y, Haller IV, Romanelli RJ, VanWormer JJ, Rodriguez CV, et al. Increasing prevalence of primary biliary cholangitis and reduced mortality with treatment. Clin Gastroenterol Hepatol. 2018;16:1342–50.e1.
4. Lleo A, Jepsen P, Morenghi E, Carbone M, Moroni L, Battezzati PM, et al. Evolving trends in female to male incidence and male mortality of primary biliary cholangitis. Sci Rep. 2016;6:25906.
5. John BV, Aitcheson G, Schwartz KB, Khakoo NS, Dahman B, Deng Y, et al. Male sex is associated with higher rates of liver related mortality in primary biliary cholangitis and cirrhosis. Hepatology. 2021;74:879–91.
6. Lammers WJ, van Buuren HR, Hirschfield GM, Janssen HL, Invernizzi P, Mason AL, et al. Levels of alkaline phosphatase and bilirubin are surrogate end points of outcomes of

patients with primary biliary cirrhosis: an international follow-up study. Gastroenterology. 2014;147(6):1338–49.e5; quiz e15.

7. Gulamhusein AF, Hirschfield GM. Primary biliary cholangitis: pathogenesis and therapeutic opportunities. Nat Rev Gastroenterol Hepatol. 2020;17(2):93–110.

8. Trivella J, John BV, Levy C. Primary biliary cholangitis: epidemiology, prognosis, and treatment. Hepatol Commun. 2023;7(6):e0179. https://doi.org/10.1097/HC9.0000000000000179.

9. Angulo P, Jorgensen RA, Lindor KD. Incomplete response to ursodeoxycholic acid in primary biliary cirrhosis: is a double dosage worthwhile? Am J Gastroenterol. 2001;96(11):3152–7.

10. Corpechot C, Poujol-Robert A, Wendum D, Galotte M, Chretien Y, Poupon RE, et al. Biochemical markers of liver fibrosis and lymphocytic piecemeal necrosis in UDCA-treated patients with primary biliary cirrhosis. Liver Int. 2004;24(3):187–93.

Chapter 85
Advanced PBC

Juan Trivella

A 55-year-old female, who hasn't seen a doctor in years, comes in with the complaint of severe itching and fatigue. She drinks only on weekends, two beers a day. She has no stigmata of chronic liver disease on exam. However, her alkaline phosphatase is elevated to 360 (fractionation shows the increase is from the liver), bilirubin is 1.8, albumin is 3.2, AST is 40, ALT is 70, Hbg is 11, platelets is 100k, and AMA is +1:160. US shows mild nodularity of liver. LSM (liver stiffness measurement) is 11 kPa on transient elastography.

Would you want a liver biopsy in this case?

This female patient with classic symptoms for PBC, a predominantly cholestatic pattern of elevated liver chemistries, and a positive AMA does not require a biopsy to make the diagnosis of PBC. Despite this, if the possibility of a concomitant diagnosis is also being considered, for example, metabolic associated steatohepatitis (MetASH), or there are concerns for overlap syndrome with autoimmune hepatitis on additional serologies, then a liver biopsy may be necessary. The combination of findings on US and elastography are concerning for progression to cirrhosis, and the thrombocytopenia could imply the development of portal hypertension. I would feel comfortable managing the patient as such and would obtain the appropriate screening per guidelines and monitor closely her liver chemistries [1].

This patient has an EGD, and there are no varices and no GAVE.

A normal endoscopy in the above scenario would not change the diagnosis of PBC or the presence of at least advanced fibrosis (given the results on elastography). The only aspect that would require further investigation is the thrombocytopenia, since initially this was believed to be secondary to portal hypertension—and

J. Trivella (✉)
Division of Gastroenterology and Hepatology, Department of Medicine, Medical College of Wisconsin, Milwaukee, WI, USA
e-mail: jtrivella@mcw.edu

although this may still be true—the normal upper endoscopy makes this possibility somewhat less likely. An alternative explanation for the low platelets would have to be ruled out.

Would you want to start ursodeoxycholic acid, even if there is advanced cirrhosis?

Yes, absolutely. UDCA improves liver chemistries, delays histological progression, and delays the development of varices. Furthermore, improved survival with the use of UDCA has been shown regardless of sex, fibrosis stage, or even in those with an inadequate response to the medication [2].

Do you monitor the AMA levels during treatment?

No, AMA titers do not correlate with disease activity, severity, or response to therapy and are devoid of prognostic significance. AMA should not be followed longitudinally since its value will not change the patient's management [3].

In this patient, ursodeoxycholic acid is started and the alkaline phosphatase doesn't drop.

Would you add OCA?

To answer this question accurately, additional clinical information is needed, but in general, OCA is indicated in patients with an inadequate response to UDCA after 1 year of monotherapy with this drug. This is exclusively for non-cirrhotics or for those with cirrhosis and a Child's Pugh score no worse than A without previous or current evidence of portal hypertension or decompensated disease [1].

What do you think about using fibrates instead of OCA?

You can consider using fibrates as an off-label add-on therapy for the management of inadequate responders. The caveat is that bezafibrate is not currently commercially available in the United States. Most of the data on the effectiveness of bezafibrate in combination with UDCA comes from Europe and Japan, where this medication has been repurposed for the treatment of PBC and cholestatic itch for years [4]. In the United States, only fenofibrate is available in retail, and data on its use for the management of inadequate responders is considerably less robust.

Although gastrointestinal and musculoskeletal side effects, like myalgias and arthralgias, are more common in patients with PBC on dual UDCA-fibrates, no significant difference in the frequency of serious side effects (including elevations of aminotransferases >5 times the ULN) has been reported when comparing the combined treatment with those on UDCA monotherapy, making this a relatively safe drug for use in PBC.

In this case, the cholesterol comes back 290. LDL is 160.

Is it unusual to see lipid levels like this in PBC, and would you start a statin?

Hyperlipidemia is very common among patients with PBC. At initial presentation, around three quarters of patients with PBC have a cholesterol level >200 mg/dL with a proportion of them also experiencing milder elevations of low-density lipoproteins (LDL) and marked elevations in high-density lipoproteins (HDL). Late-stage disease is associated with marked LDL elevations. Clinically, dyslipidemia alone does not appear to increase the risk of cardiovascular events in patients with PBC and therefore, its management should follow the same criteria that is used to treat lipid disorders in other populations with no history of PBC. In other words, statins are not contraindicated in patients with PBC and should be used as needed and according to the regular dyslipidemia guidelines used in preventive medicine and primary care [5, 6].

So, to summarize, you are going to add OCA to ursodeoxycholic acid and probably start a statin. Are there any other treatments you would start in the meantime?

If this patient is confirmed to have cirrhosis and portal hypertension and her numbers fail to normalize on combination therapy, then a conversation regarding the potential need for liver transplantation will be necessary. This is especially important if her synthetic function continues to deteriorate, or she clinically decompensates. She will also need appropriate hepatocellular carcinoma and esophageal varices screening according to guidelines. The patient will also require symptomatic management for pruritus, sicca complex, and fatigue. Lastly, she should receive appropriate screening for bone disease and liposoluble vitamin deficiencies (the latter only if jaundice is present) and her hepatitis A virus (HAV) and hepatitis B virus (HBV) vaccination status should be addressed.

References

1. Lindor KD, Bowlus CL, Boyer J, Levy C, Mayo M. Primary biliary cholangitis: 2018 practice guidance from the American Association for the Study of Liver Diseases. Hepatology. 2019;69(1):394–419.
2. Shi J, Wu C, Lin Y, Chen YX, Zhu L, Xie WF. Long-term effects of mid-dose ursodeoxycholic acid in primary biliary cirrhosis: a meta-analysis of randomized controlled trials. Am J Gastroenterol. 2006;101(7):1529–38.
3. Levy C, Bowlus CL. Role of antinuclear antibodies in primary biliary cholangitis. Am J Gastroenterol. 2020;115(10):1604–6.
4. Tanaka A, Hirohara J, Nakano T, Matsumoto K, Chazouilleres O, Takikawa H, et al. Association of bezafibrate with transplant free survival in patients with primary biliary cholangitis. J Hepatol. 2021;75:565–71.
5. Assis DN. Chronic complications of cholestasis: evaluation and management. Clin Liver Dis. 2018;22:533–44.
6. Chalifoux SL, Konyn PG, Choi G, Saab S. Extrahepatic manifestations of primary biliary cholangitis. Gut Liver. 2017;11:771–80.

Chapter 86
Autoimmune Hepatitis

Francisco Durazo

The patient is a 24-year-old female with a history of hypothyroidism who presents with weakness. She is on no medications, except oral contraceptives. Her labs reveal an ALT of 520, AST of 319, Alk phos of 80, and bilirubin of 1.0. Hepatitis panel is negative, ANA returns +1:160, and ASMA is +1:80. Gamma globulin is two times normal.

How do you manage this patient?

All things point to this being autoimmune hepatitis, but we want to send the rest of our chronic hepatitis workup for completeness. We need to do a liver biopsy to confirm the diagnosis.

Liver biopsy is consistent with AIH.

What treatment do you recommend for AIH?

We like to start with prednisone monotherapy. Once we see a definite response to steroids, with the liver enzymes improving, we add on azathioprine. We don't start azathioprine initially because we want to ensure that the hepatitis is steroid responsive. If it is not steroid responsive, we may be dealing with a different diagnosis. We start azathioprine at 50 mg. Once azathioprine is started, the goal is to taper the steroids and hopefully maintain the patient on azathioprine monotherapy. Unlike IBD, where doses of azathioprine may be 150 or 200 mg or more, in AIH hepatologists generally don't go above 50 mg. And, unlike in IBD, many hepatologists do not bother checking TPMT status before starting azathioprine.

What about the patient who has autoimmune hepatitis and cirrhosis?

We tend to avoid steroids in the patients with AIH and cirrhosis. The steroids are more likely to promote sodium retention, ascites, and decompensation. So, in

F. Durazo (✉)

Division of Gastroenterology and Hepatology, Department of Medicine, Medical College of Wisconsin, Milwaukee, WI, USA

e-mail: fdurazo@mcw.edu

cirrhotics, we generally use azathioprine monotherapy, or CellCept (mycopheno-late), or just maintenance therapy. In younger patients, AIH tends to present as a more acute hepatitis with very high transaminases and jaundice. In older patients, the disease usually presents as a more chronic hepatitis and a more subacute course, and these patients are more likely to have well-established fibrosis or cirrhosis and portal hypertension.

Chapter 87
Autoimmune Hepatitis

James Esteban

The patient is a 28-year-old female with a history of hypothyroidism due to Hashimoto's disease, who presents with weakness and anorexia for 4 weeks. She has one or two cocktails per weekend. Her only medication is levothyroxine. Her physical exam is fairly unremarkable with a BMI of 20. She has ALT of 420 U/L, AST of 300 U/L, Alk phos of 70 U/L, and a total bilirubin of 1.2 mg/dL. Her viral hepatitis panel is negative. She has elevated IgG at 2200 mg/dL, elevated titers of ANA 1:640, and anti-smooth muscle antibody of 1:160. Anti-mitochondrial antibody is negative.

This case seems fairly clear-cut, in terms of the strongly positive autoimmune markers. What is your approach to the patient with suspected autoimmune hepatitis (AIH)?

Even though the patient has classic liver biochemistries (hepatocellular) and autoantibodies, I will still obtain a liver biopsy. The liver biopsy is necessary to establish the diagnosis, evaluate concurrent liver disease (for example, NASH or alcohol), and define a baseline for future comparisons if the patient does not respond to corticosteroids and first-line immunomodulator therapy.

This patient's liver biopsy shows interface hepatitis with a dense infiltrate of plasma cells. She has minimal hepatic steatosis and hepatic fibrosis (stage 1). You start the patient on prednisone 60 mg a day, and the patient's liver enzymes start improving immediately, but the patient also complains of mood swings and insomnia.

J. Esteban (✉)
Division of Gastroenterology and Hepatology, Department of Medicine, Medical College of Wisconsin, Milwaukee, WI, USA
e-mail: jesteban@mcw.edu

How would you manage this adverse side effect?

I would see how she does on a slightly lower dose of prednisone, perhaps 40 mg a day. I will do labs weekly and try to taper her prednisone dose further as soon as her transaminases improve. I start azathioprine once I have prednisone down to 20–30 mg a day, and this may help speed up the prednisone taper.

Another option is budesonide. A 9 mg dose of budesonide is 30–40 mg of prednisone, but due to 90% first-pass metabolism in the liver, budesonide is considered a "topical" steroid and has much fewer steroid-related side effects than prednisone. Budesonide is at least as effective (possibly more effective based on trials) than prednisone in inducing and maintaining biochemical remission in non-cirrhotic patients with AIH [1].

The patient is started on budesonide 9 mg a day, and the steroid side effects cease. Her liver enzymes continue improving.

Would you add azathioprine at this point? If so, what dose do you give? Do you bother to check the TPMT status?

Once I verify a positive response to corticosteroids, I add on azathioprine (or 6-mercaptopurine, 6-MP). Since azathioprine can cause drug-induced liver injury (either related to 6-MMP metabolites or as an idiosyncratic reaction), I prefer to start azathioprine only when transaminases are normal to prevent diagnostic confusion.

I start azathioprine at 50 mg a day. I send off a thiopurine methyltransferase (TPMT) activity to identify that rare patient who will have zero or near-zero TPMT activity who will suffer from severe myelosuppression with azathioprine. Because this test takes time to result, I send it out as soon as AIH is diagnosed. The AASLD recommends sending TPMT activity [2].

The intent is for azathioprine (or 6-MP) to be the long-term, steroid-sparing maintenance regimen for AIH. For this reason, I continue to taper prednisone down to a dose of prednisone 5 mg. I try to discontinue prednisone altogether to keep patients on azathioprine (or 6-MP) monotherapy for maintenance, and I have reasonable success. Azathioprine at a dose of 50 mg is often sufficient, but I have gone up to 75–150 mg of azathioprine if patients experience small flare-ups in their transaminases. In some cases, the only way to keep patients in remission is through combination therapy of azathioprine and low-dose prednisone, 5–10 mg daily.

The patient's TPMT phenotype returns normal, and you start azathioprine 50 mg a day. However, 2 weeks later the patient develops severe pain, goes to the ER, and is found to have acute pancreatitis. Azathioprine is stopped.

Do you have any experience using mycophenolate or tacrolimus in this situation?

Mycophenolate mofetil (MMF) and mycophenolic acid (MPA) are my second-line agents for patients who do not tolerate or do not respond to azathioprine. Mycophenolate is particularly effective if the reason for withdrawing azathioprine was intolerance, rather than treatment nonresponse. However, mycophenolate is a category X drug in pregnancy, thus at our patient's age, she needs to use at least two forms of effective contraception.

Calcineurin inhibitors (CNI), like tacrolimus and cyclosporine, and biologics are also second-line agents for patients who are refractory to or intolerant of azathioprine or steroids. I almost never have had to use these agents in my non-transplant AIH patients, but there are studies showing CNIs as effective agents in normalizing transaminases.

Working in the community, we do not have much experience with mycophenolate. What is the dose you use, and what are the side effects?

You can use a bottom-up approach, starting at 500 mg BID of MMF (or 360 mg BID of MPA), and then gradually make your way up to 1000 mg BID of MMF (or 720 mg BID of MPA) based on the patient's response. You can also use a top-down approach, especially if the patient has higher transaminase levels, where you start at 1000 mg BID of MMF until you're able to induce and maintain biochemical remission, and then gradually make your way down to the minimum effective dose. The most common side effects of MMF are GI upset (e.g., nausea, vomiting, abdominal pain, diarrhea) and cytopenias.

The patient says she hopes to get pregnant in the next year or two. What options do you have?

If she hopes to get pregnant, my options are to either keep her on steroid monotherapy, since she responded to that, or use CNIs such as tacrolimus or cyclosporine instead of mycophenolate. Both are pregnancy category C. Azathioprine is category D but may be continued during pregnancy to prevent a flare-up.

For tacrolimus, a good starting dose is 0.1 mg/kg/day divided into two doses, which roughly translates to 2–3 mg BID [3]. For cyclosporine, a good starting dose is 2–3 mg/kg/day, which roughly translates to 100–150 mg BID [4]. Both tacrolimus and cyclosporine require drug-level monitoring to ensure efficacy and prevent toxicities. Drug-level monitoring requires blood testing at the same time of day, typically in the morning before taking the first dose of the day. Patients would likely need higher drug levels to induce remission (tacrolimus 6–8 ng/dL, cyclosporine 100–150 ng/dL), which could be lowered after a few months to a year of remission for maintenance (tacrolimus 4–6 ng/dL, cyclosporine 100–150 ng/dL).

The main side effects of CNIs are nephrotoxicity, neurotoxicity, and metabolic dysfunction, such as diabetes, hyperlipidemia, hypertension, and weight gain.

There are patients with AIH who have cirrhosis on their initial liver biopsy, occurring in about 30% of cases. Is this fairly uncommon in young patients presenting with AIH?

It is. Cirrhosis as the presenting phenotype of AIH is usually seen in older patients and African-Americans.

Is it true that if you have full-blown cirrhosis, you may already have burned out AIH and you may choose not to treat it?

Some patients with AIH and cirrhosis will have normal to mildly elevated transaminases and minimal inflammation on biopsy and would be labeled as "burned out" AIH. I think it would be reasonable to withhold immunosuppressive treatment for these patients because any potential benefit is not worth treatment-related side effects. These patients should continue to have periodic assessment of liver chemistries.

Some patients will have normal transaminases but will continue to have inflammatory activity on biopsy. I would treat these patients with maintenance immunosuppression to prevent progression of fibrosis (and thus portal hypertension and hepatic decompensation) and a severe, acute flare-up of AIH. We avoid azathioprine in patients with decompensated cirrhosis.

References

1. Manns M, Woynarowski M, Kreisel W, Lurie Y, Rust C, Zuckerman E, et al. Budesonide induces remission more effectively than prednisone in a controlled trial of patients with autoimmune hepatitis. Gastroenterology. 2010;139(4):1198–206.
2. Mack CL, Adams D, Assis DN, Kerkar N, Manns MP, Mayo MJ, et al. Diagnosis and management of autoimmune hepatitis in adults and children: 2019 practice guidance and guidelines from the American Association for the Study of Liver Diseases. Hepatology. 2020;72(2):671–722.
3. Hanouneh M, Ritchie MM, Ascha M, Ascha MS, Chedid A, Sanguankeo A, et al. A review of the utility of tacrolimus in the management of adults with autoimmune hepatitis. Scand J Gastroenterol. 2019;54(1):76–80.
4. Fernandes NF, Redeker AG, Vierling JM, Villamil FG, Fong TL. Cyclosporine therapy in patients with steroid resistant autoimmune hepatitis. Am J Gastroenterol. 1999;94(1):241–8.

Chapter 88
Primary Sclerosing Cholangitis

Juan Trivella

A 38-year-old male is referred because of elevated liver enzymes. He has one or two drinks a week, does not use any drugs, and is on no medications. He has mild itching, no belly pain, and no jaundice. He has an alkaline phosphatase of 240, GGT of 200, ALT of 60, AST of 45, bilirubin of 0.9, INR of 1.1, WBC of 4.3, Hgb of 11.8, platelets of 180,000, and albumin of 3.5. Ultrasound of the liver shows normal-appearing liver, normal gallbladder, and CBD of 8 mm in diameter. Hepatitis panel is negative, ANA is (+)1:16, ASMA is (−), and AMA is (−). An MRCP is performed and this demonstrates ductal narrowing both intra- and extrahepatic.

What is your diagnosis and what other tests would you want?

The presence of cholestasis and intra- and extrahepatic ductal narrowing on MRCP in a male patient who has no other previous history of biliary or liver pathology suggests the diagnosis of PSC, but careful exclusion of secondary causes of sclerosing cholangitis is required—especially in the absence of IBD. The negative AMA and the presence of intra- and extrahepatic ductal beading makes PBC unlikely. It is not uncommon to have a slight elevation of transaminases in PSC, like in the case presented above. The diagnosis of overlap AIH-PSC should be considered only when the transaminases approach five times the upper limit of normal or when these are the predominant pattern of elevation. It would also be important to order an IgG4 to exclude IgG4 sclerosing cholangitis as a potential diagnosis. A baseline CA19-9 and a colonoscopy to evaluate for inflammatory bowel disease should also be obtained [1].

J. Trivella (✉)
Division of Gastroenterology and Hepatology, Department of Medicine, Medical College of Wisconsin, Milwaukee, WI, USA
e-mail: jtrivella@mcw.edu

What is the current role of colonoscopy in PSC, both IgG4 positive and negative?

In patients with PSC without a known history of IBD, a diagnostic colonoscopy with histologic sampling should be performed at the diagnosis of PSC and then every 5 years if IBD is not initially detected, or earlier if the patient develops gastrointestinal symptoms to suggest IBD. Colon cancer surveillance should begin at age 15 years in patients with PSC and IBD and should be repeated yearly, given their higher risk for developing colorectal cancer.

Is that true for IgG4 sclerosing cholangitis?

No. Although there is paucity of data regarding the course of IgG4 sclerosing cholangitis, given its rarity, no strong association with IBD and/or colorectal cancer has been established. Therefore, surveillance colonoscopy is not currently recommended for these patients.

What is the role of ursodeoxycholic acid in PSC?

The efficacy of UDCA in PSC has not been consistent, despite this being the most studied drug for this particular disease. Low-dose UDCA (13–15 mg/kg/day) has shown an improvement in ALP (in those with baseline elevated ALP) but has shown no benefits on liver histology or transplant-free survival. High-dose UDCA (28–30 mg/kg/day) should be avoided in patients with PSC, given the high risk for serious adverse events.

Intermediate-dose UDCA (17–23 mg/kg/day) has shown both ALP and histological improvement in a proportion of patients with PSC, but research has failed to demonstrate a statistically significant reduction in the need for liver transplantation, cholangiocarcinoma, or overall mortality. This is with the caveat that most of these reports have been underpowered. Medical societies like the AASLD currently support trials of intermediate-dose UDCA in PSC patients with baseline elevated ALP. This medication can be continued lifelong if the patient experiences improvement of symptoms and/or a meaningful alkaline phosphatase reduction after 12 months of treatment [1].

How do you do surveillance studies in PSC?

Cholangiocarcinoma and gallbladder carcinoma surveillance should be performed annually and include MRI/MRCP and a CA19-9. Surveillance is currently not recommended for patients with PSC who are younger than 18 years of age or in those with exclusively small duct PSC.

In this case, the patient remains stable for a couple of years, with a stable MRCP and CA19-9, and then, without explanation, his alkaline phosphatase goes up to 350, and his bilirubin goes up to 3. Another MRCP is performed, and there's a dominant stricture in the common bile duct.

How would you manage this?

This patient was found to have a relevant stricture on MRI/MRCP and should receive an ERCP. ERCP is indicated for the evaluation of relevant strictures as well as for the evaluation of new onset or worsening of pruritus, unexplained weight loss, worsening serum liver chemistry abnormalities, rising CA19-9, recurrent bacterial cholangitis, or progressive ductal dilatation on MRI/MRCP surveillance.

On ERCP brushings of the stricture are performed. Cytology returns suspicious and FISH cytology is pending.

The first step should be to wait for the FISH analysis to return. If negative, then the patient should receive a repeat ERCP in 3 months. If positive, this case should be discussed with a multidisciplinary team that includes pancreaticobiliary and transplant surgery. Depending on the location of the stricture (intrahepatic vs. hilar vs. distal CBD), this patient may qualify for resection or liver transplantation.

Can you do a liver transplant in a PSC patient who has a cholangiocarcinoma?

The management of cholangiocarcinoma in patients with PSC depends on several factors. The size and the location of the primary tumor in the biliary tree is one of them. Well-selected patients with PSC and perihilar early-stage cholangiocarcinoma can be considered for liver transplantation and can even qualify for exception points after a rigorous process that involves close monitoring for metastatic disease, neoadjuvant chemoradiation, and pretransplant staging laparoscopy. This is commonly referred to as the "Mayo protocol" and has shown an overall survival of around 65% and a recurrence-free survival close to 80% at 5 years [2].

Early studies evaluating liver transplantation in patients with intrahepatic cholangiocarcinoma showed a posttransplant recurrence in up to 25% and an overall survival of about 40% at 5 years, making this approach undesirable for quite some time. Most recently, retrospective data looking at liver explants of patients with PSC and an incidentally found, small (<3 cm), solitary intrahepatic cholangiocarcinoma showed an overall survival of around 61% and a recurrence-free survival of 75% at 5 years. This has prompted different centers around the country to develop prospective research protocols to reevaluate LT as a possibility for those with a single small liver lesion. Results from these trials are eagerly awaited.

Distal cholangiocarcinomas are best treated with surgical resection when possible, removing the bile duct, gallbladder, head of the pancreas, and the first portion of the duodenum (pancreaticoduodenectomy). There is currently no role for liver transplantation in patients with distal cholangiocarcinoma.

References

1. Bowlus CL, Arrivé L, Bergquist A, Deneau M, Forman L, Ilyas SI, Lunsford KE, Martinez M, Sapisochin G, Shroff R, Tabibian JH, Assis DN. AASLD practice guidance on primary sclerosing cholangitis and cholangiocarcinoma. Hepatology. 2023;77(2):659–702. https://doi.org/10.1002/hep.32771.
2. Rosen CB, Heimbach JK, Gores GJ. Surgery for cholangiocarcinoma: the role of liver transplantation. HPB (Oxford). 2008;10(3):186–9. https://doi.org/10.1080/13651820801992542.

Chapter 89
PBC-AIH Overlap

Juan Trivella

A 35-year-old female is referred for lethargy and elevated LFTs. Her alkaline phosphatase is 320, AST is 289, ALT is 391, and bilirubin is 1.2. He is in no ETOH or meds. AMA +1:320, ANA +1:160, ASMA +1:80, IgG 2200.

What is your diagnosis, and do you want a liver biopsy?

The information provided suggests a diagnosis of PBC-AIH overlap syndrome. Although there is no standardized definition, this clinical entity is commonly characterized by clinical, histologic, and serologic features of both autoimmune hepatitis and PBC, ensuing either simultaneously or sequentially.

According to the Paris criteria, which has a sensitivity of 92% and specificity of 97% for the diagnosis of overlap syndrome, two out of three key features for the diagnosis of PBC and AIH, respectively, should be met to establish the diagnosis. One of these is the presence of interface hepatitis and/or the presence of florid bile duct lesions on histology. A liver biopsy in the case presented is not only indicated to establish the diagnosis of overlap syndrome but also to exclude other potential explanations for her elevated liver chemistries and to stage the fibrosis status of her liver [1].

Liver biopsy is performed and shows granulomas with bile duct inflammation and also mild interface hepatitis with lymphocytes and plasma cells.

Would you start the patient on ursodeoxycholic acid alone, steroids alone, or a combination?

The therapeutic approach for overlap syndrome has not been completely defined because its low prevalence prevents the performance of large randomized clinical trials. Most agree that the treatment should be directed toward the predominant

J. Trivella (✉)
Division of Gastroenterology and Hepatology, Department of Medicine, Medical College of Wisconsin, Milwaukee, WI, USA
e-mail: jtrivella@mcw.edu

© The Author(s), under exclusive license to Springer Nature Switzerland AG 2023
W. H. Sobin et al. (eds.), *Managing Complex Cases in Gastroenterology*,
https://doi.org/10.1007/978-3-031-48949-5_89

component, particularly when patients do not completely meet Paris criteria. The rationale for this approach comes from the premise that rather than being two separate disorders occurring in parallel, overlap syndrome appears to be the result of a single disease with atypical features. In these circumstances, steroids or UDCA induce biochemical response when selected toward the predominant phenotype. In those who meet Paris criteria, combination therapy with immunosuppression and UDCA has proven to be superior in achieving biochemical response than either of them alone. Since this patient meets all Paris criteria, then combination therapy would be more appropriate [2, 3].

What steroid would you use?

Both prednisone and prednisolone can be used for the management of overlap syndrome in combination with UDCA. Steroids should be tapered slowly to about 10 mg daily after 4 weeks of treatment to decrease the risk of adverse events.

Would you add azathioprine as you attempt to taper steroids?

Yes, I would attempt this. Given the low prevalence of PBC-AIH overlap syndrome, guidelines for its long-term treatment lack robust evidence. Despite this, azathioprine has successfully been used as the long-term immunosuppressive agent of choice for those with AIH. It would be reasonable to extrapolate this information to patients with overlap syndrome, especially when considering the adverse events that are commonly associated with long-term steroid use.

References

1. Lindor KD, Bowlus CL, Boyer J, Levy C, Mayo M. Primary biliary cholangitis: 2018 practice guidance from the American Association for the Study of Liver Diseases. Hepatology. 2019;69(1):394–419.
2. Chazouilleres O, Wendum D, Serfaty L, Montembault S, Rosmorduc O, Poupon R. Primary biliary cirrhosis–autoimmune hepatitis overlap syndrome: clinical features and response to therapy. Hepatology. 1998;28:296–301.
3. Kuiper EM, Zondervan PE, van Buuren HR. Paris criteria are effective in diagnosis of primary biliary cirrhosis and autoimmune hepatitis overlap syndrome. Clin Gastroenterol Hepatol. 2010;8:530–4.

Chapter 90
Immune-Tolerant Chronic HBV

James Esteban

A 24-year-old male, born in the United States and whose parents emigrated from Taiwan, is evaluated in the clinic for a hepatitis B infection. This was detected when he went to donate blood at a blood drive. He has no history of intravenous drug use, tattoos, or blood transfusions. He is in a monogamous sexual relationship with a female spouse. He is asymptomatic and has normal transaminases. He is hepatitis B surface antigen (HBsAg) positive with an HBV DNA of 10 million IU/mL. His total hepatitis B core antibody (anti-HBc total) is positive, and the anti-HBc IgM is negative. He is hepatitis B envelope antigen positive (HBeAg).

How would you describe the phase of the patient's hepatitis B infection?

We first have to establish the chronicity of hepatitis B infection. Chronic hepatitis B is the presence of hepatitis B surface antigen and HBV viremia for at least 6 months. The absence of significant hepatocellular liver injury and anti-HBc IgM strongly suggests chronic hepatitis B. I would make sure to repeat HBV serologies, HBV DNA, and liver enzymes in the next 3–6 months to verify chronic hepatitis B.

After we have established chronic hepatitis B, we need to determine the phase of HBV infection the patient is experiencing. In the immune-tolerant phase, there is normal ALT, minimal to no hepatic inflammation, and high HBV DNA viral load. Immune-tolerant hepatitis B is commonly seen in perinatally or vertically acquired infection, which is potentially the route of transmission for our patient. These patients are typically HBeAg-positive.

J. Esteban (✉)
Division of Gastroenterology and Hepatology, Department of Medicine, Medical College of Wisconsin, Milwaukee, WI, USA
e-mail: jesteban@mcw.edu

© The Author(s), under exclusive license to Springer Nature Switzerland AG 2023
W. H. Sobin et al. (eds.), *Managing Complex Cases in Gastroenterology*, https://doi.org/10.1007/978-3-031-48949-5_90

It is my impression that immune-tolerant chronic hepatitis B refers to the fact that the immune system does not recognize the hepatitis B virus as a foreign invader. This is a unique situation where the virus keeps replicating, undisturbed by the immune system, and you can have hundreds of thousands, or even millions of viral particles present with totally normal liver enzymes. If you were to do a liver biopsy, there would be no signs of liver damage. Is that correct?

This is the expected finding. The immune-tolerant phase of chronic HBV is thought to be the result of reduced responsiveness of immunologic T cells to the virus, which leads to unrestricted hepatitis B viral replication and, thus, high HBV DNA viral load. Liver injury in chronic hepatitis B is the result of immune-mediated (e.g., cytotoxic T cells, NK cells, and neutrophils) cell and tissue injury. Therefore, a hypoactive immune response also means that there is little to no liver injury, which explains the typically normal transaminases in immune-tolerant chronic hepatitis B.

Would you start antiviral therapy?

AASLD [1] and EASL [2] do not recommend starting antiviral treatment in immune-tolerant chronic hepatitis B infection, unless the patient has any of the following:

1. Cirrhosis
2. Extrahepatic manifestations (usually immune-mediated) of HBV infection such as vasculitis, purpura, polyarteritis nodosa, arthralgias, neuropathy, and glomerulonephritis
3. Receiving immunosuppressive therapy
4. Pregnant women with HBV DNA >200,000 IU/mL in the third trimester to help prevent mother-to-child transmission of HBV (tenofovir disoproxil fumarate is the preferred antiviral medicine in pregnancy)

We are not starting antiviral therapy. How would you monitor this patient after this initial encounter?

In these patients, liver chemistries and HBV DNA should be monitored every 3–6 months to determine if they are transitioning to the immune-active or chronic inactive phases of infection. Increasing transaminases warrants more frequent monitoring. Patients should meet criteria for immune-active chronic hepatitis B (ALT $>2 \times$ ULN and HBV DNA >20,000 IU/mL if HBeAg-positive and >2000 if HBeAg-negative) for at least 3–6 months before committing to antiviral therapy, since it is possible that increased immunologic activity may lead to viral clearance and entry into the chronic inactive phase of infection.

Some patients will have elevated transaminases that are less than 2× the upper limit of normal. In addition to further testing to ensure that they do not have other causes of liver disease, such as metabolic dysfunction or alcohol-associated fatty liver diseases, liver biopsy and/or elastography should be considered for these patients because significant inflammation or fibrosis will warrant antiviral therapy.

What other issues need to be addressed for this patient?

Certain subpopulations of patients with chronic hepatitis B should undergo regular screening for hepatocellular carcinoma (HCC) with abdominal imaging (e.g., ultrasound, CT or MRI) and a-fetoprotein every 6 months. Subpopulations who should undergo regular HCC screening are:

1. All patients with cirrhosis
2. Asian and Black men above 40 years old, irrespective of cirrhosis
3. Asian women above 50 years old, irrespective of cirrhosis
4. First-degree relatives with HCC, irrespective of cirrhosis

Patients with immune-tolerant chronic hepatitis B are highly viremic and are therefore very contagious. Sexual partners and household members of the patient should be screened for chronic hepatitis B with HBsAg and anti-HBs testing. Uninfected and nonimmune sexual partners and household members should complete the hepatitis B vaccine series, followed by repeat anti-HBs testing to ensure an adequate response to the vaccine.

The patient should also be counseled the following:

1. Use barrier contraception if their sexual partner is not vaccinated or naturally immunized
2. Not to share toothbrushes and razors
3. Not to share injection equipment, including glucose testing equipment for diabetics
4. Cover all open cuts and scratches
5. Clean blood spills with bleach solution
6. Not to donate blood, organs, or sperm

Is there a certain age when you would start antivirals in a patient with immune-tolerant phase chronic hepatitis B?

AASLD [1] recommends liver biopsy in patients with immune-tolerant chronic hepatitis B aged 40 years and above, especially those infected at a young age and with very elevated HBV viral load (HBV DNA >1 million IU/mL) to assess severity of inflammation and fibrosis. Immune-tolerant hepatitis B patients with at least moderate inflammation and/or stage 2 fibrosis should receive antiviral therapy. These patients could alternatively undergo noninvasive testing of hepatic fibrosis through elastography first. Patients with significant fibrosis (i.e., F2 or greater) on elastography should warrant antiviral therapy.

EASL [2] is more aggressive and recommends antiviral therapy in patients with immune-tolerant hepatitis B age 30 years and above, regardless of the severity of liver histologic lesions.

References

1. Terrault N, Lok ASF, McMahon BJ, Chang KM, Hwang JP, Jonas MM, et al. Update on prevention, diagnosis, and treatment of chronic hepatitis B: AASLD 2018 hepatitis B guidance. Hepatology. 2018;67(4):1560–99.
2. European Association for the Study of the Liver. EASL 2017 clinical practice guidelines on the management of hepatitis B virus infection. J Hepatol. 2017;67(2):370–98.

Chapter 91
Immune-Active Chronic HBV

James Esteban

A 30-year-old Asian male has had a diagnosis of chronic hepatitis B since his teen years. His mother also has chronic hepatitis B. He previously had normal transaminases, HBV viral load ranging from 10 to 20 million IU/mL, and positive HBeAg. On routine testing 3 months ago, he was found to have elevated transaminases (ALT of 140, AST of 80). His HBV DNA remains elevated, but at a lower level than previously, currently at around 100,000 IU/mL. On repeat testing today, he continues to have elevated transaminases (ALT of 120, AST of 80) and elevated HBV DNA (90,000 IU/mL). He remains HBeAg-positive.

The fact that his liver chemistries increased to more than twice the upper limit normal while maintaining significant hepatitis B viremia indicates that he has evolved into immune-active chronic hepatitis B. Can you explain the significance of the positive HBeAg and the usual transition to negative HBeAg?

The hepatitis B envelope antigen (HBeAg) is a hepatitis B viral protein that indicates active viral replication. Thus, patients who are HBeAg-positive typically have very high titers of HBV DNA in serum. HBeAg-positive infection, particularly in younger persons, will have normal or near-normal transaminases, because HBV does not have a direct cytopathic effect and does not cause liver inflammation on its own. This is known as the immune-tolerant phase of chronic hepatitis B infection, where the body's T-cell-mediated response to the virus is thought to be blunted.

J. Esteban (✉)

Division of Gastroenterology and Hepatology, Department of Medicine, Medical College of Wisconsin, Milwaukee, WI, USA

e-mail: jesteban@mcw.edu

The body may attempt to clear the virus at some point through an immune-mediated and inflammatory response, which leads to hepatic injury and inflammation, causing a rise in transaminases and eventually hepatic fibrosis if left unabated. HBV DNA titers remain elevated, but typically not at the same magnitude as in the immune-tolerant phase. This is known as the immune-active phase of chronic hepatitis B infection.

The immune-active phase of chronic hepatitis infection is defined by the AASLD as [1]:

1. HBsAg-positive for at least 6 months
2. ALT or AST > 2× upper limit of normal, defined as 35 U/L in males and 25 U/L in females
3. HBV DNA >20,000 IU/mL in HBeAg-positive hepatitis B and >2000 IU/mL in HBeAg-negative hepatitis B

The immune-active phase can lead to a couple of possible outcomes. The patient can continue to have viral replication (HBeAg-positive, high HBV DNA) with continuing liver injury and inflammation, and this warrants antiviral therapy. On the other hand, the immune system may succeed in suppressing the infection, which can lead to loss of HBeAg and low HBV DNA viral loads (defined as <2000 IU/mL), indicating suppression of viral replication and improving liver chemistries. This is known as the inactive phase of chronic hepatitis B infection. Spontaneous HBeAg seroconversion, which is a way of saying that HBeAg is lost and anti-HBe antibodies have appeared, occurs in 15% of cases per year [2]. Some patients may lose hepatitis B surface antigen (HBsAg) altogether, representing a functional cure of the infection, but this occurs much more rarely at a rate of 1–2% per year [3].

A few patients will have lost HBeAg but will continue to have active viral replication (i.e., high HBV DNA) and hepatic inflammation (i.e., ALT >2× ULN). These patients have HBeAg-negative, immune-active chronic hepatitis B, and typically mutations in the precore or basal core promoter region of the HBV genome.

You decide that the patient has immune-active chronic hepatitis B and will need antiviral therapy. What are the options and what would you recommend for the patient?

AASLD [1] and EASL [4] recommend antiviral therapy in patients with immune-active hepatitis B (Fig. 91.1). (Note: "Chronic hepatitis B" is the EASL nomenclature for immune-active hepatitis B, while "chronic HBV infection" is the EASL nomenclature for immune-tolerant hepatitis B) Antiviral therapy is also recommended in all patients with cirrhosis and in patients who have significant inflammation or fibrosis on liver biopsy or elastography, regardless of ALT and HBV DNA titers.

Patients who have elevated transaminases, but do not quite meet criteria for immune-active hepatitis B, should undergo further evaluation for other liver diseases. They should also be considered for liver biopsy or elastography. The presence of significant hepatic inflammation and fibrosis stage 2 or greater warrants antiviral treatment. Antiviral therapy is not recommended in most patients with immune-tolerant hepatitis B, and this is discussed in a separate chapter.

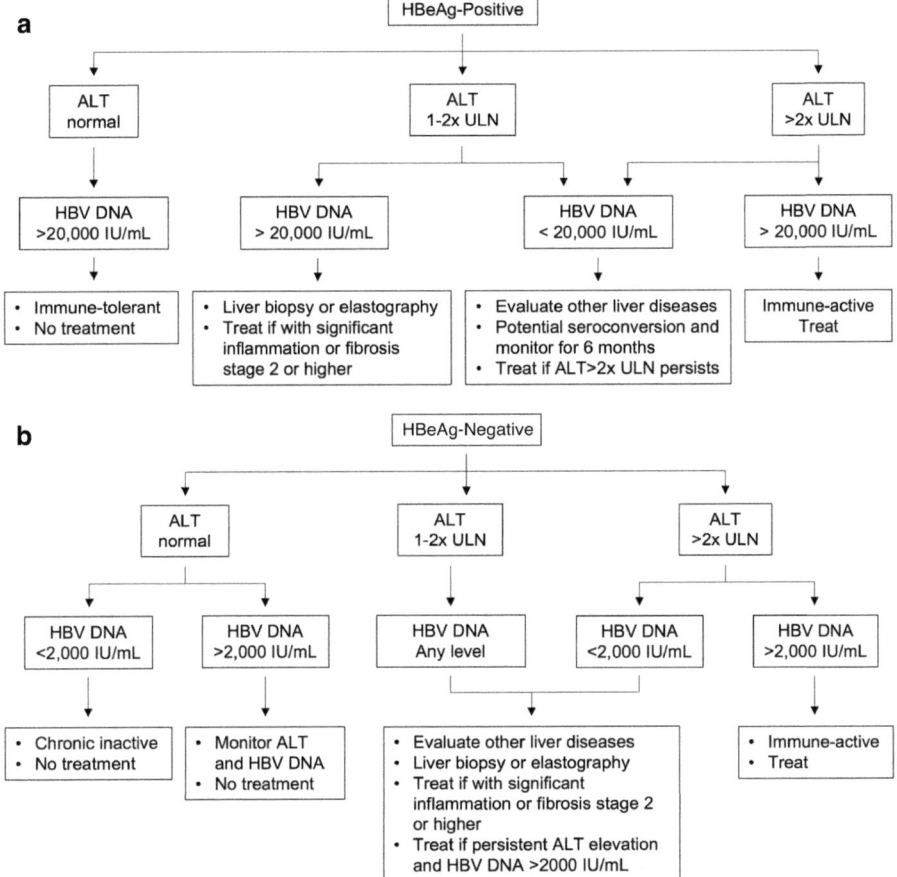

Fig. 91.1 Treatment algorithm for chronic hepatitis B according to HBeAg status. (**a**) HBeAg-positive. (**b**) HBeAg-negative

The two treatment options for chronic hepatitis B include pegylated interferon (PEG-IFNa) and nucleos(t)ide analogs (NA). Earlier generation NAs (lamivudine, telbivudine, adefovir) have a low genetic barrier to resistance. Newer NAs (entecavir, tenofovir disoproxil fumarate [TDF], tenofovir alafenamide [TAF]) have high genetic barriers to resistance and are the recommended first-line antiviral therapy for chronic hepatitis B. In all honesty, we can choose either entecavir, TDF, or TAF for our patient.

PEG-IFNa has the advantages of finite treatment duration (48 weeks) and slightly higher rates of HBsAg loss, but significant side effects limit its wider use in clinical practice, relative to entecavir and tenofovir. PEG-IFNa is contraindicated in decompensated cirrhosis and acute liver failure.

The patient has normal kidney function. He underwent vibration-controlled transient elastography (VCTE or FibroScan®), which showed liver stiffness of 5 kPa (F0). You recommend starting the patient on tenofovir disoproxil fumarate (TDF) 400 mg once daily.

The patient asks about the effectiveness of TDF and possible long-term side effects.

The effectiveness of TDF and other NAs in clinical trials are summarized below [4]:

	Entecavir	TDF	TAF
HBeAg-positive			
Anti-HBe seroconversion	21%	21%	10%
HBV DNA suppression	67%	76%	64%
ALT normalization	68%	68%	72%
HBsAg loss	2%	3%	1%
HBeAg-negative			
Anti-HBe seroconversion	N/A	N/A	N/A
HBV DNA suppression	90%	93%	94%
ALT normalization	78%	76%	83%
HBsAg loss	0%	0%	0%

Long-term treatment with NA, specifically due to result of suppression of viral replication, halts the progression of liver disease, improves hepatic fibrosis (potentially even regression of cirrhosis) and hepatic recompensation in cases of decompensated cirrhosis, reduces the need for liver transplantation, and reduces the risk of HCC [5].

TDF has been associated with renal dysfunction, including Fanconi syndrome, and bone mineral density loss. Entecavir or TAF are preferred in older patients (age >60 years), patients with established osteopenia or osteoporosis or at risk for these conditions (e.g., long-term use of corticosteroids), and patients with renal dysfunction (e.g., estimated GFR <60 mL/min/1.73 m^2, established albuminuria).

After 9 months on TDF, he becomes HBeAg-negative and develops anti-HBe. His transaminases normalize and HBV DNA becomes undetectable.

Would you consider stopping TDF in this patient now or in the near future?

I would have him continue TDF for an additional 12 months as consolidation therapy. If transaminases remain normal and HBV DNA remain undetectable at the end of consolidation therapy—assuming repeat VCTE or FibroScan® continues to show absence of significant fibrosis, he does not have extrahepatic manifestations, and he is not receiving immunosuppressive therapy of any kind—then, yes, I will consider discontinuing TDF. I would obtain transaminases and HBV DNA every 3 months for at least a year to make sure that he does not experience a relapse and hepatitis flare-up.

The majority of initially HBeAg-positive patients who seroconvert remain in remission [6]. Treatment discontinuation is discussed in more detail in another chapter.

References

1. Terrault N, Lok ASF, McMahon BJ, Chang KM, Hwang JP, Jonas MM, et al. Update on prevention, diagnosis, and treatment of chronic hepatitis B: AASLD 2018 hepatitis B guidance. Hepatology. 2018;67(4):1560–99.
2. Dusheiko G, Agarwal KM, Maini MK. New approaches to chronic hepatitis B. N Engl J Med. 2023;388(1):55–69.
3. Yeo YH, Ho HJ, Yang HI, Tseng TC, Hosaka T, Trinh HY, et al. Factors associated with rates of HBsAg Seroclearance in adults with chronic HBV infection: a systematic review and meta-analysis. Gastroenterology. 2019;156(3):635–646.e9.
4. European Association for the Study of the Liver. EASL 2017 clinical practice guidelines on the management of hepatitis B virus infection. J Hepatol. 2017;67(2):370–98.
5. Su TH, Hu TH, Chen CY, Huang YH, Chuang WL, Lin CC, et al. Four-year entecavir therapy reduces hepatocellular carcinoma, cirrhotic events and mortality in chronic hepatitis B patients. Liver Int. 2016;36(12):1755–64.
6. Papatheodoridis G, Vlachogiannakos I, Cholongitas E, Wursthorn K, Thomadakis C, Touloumi G, et al. Discontinuation of oral antivirals in chronic hepatitis B: a systematic review. Hepatology. 2016;63(5):1481–92.

Chapter 92
HBV Treatment Discontinuation

James Esteban

A 42-year-old former IV heroin user with immune-active, HBeAg-positive, chronic hepatitis B was treated with tenofovir disoproxil fumarate (TDF). After 6 months of treatment, he had normal liver chemistries and undetectable HBV DNA. He was still HBeAg-positive. Shortly after, he ran out of TDF and went about 6 months without medication before returning to the office with malaise, jaundice, and right upper quadrant tenderness. His current labs are ALT of 350, AST of 240, total bilirubin of 4 mg/dL, and HBV DNA of 25 million IU/mL. He continues to be HBeAg-positive.

Are patients with chronic hepatitis B able to come off antiviral therapy without risk of relapse?

It is clear that our patient relapsed after treatment interruption of tenofovir.

Patients who are HBeAg-positive can potentially stop nucleos(t)ide analog (NA) therapy after a finite duration of treatment. HBeAg-positive chronic hepatitis B patients being considered for treatment discontinuation should, at minimum, have achieved HBeAg seroconversion (i.e., HBeAg loss with appearance of anti-HBe), normal liver chemistries, and undetectable HBV DNA. They should then continue NA therapy for an additional 12 months (consolidation therapy) before NA discontinuation.

Liver chemistries, HBV DNA, and signs and symptoms of hepatic decompensation should be followed very closely (i.e., every 3 months) for the first year after treatment discontinuation. Available data indicate that, at 12 months after treatment discontinuation, initially HBeAg-positive patients will remain in virologic remission, biochemical remission, and HBeAg-negative in 60%, 75%, and 90% of cases, respectively [1].

J. Esteban (✉)
Division of Gastroenterology and Hepatology, Department of Medicine, Medical College of Wisconsin, Milwaukee, WI, USA
e-mail: jesteban@mcw.edu

The AASLD recommends that patients who are HBeAg-negative should remain on NA therapy indefinitely or until HBsAg is lost, based on data indicating high rates of virologic (60%) and biochemical (45%) relapse [1, 2]. However, there is evidence that NA therapy can be safely discontinued in select HBeAg-negative patients with reasonably low risk of virologic relapse and hepatitis flare, especially if patients have undetectable HBV DNA for at least 2–3 years while on treatment [1, 3]. As with HBeAg-positive patients, these patients should undergo frequent monitoring after stopping NA therapy. Interestingly, HBeAg-negative patients who stop NA therapy may have a greater chance for HBsAg loss (up to 30%) if quantitative HBsAg titers are <1000 IU/mL at treatment discontinuation [4, 5]. Unfortunately, quantitative HBsAg testing is not widely available in the United States.

Patients with cirrhosis, irrespective of HBeAg status, should remain on antiviral treatment indefinitely due to increased risk of fatal acute-on-chronic liver failure.

How would you manage this situation? Do you restart the same antiviral or do you need to start something different because of concerns about resistance?

Since he continues to have immune-active, HBeAg-positive, chronic hepatitis B, I will retreat and resume tenofovir. Entecavir and tenofovir are NAs with high genetic barriers to resistance, and reported antiviral resistance to these agents is uncommon (1% or less) [6]. The likelihood of resistance is proportionate to the duration of treatment, and our patient has only been on treatment for a few months. Antiviral-resistant viruses are in general also "less fit" for replication than their wild-type counterparts.

If he develops virological failure to tenofovir, defined as less than tenfold reduction in HBV DNA at 3 months of treatment, or virological breakthrough, defined as tenfold or more increase from the lowest HBV DNA level, then I would first ascertain that he is adhering to treatment. I will obtain HBV genotype and antiviral resistance testing only after I am able to determine that he is adherent.

Switching to entecavir is the next step if he is tenofovir-resistant. Conversely, switching to tenofovir is the next step if a patient is entecavir-resistant. Entecavir should not be used if a patient is resistant to lamivudine or telbivudine. Combination therapy with entecavir and tenofovir is typically not needed, since the individual agents are highly effective on their own, but should be considered in cases of documented multidrug resistance or persistent plateauing viremia after 12 months or more of treatment.

If our patient was HBeAg-negative at the start of NA treatment, how would you manage the situation?

Experts recommend delaying retreatment of relapse in HBeAg-negative patients for as long as possible, because this potentially increases the likelihood of spontaneously losing HBsAg and achieving functional cure [4, 5, 7]. These patients should be followed up very closely. Some indications for retreatment include severe (e.g., ALT >10× ULN for more than 1 week) or persistent (e.g., ALT >2× ULN for more than 3 months) hepatitis flare or jaundice [5, 7]. My choice of NA therapy and decision to pursue antiviral resistance testing would be similar to HBeAg-positive patients.

References

1. Papatheodoridis G, Vlachogiannakos I, Cholongitas E, Wursthorn K, Thomadakis C, Touloumi G, et al. Discontinuation of oral antivirals in chronic hepatitis B: a systematic review. Hepatology. 2016;63(5):1481–92.
2. Terrault N, Lok ASF, McMahon BJ, Chang KM, Hwang JP, Jonas MM, et al. Update on prevention, diagnosis, and treatment of chronic hepatitis B: AASLD 2018 hepatitis B guidance. Hepatology. 2018;67(4):1560–99.
3. European Association for the Study of the Liver. EASL 2017 clinical practice guidelines on the management of hepatitis B virus infection. J Hepatol. 2017;67(2):370–98.
4. van Bömmel F, Berg T. Risks and benefits of discontinuation of nucleos(t)ide analogue treatment: a treatment concept for patients with HBeAg-negative chronic hepatitis B. Hepatol Commun. 2021;5(1):1632–48.
5. van Bömmel F, Stein K, Heyne R, Petersen J, Buggisch P, Berg C, et al. A multicenter randomized-controlled trial of nucleos(t)ide analogue cessation in HBeAg-negative chronic hepatitis B. J Hepatol. 2023;78(5):926–36.
6. Tenney DJ, Rose RE, Baldick CJ, Pokornowski KA, Eggers BJ, Fang J, et al. Long-term monitoring shows hepatitis B virus resistance to entecavir in nucleoside-naïve patients is rare through 5 years of therapy. Hepatology. 2009;49(5):1503–14.
7. Hadziyannis SJ, Sevastianos V, Rapti I, Vassilopoulos D, Hadziyannis E. Sustained responses and loss of HBsAg in HBeAg-negative patients with chronic hepatitis B who stop long-term treatment with Adefovir. Gastroenterology. 2012;143(3):629–36.

Chapter 93
Differentiating Acute HBV from an Acute Exacerbation of Chronic HBV

James Esteban

A patient presents with fever and elevated transaminases—ALT of 350, AST of 260, and total bilirubin of 5 mg/dL. He has no past history of hepatitis but did use intravenous heroin several times, about 10 years ago. One month before the presentation, he got a tattoo in a parlor. Labs show a positive hepatitis B surface antigen (HBsAg), positive hepatitis B core antibody (anti-HBc) IgM and total, and elevated HBV DNA of greater than 20 million IU/mL.

Are you able to say if this is a case of acute hepatitis B infection or an exacerbation of chronic hepatitis B infection?

Chronic hepatitis B is defined as the persistence of HBsAg or positive HBV DNA for at least 6 months [1, 2]. Without prior HBV serologic testing, we have not established HBV chronicity for this patient. I would make sure to look for signs of liver disease chronicity and portal hypertension on the physical exam and abdominal ultrasound.

The presence of anti-HBc IgM is a strong indicator of acute hepatitis B infection, but some patients with chronic hepatitis B who are experiencing an acute flare-up or exacerbation may also be anti-HBc IgM-positive.

Would you start antiviral therapy?

First, I would examine him for hepatic encephalopathy, obtain hepatitis B envelope antigen (HBeAg), and antibody (anti-HBe), check his international normalized ratio (INR), and obtain abdominal ultrasound to determine if he has cirrhosis and portal hypertension.

J. Esteban (✉)
Division of Gastroenterology and Hepatology, Department of Medicine, Medical College of Wisconsin, Milwaukee, WI, USA
e-mail: jesteban@mcw.edu

If he has acute liver failure, defined as severe liver injury with hepatic synthetic dysfunction (coagulopathy, INR > 1.5), and hepatic encephalopathy within 26 weeks of disease onset, in a person without a history of cirrhosis, I will start antiviral therapy in addition to getting him evaluated for liver transplantation.

If he does not have acute liver failure, I would follow him up closely and obtain liver chemistries and INR frequently (every 1–2 weeks for 1–2 months). If he has persistent hyperbilirubinemia (total bilirubin > 3 mg/dL) or coagulopathy (INR > 1.5), which indicate severe disease, for greater than 4 weeks, then I will start antiviral therapy because he has a protracted course of severe acute HBV infection.

The preferred antiviral therapies are the nucleos(t)ide analogs entecavir, tenofovir disoproxil fumarate, and tenofovir alafenamide. Interferon is contraindicated in acute hepatitis B infection due to risk of exacerbating liver inflammation.

If he has neither of these, then close monitoring and expectant management are appropriate. More than 95% of immunocompetent patients with acute hepatitis B infection will recover spontaneously and lose HBsAg over time. In a large clinical trial of patients with severe acute hepatitis B infection, lamivudine was no better than placebo in terms of biochemical improvement and rates of HBsAg loss (both ~93% at 12 months) [3].

He is HBeAg-positive and anti-HBe-negative. His INR is 1.3. On exam, he was alert and oriented. He did not have spider angiomas, abdominal distention, fluid wave, or asterixis. Abdominal ultrasound shows a normal-appearing liver, without splenomegaly or ascites. You decided that he does not require immediate initiation of antiviral therapy. You monitor his liver chemistries and INR weekly. In week 4, his liver chemistries showed the following: ALT of 120, AST of 100, total bilirubin of 1.8 mg/dL, and INR of 1.2.

How would you follow him up?

I would continue following his liver chemistries, and I will, in addition, be following his HBsAg, anti-HBs, HBeAg, anti-HBe, and HBV DNA periodically because we need to know if he will "clear" the HBV infection or if he will go on to develop chronic hepatitis B infection. I will obtain hepatitis B serologies at 3 and/or 6 months. If he remains HBsAg positive at 6 months or more, then we have established that he has chronic hepatitis B infection. Management of chronic hepatitis B is discussed in other chapters in the book.

References

1. Terrault N, Lok ASF, McMahon BJ, Chang KM, Hwang JP, Jonas MM, et al. Update on prevention, diagnosis, and treatment of chronic hepatitis B: AASLD 2018 hepatitis B guidance. Hepatology. 2018;67(4):1560–99.
2. European Association for the Study of the Liver. EASL 2017 clinical practice guidelines on the management of hepatitis B virus infection. J Hepatol. 2017;67(2):370–98.
3. Kumar M, Satapathy S, Monga R, Das K, Hissar S, Pande C, et al. A randomized controlled trial of lamivudine to treat acute hepatitis B. Hepatology. 2007;45(1):97–101.

Chapter 94
Acute HBV and Risk of HBV Reactivation

James Esteban

A 25-year-old male gets acute hepatitis B from a sexual encounter. He completely clears the infection spontaneously, without treatment.

Is there a need for extended follow-up of any kind?

Clearance of hepatitis B surface antigen (HBsAg) and formation of hepatitis B surface antibody (HBsAb) defines functional cure. Loss of HBsAg is associated with durable suppression of viral replication. Thus, he will not require extended follow-up [1].

What if, 25 years from now, he needs to receive rituximab-based regimen for lymphoma, will he need special precautions?

After entry into the hepatocyte, hepatitis B virus (HBV) translocates into the nucleus, where the double-stranded HBV DNA (dsDNA) is repaired into an extremely stable covalently closed circular DNA (cccDNA). cccDNA persists in hepatocytes long after loss of HBsAg. HBV dsDNA may also integrate with the human genome as HBV integrated or iDNA. The persistence of cccDNA and iDNA in hepatocytes, despite complete suppression of HBV replication and even loss of HBsAg, is the reason why true virologic cure is not achievable in hepatitis B infection with current medical therapies.

Immunosuppressive therapy may release immunologic control over HBV, leading to resumption of transcription of HBV cccDNA and/or iDNA. This leads to reappearance of HBsAg and HBV DNA in serum and hepatitis flares in some cases. This is called HBV reactivation. Risk of HBV reactivation varies by intensity of immunosuppression. B-cell depleting agents such as rituximab, or prolonged use of

J. Esteban (✉)
Division of Gastroenterology and Hepatology, Department of Medicine, Medical College of Wisconsin, Milwaukee, WI, USA
e-mail: jesteban@mcw.edu

© The Author(s), under exclusive license to Springer Nature Switzerland AG 2023
W. H. Sobin et al. (eds.), *Managing Complex Cases in Gastroenterology*,
https://doi.org/10.1007/978-3-031-48949-5_94

Table 94.1 Risk of HBV reactivation according to immunosuppressive agent and HBsAg status

	HBsAg+/ HBcAb+	HBsAg−/ HBcAb+
B-cell depleting therapy (e.g., rituximab, belimumab, alemtuzumab, etc.)	High	High
High-dose steroids (pred >20 mg/day × >4 weeks)	High	Moderate
Med-dose steroids (pred 10–20 mg/day × >4 weeks)	Moderate	Low
Low-dose steroids (pred <10 mg/day), intra-articular steroids	Low	Low
Anthracycline-based systemic chemotherapy	High	Moderate
Non-anthracycline systemic chemotherapy	Moderate	Moderate
Immune checkpoint inhibitors (e.g., pembrolizumab, nivolumab, ipilimumab)	High	Moderate
Anti-TNF agents (e.g., infliximab, adalimumab, certolizumab, golimumab)	High	Moderate
Cytokine therapies (e.g., ustekinumab, abatacept, natalizumab, vedolizumab)	Moderate	Moderate
TK inhibitors (e.g., imatinib, nilotinib)	Moderate	Moderate
Proteosome inhibitors (e.g., bortezomib)	Moderate	Moderate
Histone deacetylase inhibitors (e.g., romidepsin)	Moderate	Moderate
Calcineurin inhibitors (e.g., tacrolimus, cyclosporine)	Moderate	Moderate
Antimetabolites (e.g., 6-MP, azathioprine, methotrexate, mycophenolate)	Low	Low

High risk, >10% risk of HBV reactivation; Moderate risk, 1–10% risk of HBV reactivation; Low risk, <1% risk of HBV reactivation

high-dose corticosteroids, are associated with the highest risk of HBV reactivation (>10%). Patients with a history of hepatitis B infection, i.e., HBsAg and hepatitis B core antibody (HBcAb) positive, who will be receiving high-risk immunosuppressive agents (Table 94.1), should be provided with antiviral prophylaxis with nucleos(t)ide analogs such an entecavir, tenofovir disoproxil fumarate, or tenofovir alafenamide to prevent HBV reactivation [2, 3].

Some immunosuppressive agents, such as tumor necrosis factor inhibitors or cytokine inhibitors, have a lower, but not negligible, risk of HBV reactivation. Some patients who will be receiving these agents may be offered on-demand therapy (Fig. 94.1), where we periodically check (typically every 3 months) HBV DNA, transaminases, and HBsAg for HBV reactivation or a hepatitis flare (i.e., ALT >3× upper limit of normal). Patients would then be promptly treated with nucleos(t)ide analogs upon diagnosis of HBV reactivation.

In patients who are HBsAg positive, reactivation may be defined as:

- 100× increase in HBV DNA
- HBV DNA 1000 IU/mL if previously undetectable
- HBV DNA 10,000 IU/mL if previous level unknown

In patients who are HBsAg negative and HBcAb positive, reactivation may be defined as:

- Any detectable HBV DNA
- Reverse seroconversion to HBsAg positive

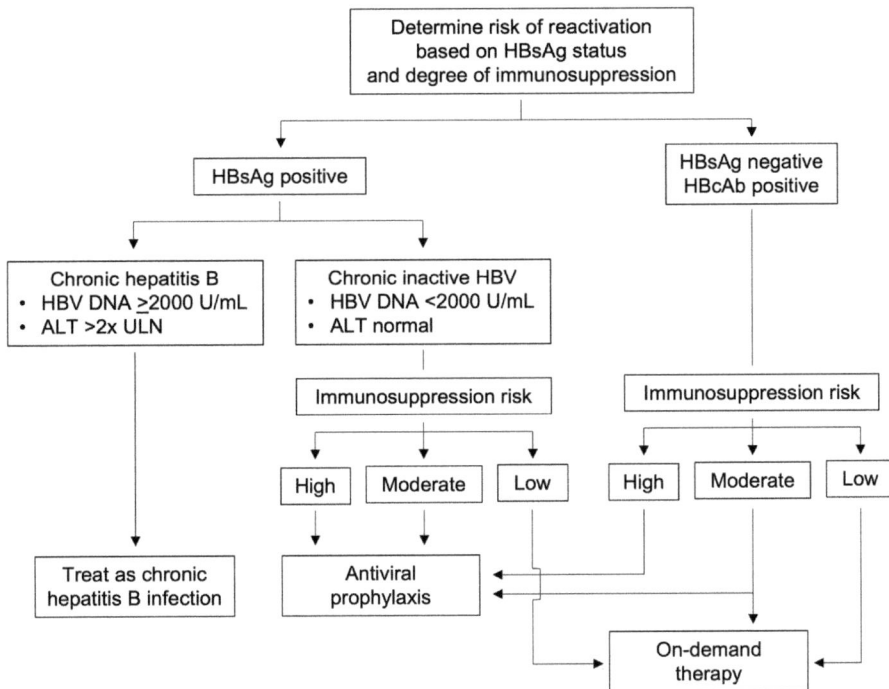

Fig. 94.1 Algorithm for prevention and management of HBV reactivation in patients receiving immunosuppressive therapy

References

1. Terrault N, Lok ASF, McMahon BJ, Chang KM, Hwang JP, Jonas MM, et al. Update on prevention, diagnosis, and treatment of chronic hepatitis B: AASLD 2018 hepatitis B guidance. Hepatology. 2018;67(4):1560–99.
2. Reddy KR, Beavers KL, Hammond SP, Lim JK, Falck-Ytter Y, AGA Institute. American Gastroenterological Association Institute guideline on the prevention and treatment of hepatitis B virus reactivation during immunosuppressive drug therapy. Gastroenterology. 2015;1480:215–9.
3. Loomba R, Liang TJ. Hepatitis B reactivation associated with immune suppressive and biological modifier therapies: current concepts, management strategies, and future directions. Gastroenterology. 2017;152(6):1297–309.

Chapter 95
Complicated HCV

Kia Saeian

Patient is a 35-year-old female with a history of IV drug abuse from age 18–25 who comes in with jaundice and weakness. She is overweight with a BMI of 33 and has no history of significant alcohol use. On exam, she has no stigmata of chronic liver disease. Her liver enzymes are as follows: ALT of 240, AST of 150, bilirubin of 3.2, and Alk phos of 120. Her US shows marked steatosis of the liver. Hepatitis panel is positive for HCV ab, and her HCV PCR is (+) 1.2 million. ANA returns positive at 1:640.

What is your impression, and how would you manage this patient?

One of the first things I would like to do is check the gamma globulin level to corroborate the positive ANA and substantiate the impression of AIH. I would consider doing a liver biopsy. There would be two reasons to consider a liver biopsy. First, would be to confirm a diagnosis of AIH, assuming her IgG level comes back elevated. Personally, I like to have a biopsy confirmation of AIH before initiating therapy, although not everyone agrees.

The second would be to evaluate for fibrosis from HCV. Since her HCV exposure was probably over 10 years ago, there is a good chance she could have fibrosis from the chronic HCV. Most of the time with HCV we don't need a liver biopsy, we simply treat the HCV, but in this case, we might.

An interesting question in this case is whether the patient has two distinct disorders—**both** HCV and AIH (as well as potentially NAFLD). This question comes up because some patients with HCV may have a positive ANA and features of autoimmune disease without having AIH. The distinction used to be much more of a quandary when we used interferon to treat HCV, because interferon would dramatically exacerbate AIH.

K. Saeian (✉)
Division Gastroenterology and Hepatology, Department of Medicine, Medical College of Wisconsin, Milwaukee, WI, USA
e-mail: ksaeian@mcw.edu

W. H. Sobin et al. (eds.), *Managing Complex Cases in Gastroenterology*, https://doi.org/10.1007/978-3-031-48949-5_95

Now in this case, even if the patient has AIH, I don't think it is urgent that we start corticosteroids immediately, seeing how there is only a moderate level of trans-aminase elevation. You can argue to hold off on biopsy, treat the HCV first, and see what happens with the autoimmune findings.

The other interesting question about this case is the interplay between HCV and NAFLD. I would check the HCV genotype, and if it is genotype 3, it might also explain the degree of fat in the liver. Her BMI alone is probably adequate to explain it, but genotype 3 has been associated with more significant steatosis.

You talk about fibrosis, if you weren't going directly to biopsy, would you do a FibroScan®?

I do use the FibroScan®, although I do not use it as liberally as some. But the fact is that it's available and it's pretty easy to do. Now I perform a significant proportion of the liver biopsies done in our institution, and I have a healthy appreciation for the potential complications associated with liver biopsy. Therefore, I don't rush into doing liver biopsies as quickly as some others do. So, if the only reason for doing a liver biopsy is to establish the diagnosis of fibrosis, I would try FibroScan® first.

However, there are confounding issues, like obesity, that can make FibroScan® less reliable. In the aforementioned patient, because she has a BMI of 33, FibroScan® would be of limited benefit. But if I have a case of chronic HCV (uncomplicated by autoimmune features), where the patient is not obese and doesn't have other con-founding factors, I have a very low threshold to spend the few minutes doing the FibroScan®. Then, if I don't see any indication of fibrosis, I can treat their hepatitis C and not need to arrange for follow-up, because I'm comfortable that fibrosis is absent, and surveillance for HCC unnecessary.

What about the utility of FibroScan® in congestive heart failure? What if you have a patient with congestive heart failure and elevated liver enzymes, will you get a FibroScan® in that setting?

I would absolutely not use it in that setting because you're likely to get a false reading. If you look at the concept of elastography, it's based on elasticity of the tissue, and if you have elevated back pressures from CHF, pulmonary hypertension, or hepatic vein obstruction, you lose that elasticity. Whether or not fibrosis is pres-ent, the FibroScan® will imply advanced fibrosis.

Chapter 96
Acute Liver Failure

Kia Saeian

A patient presents with acute liver failure. A 27-year-old female college student, who had complained to her roommate that she felt weak and nauseated for several days, is now found lying in bed in her dorm room, extremely lethargic. The roommate calls her parents who urge her to call an ambulance. She is sent to the ER. On the physical exam, she is responsive but keeps drifting off to sleep. Her BP is 90/70, pulse is 90, and temperature is 99. She has no signs of portal hypertension on exam. Liver and spleen are not palpable.

WBC, 12,000; Hbg 11.5; platelets, 180,000; AST, 1700; ALT, 2200; ALK phos, 140; Bili, 8; INR, 2.5

How would you address this problem?

This pattern of enzymes is suggestive of zone three necrosis, and a common cause of this is acetaminophen overdose, even though there isn't a history of her taking that. The other things you would think about in a young woman like this (not necessarily involving zone 3 necrosis) are acute presentations of autoimmune hepatitis, other drug induced injuries, or an unknown viral infection. Those are the most likely explanations for her presentation.

The fact that she is already presenting with synthetic dysfunction and encephalopathy qualifies her as having acute liver failure, so she absolutely must be at a transplant center. Even if you think she has autoimmune hepatitis and you're going to treat her, you absolutely need to be prepared for the possibility of transplantation, and that needs to be done pronto because these patients can deteriorate very rapidly.

K. Saeian (✉)
Division of Gastroenterology and Hepatology, Department of Medicine, Medical College of Wisconsin, Milwaukee, WI, USA
e-mail: ksaeian@mcw.edu

© The Author(s), under exclusive license to Springer Nature Switzerland AG 2023
W. H. Sobin et al. (eds.), *Managing Complex Cases in Gastroenterology*, https://doi.org/10.1007/978-3-031-48949-5_96

Now, we've had some patients present like this who turned out to have autoimmune hepatitis who we've been able to treat and have them recover without transplant. But once they've developed encephalopathy, it's more unlikely that they will turn around and improve quickly enough to avoid listing them.

We have a specific liver failure protocol in which we screen for the routine viral hepatidites—HAV, HBV, HCV. We also include lab tests looking for alternative viruses like CMV, EBV, and hepatitis E. In addition, we would certainly do toxicology screens and check the autoimmune markers.

We also monitor the AFP because it can be a marker of the ability of the liver to regenerate. Factor V can also be a marker so we monitor that as well. If the patient becomes acidotic, that is a poor prognostic factor and we get even more concerned. So that's our lab work.

In terms of the imaging studies, we get a CT scan of the head to make sure there is no midline shift or cerebral edema, which would necessitate more aggressive measures, including hypernatremia, hypothermia, and occasional osmotic diuresis with mannitol, although we don't use that or hyperventilation as frequently as we used to.

We would consider initiating n-acetyl-cysteine (NAC) even in the absence of known acetaminophen overdose. The evidence is less robust in ALF not related to acetaminophen, but there is some decent data that it can help in that setting.

Directing our attention to the alkaline phosphatase, it is not elevated in proportion to the transaminases in this patient. In cases of viral hepatitis and autoimmune hepatitis, usually the alkaline phosphatase elevation is proportional to the transaminase elevation. But it is possible that the alk phos is on a slower upward course, it's still early on, and it could take longer for that alk phos to get transcribed.

The elevated bilirubin/alkaline phosphatase ratio raises the possibility of Wilson's disease. However, if this was Wilson's, I would expect her Hbg to be lower, and the alkaline phosphatase might be even lower than it is in this case. Regardless, if this was acute Wilson's, you're probably headed for transplant.

However, in cases of zone 3 necrosis of the liver, the transaminases tend to be proportionally higher than the alkaline phosphatase. Other things that could cause zone 3 injury include hypotension and heat stroke. Heat stroke can sometimes fool you, although in this case, the AST being lower than the ALT makes that less likely.

Would you start steroids in this patient with acute liver failure?

We are reluctant to start steroids. Our transplant surgeons prefer to avoid steroids in a patient headed for transplant. We would certainly wait for our autoimmune markers to come back. But even if the ANA came back elevated, I would want to see an elevated IgG as well, because we do see elevated ANA in a number of cases that are not autoimmune liver disease. And even with an elevated ANA and IgG, I would prefer to have a liver biopsy before starting steroids for AIH.

Now if this patient was somewhat more stable, not encephalopathic, and time was more on our side, I would consider doing a liver biopsy. We have done transjugular liver biopsies in some patients with an INR in this range. If a biopsy confirmed the diagnosis of AIH, I would be much more inclined to start steroids.

Chapter 97
Delayed Presentation of Tylenol Overdose

Kia Saeian

A patient with a history of taking a large dose of Tylenol 5 days earlier is brought into the hospital now. She is lethargic on presentation, ALT is 3000, AST is 2400, INR is 2.5, bilirubin is 2.2, and Alk phos is 140.

Is there any role for NAC at this late point?

I think almost everyone would give it, even 5 days after the overdose. The question of whether it will benefit the patient is a valid one, because we don't have many studies on initiating NAC in this subset of patients who are presenting this late in the clinical course. One thing about this case is that it's unusual for the numbers to be this high on day five. The numbers tend to peak on day three, so it is possible that the transaminases might have been higher, say even 10,000, and are now trending down. The patient may be recovering from the injury, but the fact that the numbers decrease is not necessarily a good sign. It could be a sign of fulminant hepatic necrosis.

The traditional teaching now is that you give NAC until the transaminases drop below 1000. I would treat her as someone we might possibly be able to salvage, so in this patient, even though it may be too late, we would start NAC and continue until the numbers dropped to at least below 1000. The one reassuring thing in this case is that the bilirubin is not extremely high. Treatment with NAC is generally very safe, but some patients do develop nausea and vomiting, particularly with the oral formulation.

K. Saeian (✉)
Division of Gastroenterology and Hepatology, Department of Medicine, Medical College of Wisconsin, Milwaukee, WI, USA
e-mail: ksaeian@mcw.edu

© The Author(s), under exclusive license to Springer Nature Switzerland AG 2023
W. H. Sobin et al. (eds.), *Managing Complex Cases in Gastroenterology*,
https://doi.org/10.1007/978-3-031-48949-5_97

405

There are some centers that use fomepizole to treat severe episodes of acetaminophen toxicity. Fomepizole is a competitive inhibitor of alcohol dehydrogenase, which inhibits formation of toxic acetaminophen (APAP) metabolites; I have never used it, but based on its mechanism of action, it would make sense to use it in those who have concomitant acetaminophen and alcohol toxicity.

Chapter 98
Candidates for Liver Transplant?

Veronica Loy

A GI fellow who left your training program to join a group GI practice several weeks ago asks to set up a meeting. He took over the practice of a retiring gastroenterologist and wants to discuss management of several patients. There were four patients with ESLD who he thinks may warrant liver transplant evaluation. The practice is located in a rural area, one and a half hours away from your academic transplant center.

Do you think any of these patients are liver transplant candidates?

1. *A 58-year-old male with alcoholic cirrhosis who has been abstinent 3 years is living in a shelter. He has been treated for encephalopathy, recurring ascites, and varices. He takes his meds as prescribed and manages to have a friend drive him to the hospital for all his office visits and procedures. He is on public assistance. The former doctor did not refer him for transplant evaluation because of his lack of social and financial support.*

    This is a difficult case. I think that the first concern is both financial and social support, and we need to consider why those are so important in the posttransplant period. As we know, if the patient does not have access to the immunosuppressive medications for life, then the organ will be rejected. If that's the case, you've done the patient a disservice as well as the organ donor and another potential recipient did not receive the organ. It is critical that we have a multidisciplinary approach to assessing both financial support and social support. Our program has our own financial liaison as well as a social worker, who hone in, and try every avenue, to make sure that they can assure coverage for these medicines.

V. Loy (✉)
Division of Gastroenterology and Hepatology, Department of Medicine, Medical College of Wisconsin, Milwaukee, WI, USA
e-mail: vloy@mcw.edu

W. H. Sobin et al. (eds.), *Managing Complex Cases in Gastroenterology*,
https://doi.org/10.1007/978-3-031-48949-5_98

In this patient's case, he has been taking his prescribed meds, he must have public assistance, and Medicaid usually will cover these meds. Coverage and compliance don't seem to be a problem for him, so that bodes well.

However, the second thing we have to worry about is the infection risk. And unfortunately, staying in shelters, most of the time, is something that the transplant committee is really going to struggle with as far as reliable housing and infection risk. It's even a struggle for patients living in a nursing home because of an increased risk of posttransplant infection. Typically, we prefer people that have individualized housing. I think every transplant center is probably a little different on how they would view this case. I'm pretty confident that in our center living in a shelter would not be considered reliable housing.

What makes things more complicated is that there is a recent law about discrimination and access to an organ transplant. Transplant programs must be careful with the reasons for declining to list someone for transplant. The psychosocial issues, especially for people with mental health or developmental delays, are really challenging. There have been lawsuits when some of these patients were declined. In this patient's case, infection risk of rejection is a realistic reason for declining to list the patient.

2. *A 57-year-old female has NASH cirrhosis. She has had treatment for esophageal varices and recurring ascites. Her BMI is 35. The previous doctor pushed her to diet and lose weight. He insisted that she lose at least 20 lbs. She was not having much success, losing only about 5 lbs. The doctor did not refer her for liver transplant, thinking that she was not a candidate because of her obesity.*

This is a very timely topic. What we know about organ transplant is that the extremes of weight don't do as well. The super obese or the very sarcopenic patients don't do well. In this case, the patient has a BMI of 35; that's not a big problem, and that patient certainly should be considered as a transplant candidate. Once you're heading towards a BMI of 40, 45, or 50, that becomes more challenging and controversial. It depends on where the person holds their weight. If it's all abdominal fat, that is more of a problem, especially if it's a dual organ transplant, like a liver-kidney, because the abdominal weight may cause problems with the kidney. But if they're carrying all their weight in their legs and their glutes, then that's not really prohibitive to transplant. There are some really good studies looking at outcomes in obese patients after transplant and they do quite well as long as they're not in the far extremes. In fact, obese patients tend to do better than sarcopenic patients who have no muscle mass, very low BMIs, and poor nutrition. The outcomes relate mostly to nutrition and functional status. If you have a morbidly obese patient that has good nutrition and a good functional status, that's helpful, but many centers are doing bariatric surgery along with the transplant if their weight is extreme. Some do it in the pre-op period, some at the time of transplant, and others after they've recovered from the transplant. There's a little bit of controversy over which is the best way to do it. But a lot of people are looking into bariatric surgery as it relates to liver transplant, particularly in NASH patients.

The Mayo Clinic has done a really nice study where they compared patients who, like this patient, were told they had to lose weight prior to transplant. And those patients did lose weight and were transplanted, and they were compared with a group of patients who had bariatric surgery and then were transplanted. It turned out that those patients who had bariatric surgery and then were transplanted actually did much better than those that lost weight on their own and then got their transplant. That group tended to gain back a lot of their weight after transplant. And progression to NASH cirrhosis posttransplant happens very quickly in those who gain their weight back. So, I think, as we move forward in the next decade, it probably will become the standard of care that these patients with NASH cirrhosis have some sort of bariatric procedure along with their transplant.

3. *A 49-year-old male alcoholic presented with a GI bleed and required an ICU admission with banding of varices. He was discharged from the hospital, but over the next 3 months, he has had repeat admissions with banding and then bleeding from post-banding ulcers, ascites, and SBP. He has also had encephalopathy controlled with lactulose. He has been abstinent since the first admission. The previous doctor would not refer him for transplant because he has only been abstinent for 3 months.*

I am really passionate about this one. Using duration of sobriety or abstinence alone has been shown time and time again to not predict recidivism posttransplant. And so, in this patient, I would absolutely encourage referring to a transplant center. And at that center, there'll be a multidisciplinary approach with a psychology evaluation and a social work evaluation and really assess this patient's commitment to lifelong sobriety and their social support. Many centers are integrating alcohol and drug addiction counseling along with their clinic visits, and that's been shown to improve the chances of patients having lifelong sobriety.

It's very important not just to use time alone as a reason not to refer someone for transplant. It doesn't predict posttransplant alcohol use. Even those who have 6 months or a year of sobriety have the same recidivism rate as those who have no sobriety. So, time should really not be a factor.

4. *A 72-year-old female with NASH cirrhosis has ESLD. She has encephalopathy requiring lactulose and rifaximin. She has had a prior TIPS procedure for variceal bleeds and gastric varices. Because the encephalopathy is hard to control, the TIPS needed to be narrowed, and now the patient has chronic GI bleeding from GAVE. The previous doctor would not refer her for liver transplant evaluation because he thought she was too old.*

Once again, similar to our last discussion, this is a misconception that many people have; it's really an outdated thought. There is actually no age cutoff for transplant. Most transplant centers look at the physiological age, so the health of the patient, their functional status, their cardiac comorbidities, and pulmonary comorbidities are far more important than the age alone. So, this patient, depending on her other medical comorbidities could certainly be considered for transplant.

Chapter 99
Frustrations with Waiting for a Transplant

Veronica Loy

*A 57-year-old male with alcoholic cirrhosis is referred for liver transplant evalua-
tion. He was diagnosed 2 years earlier and has been abstinent since. He was found
on index endoscopy to have esophageal varices, which were banded and remain
obliterated on a recent endoscopy. He has been plagued with recurring ascites.
Initially diuretics were used but when doses needed to be increased, he developed
renal insufficiency. He now comes in for weekly paracentesis during which 5–7
liters of fluid is usually removed. He has had one episode of SBP and remains on
prophylactic ciprofloxacin. He has had several episodes of hepatic encephalopathy:
the first when his creatinine was elevated and the second when he had SBP. He was
placed on lactulose, which he takes regularly, except when he is in situations where
he needs to avoid having diarrhea. When he doesn't take his lactulose, he gets very
sleepy. His INR is 1.9, albumin is 3.4, bilirubin is 1.3, AST is 30, ALT is 50, Alk phos
is 90, creatinine is 1.2, Na is 136, and MELD is 16. His local gastroenterologist tells
him that with his MELD score, he probably won't qualify for a liver transplant for
a while.*

1. **How do you deal with patients who are suffering from complications of cirrhosis but can't qualify for a transplant for protracted periods because
   their MELD is not high enough?**

   This is an ongoing, common problem. But I would advocate for evaluation
   and, if possible, listing for transplant. We understand that with the MELD score
   of 16, they're not likely to get an organ quickly. However, the medical condition
   can deteriorate very quickly for these patients. We know that people with diuretic

V. Loy (✉)
Division of Gastroenterology and Hepatology, Department of Medicine, Medical College of
Wisconsin, Milwaukee, WI, USA
e-mail: vloy@mcw.edu

© The Author(s), under exclusive license to Springer Nature
Switzerland AG 2023
W. H. Sobin et al. (eds.), *Managing Complex Cases in Gastroenterology*,
https://doi.org/10.1007/978-3-031-48949-5_99

resistant or diuretic refractory ascites have a 50% 2-year mortality, which is very high. We tend to see them develop SBP and liver decompensation, or they have a bleed after a paracentesis and their liver decompensates, so these complications can happen very quickly. Therefore, the benefit of listing them early. I feel that even though the MELD is on the low side, at 16, I advocate listing if it's over 15. But sometimes, we see these patients with a MELD score of eight, and I still think with diuretic resistant or refractory ascites or patients with varices that we should try to get them on the transplant list because things change quickly and it allows the patient and their family time to be educated and learn and understand.

And we can work on other things. Often, during the transplant evaluation, we uncover other risks that we need to mitigate, like maybe they need to stop smoking. And we can work on these things for the best results with transplant. Also, if this patient did not have a history of encephalopathy, I would look into doing a TIPS at this time, but because of the encephalopathy, I won't.

Additionally, there are other avenues to help get a patient a liver transplant sooner, such as living donor liver transplantation. A patient needs to be assessed early to see if they might qualify for this.

In summary, I would try to get the patient listed, and then, I would continue to do what this gastroenterologist is doing with the repeated paracentesis, low sodium diet, and antibiotic prophylaxis.

2. **What do you think about a system where the sicker, higher risk patients are the ones who are having this aggressive operation? Wouldn't you rather your patient receives the transplant when they are less sick?**

The system is not always logical but it's meant to be fair. The people who need the transplant the most have access to the transplant. However, we do know that, in terms of posttransplant outcomes, there is a tipping point at which patients have worse survival after transplant because they were so sick going into the transplant. The ideal time to get a transplant is probably at a MELD of 24–30 instead of a MELD of 40. These patients are not as sarcopenic; they can recover quicker. They don't have as many complications, they're not as immunocompromised.

I agree it would be phenomenal to offer a transplant when a patient is less sick, and I think we're making some progress toward transplanting patients at a lower MELD. Ideally, anyone who needs a transplant would have access to it, but the real issue is an organ donor shortage. The demand far outstrips the resources.

One way we're making progress is by using other types of liver donations besides just brain-dead donors. In some of these patients with the lower MELD scores, there might be the option of using a living donor transplant, if they qualify. However, patients with a lot of portal hypertension, like this one, are generally not ideal candidates for a living donor transplant, they often need a whole donor graft.

Another potential source of livers is to use not only brain-dead donors but also donations after cardiac death. Another group is the hepatitis C-positive donors. We're using them a lot more now because we can eradicate hepatitis C easily after the transplant. Another new thing that's happened in the last couple of years is the machine perfusion-donor livers. Here, they take organs that previously would have been discarded because of their questionable quality. This may be the case if a liver had a lot of steatosis or the donor was elderly. There is now available hypothermic and normothermic machine perfusion for these donor organs, which can optimize the graft allowing for transplant in some cases where previously they would've gone unused. The transplant surgeon will take the donor liver and hook it up to this perfusion device, and they're able to monitor the liver and see if this liver will work in the recipient. Another technique is to do organ procurement the traditional way, then put the liver in the cooler and get on the airplane, and then when they get back to their own hospital, hook it up to a pump. This is something they've been doing with kidneys for some time now.

3. **What percentage of patients develop HCC or develop medical complications that make them inoperable while waiting to be transplanted?**

This is very common because of problems waiting for access to a donor. There is only so long that you can keep someone's cancer within Milan criteria. There's only so long that you can keep someone with end-organ failure alive before they get an infection that prohibits transplant.

Many patients will develop hemodynamic instability with which there's no way they could survive a transplant. What is the waiting list mortality rate? It's variable across the country, depending on access to grafts. But nationwide, I would guess the wait list mortality rate is about 20%.

With HCC in particular, there have been some changes in organ allocation. So, some patients who are listed with MELD exception points, depending on where they live, may have better access to organs, while others have less access to organs. We've seen that some of our patients with tumor exception points are on our wait list for up to 200, even 300 days. But keeping cancer in check for a year is quite challenging.

Chapter 100
Complications Posttransplant

Veronica Loy

A 57-year-old female receives a liver transplant for PBC. She is started on predni-sone, tacrolimus, and mycophenolate. Within the first 3 months, she develops mul-tiple medical problems. She has developed hypertension, which was not present previously, she progressed from having prediabetes to diabetes, and her creatinine has risen from 1.4 to 1.8.

Can you discuss the contribution of her antirejection meds to these different medical problems and how you might manage the antirejection meds per. se.

When transplants were initiated in the late 1960s and early 1970s, the main cause of death was acute cellular rejection. Things have come a really long way, thanks to our superior antirejection meds. We have available calcineurin inhibitors, mycophe-nolate, and azathioprine and prednisone. We are at a point where patients are living a long time. The expectation is that survival at 10 years should be 70% or more. Transplant rejection still remains a concern; up to 30% of patients may develop rejection, but we can manage that much better now.

Now the major problems we are dealing with are the side effects from long-term use of these antirejection medications. One concern is new cancers, and we encoun-ter a lot of these, particularly skin cancers. Depending on the etiology of the patient's disease, we have to be very careful looking for other types of new malignancies. Of course, infections are a big concern.

This case points out two other very challenging side effects of antirejection meds, the metabolic syndrome and hypertension. Cardiovascular events, heart attack and stroke, are all happening at a far greater rate in transplant recipients com-pared with their nontransplant recipient counterparts.

V. Loy (✉)

Division of Gastroenterology and Hepatology, Department of Medicine, Medical College of Wisconsin, Milwaukee, WI, USA
e-mail: vloy@mcw.edu

W. H. Sobin et al. (eds.), *Managing Complex Cases in Gastroenterology*, https://doi.org/10.1007/978-3-031-48949-5_100

Additionally, data shows that at 5–10 years posttransplant, the rate at which people have kidney disease, CKD3 or CKD4, approaches almost 70%. Historically, it's a very high percentage of people who receive the transplant of a heart or a liver who ultimately end up needing to talk about going on dialysis or having a kidney transplant.

The long-term effects of immunosuppression are a big problem. How can we manage this? I think looking at strategies for minimizing immunosuppression is very important. The level of immunosuppression that the patient is maintained on in the immediate posttransplant period will predict how they do 10 years later. So, the goal is to work on minimizing medication without putting the patient at risk of rejection. There's a lot of research in the area. The strategy used in this patient's case of using three drugs rather than using a high-dose calcineurin inhibitor alone is an important step. With the calcineurin inhibitors, we're worrying most about renal insufficiency, but they also contribute to hypertension, hyperlipidemia, and diabetes. By using mycophenolate and prednisone, we may be reducing the risk of kidney damage, but there is a trade-off with some of these other problems and metabolic conditions.

There's also another class of agents, the mTOR inhibitors, which are sometimes used with a strategy of minimizing the dose of calcineurin inhibitor. The hope is that this will prevent renal insufficiency and may possibly help reduce the recurrence of cancers. In this patient, I might have titrated some of the dosages of medicines she was on to try to avoid some of these complications.

Now there is ongoing research about immunosuppression withdrawal. There are ongoing trials to determine which patients could actually come off immunosuppression completely. I don't think it's yet at the point where I would feel comfortable doing that, although some hepatologists have moved in this direction. I would work, instead, on managing the comorbidities, trying to help the patient have better control of the hypertension, the diabetes, and the lipids. And ultimately, if renal function continues to decline, getting a nephrologist involved early on.

After 3 months, the patient comes in complaining of some increased fatigue and weakness, and liver enzymes show a significant increase from her posttransplant baseline. Her AST increased from 30 to 90, the ALT from 40 to 120, the Alk phos from 100 to 160, and the bilirubin from 1.3–2.3. She is not taking any OTC meds—nothing but what has been prescribed for her.

What are some possible explanations for this and how would you manage it?

You would certainly worry about rejection here, especially if you previously decided to reduce immunosuppression. The other common problem I always want to rule out in a patient like this is infection. CMV is very common; even far posttransplant and any infection is going to cause a rise in the liver enzymes and perhaps a cholestatic liver injury, which this patient has. Any infection, including c diff, is a possibility, so I would screen for infection.

I also usually get some imaging to make sure that there's no problem with the bile duct. You know that's very common posttransplant as well.

The other thing I would worry about in this patient is the possibility of PBC recurrence posttransplant or even autoimmune hepatitis. The rate of recurrence of PBC posttransplant is high.

In addition to rejection, I would work the patient up for infection, recurrent disease, any bile duct injury, or steatosis of the liver. For this patient, you're probably going to do a liver biopsy at some point. I wouldn't send someone for a biopsy based on one set of labs, but if the problem were to persist for a couple of weeks or even a month or if the labs were quickly deteriorating, I would get this patient in for a biopsy.

A liver biopsy is done that reveals lymphocytic infiltration within portal tracts, mild inflammation of bile ducts, and lymphocytic infiltration of portal and hepatic venules. A Doppler US shows normal blood flow without thrombosis but suggests extrahepatic biliary dilation. An MRCP is done that shows a mild extrahepatic stricture of questionable significance.

This looks like rejection, but the management of rejection depends on the severity of the rejection and which drugs and at what dosages the patient was on prior to developing the rejection. The pathologist will generally give you the level of rejection based on the Banff criteria. They're going to tell you, is this mild, moderate, or severe rejection?

If it is mild, sometimes just increasing immunosuppression is enough. If a patient was on cyclosporine only, then switching them to tacrolimus or adding mycophenolate would be my strategy for managing mild rejection. For moderate and severe rejection, it's going to take more than that. Usually, you're going to need to use an IV dosage of solumedrol, and if it's refractory to that, sometimes even more aggressive IV therapies for acute cellular rejection are required. And then, once they are improved, you need to increase their outpatient regimen as well.

This patient's case is tough because presumably she's still taking prednisone, tacrolimus, and mycophenolate. We're not given the dosage, but you may have to increase the prednisone and increase the trough level of the tacrolimus.

When you see patients coming from a different transplant center, what initial therapy might you be less pleased with?

I think the etiology of disease is very important to consider. For autoimmune hepatitis, PSC, and PBC, a lot of those patients are tapered completely off prednisone. But realize that they have an immune-mediated indication for transplant, and most of these do recur posttransplant. So, I think that these patients should be maintained on at least a low dose of prednisone. Oftentimes, I'll see that they're not.

Now another drug that has fallen out of favor is cyclosporine, but depending on where and how long-ago patients were transplanted, we may see them on cyclosporine. It's not as strong an immunosuppressive agent, and it causes more renal insufficiency and comorbid problems than tacrolimus. If patients are on cyclosporine, I'll often switch it. Some patients get started on cyclosporine because they have mental status alteration posttransplant while taking tacrolimus and may be labeled with

PRES (posterior reversible encephalopathy syndrome), which is occasionally a side effect of tacrolimus. But in many cases, the mental changes are unrelated and self-limited and not a reason to give up on tacrolimus.

I think that having patients on tacrolimus instead of cyclosporine is important, whenever possible. Some patients are on mTOR inhibitors, which are not as strong immune suppressing drugs. If a patient is on an mTOR inhibitor alone, like sirolimus or everolimus, they are far more likely to have rejection than a patient who is on an mTOR inhibitor, along with a calcineurin inhibitor. While it's pretty unusual to be on monotherapy with an mTOR inhibitor, I do see it from time to time. Those are some of the drug choices that are occasionally problematic.

Index